Advances in Arrhythmia Analyses: A Case-Based Approach

Guest Editors

MELVIN SCHEINMAN, MD
MASOOD AKHTAR, MD

CARDIAC ELECTROPHYSIOLOGY CLINICS

www.cardiacEP.theclinics.com

Consulting Editors
RANJAN K. THAKUR, MD, MPH, FHRS
ANDREA NATALE, MD, FACC, FHRS

June 2010 • Volume 2 • Number 2

SAUNDERS an imprint of ELSEVIER, Inc.

W.B. SAUNDERS COMPANY
A Division of Elsevier Inc.

1600 John F. Kennedy Boulevard • Suite 1800 • Philadelphia, Pennsylvania 19103-2899

http://www.theclinics.com

CARDIAC ELECTROPHYSIOLOGY CLINICS Volume 2, Number 2
June 2010 ISSN 1877-9182, ISBN-13: 978-1-4377-1799-0

Editor: Barbara Cohen-Kligerman

Cardiac Electrophysiology Clinics (ISSN 1877-9182) is published quarterly by Elsevier Inc., 360 Park Avenue South, New York, NY 10010-1710. Months of issue are March, June, September, and December. Subscription prices are $167.00 per year for US individuals, $250.00 per year for US institutions, $84.00 per year for US students and residents, $187.00 per year for Canadian individuals, $299.00 per year for Canadian institutions, $239.00 per year for international individuals, $299.00 per year for international institutions and $120.00 per year for Canadian and foreign students/residents. To receive student/resident rate, orders must be accompanied by name of affilliated institution, date of term, and the signature of program/residency coordinator on institution letterhead. Orders will be billed at individual rate until proof of status is received. Foreign air speed delivery is included in all Clinics subscription prices. All prices are subject to change without notice. **POSTMASTER:** Send address changes to Cardiac Electrophysiology Clinics, Elsevier Health Sciences Division, Subscription Customer Service, 3251 Riverport Lane, Maryland Heights, MO 63043. **Customer Service: 1-800-654-2452 (US and Canada). From outside of the US and Canada, call 314-477-8871. Fax: 314-447-8029. E-mail: JournalsCustomerService-usa@elsevier.com (for print support); JournalsOnlineSupport-usa@elsevier.com (for online support).**

Reprints. For copies of 100 or more of articles in this publication, please contact the Commercial Reprints Department, Elsevier Inc., 360 Park Avenue South, New York, NY 10010-1710. Tel.: 212-633-3812; Fax: 212-462-1935; E-mail: reprints@elsevier.com.

Printed and bound by CPI Group (UK) Ltd, Croydon, CR0 4YY

Transferred to Digital Print 2011

The cover illustration shows the typical intracardiac electrograms demonstrating "lower loop reentry." The figure also shows a schematic of the circuit with looping of the wave front around the inferior vena cava and impulse collision over the lateral wall of the right atrium. This and other flutter circuits are discussed in the text in the section on Atrial Fibrillation/Atrial Flutter. Artwork by David Criley.

Contributors

CONSULTING EDITORS

RANJAN THAKUR, MD, MPH, FHRS
Professor of Medicine and Director, Arrhythmia Service, Thoracic and Cardiovascular Institute, Sparrow Health System, Michigan State University, Lansing, Michigan

ANDREA NATALE, MD, FHRS
Executive Medical Director of the Texas Cardiac Arrhythmia Institute at St David's Medical Center, Austin, Texas; Consulting Professor, Division of Cardiology, Stanford University, Palo Alto, California; Clinical Associate Professor of Medicine, Case Western Reserve University, Cleveland, Ohio; Senior Clinical Director, EP Services, California Pacific Medical Center, San Francisco; Department of Biomedical Engineering, University of Texas, Austin, Texas

GUEST EDITORS

MELVIN SCHEINMAN, MD
Professor of Medicine, Section of Cardiac Electrophysiology, Division of Cardiology, Department of Medicine, University of California, San Francisco, California

MASOOD AKHTAR, MD, FACC, FACP, FAHA, MACP
Clinical Professor of Medicine, Aurora Sinai St Luke's Medical Center, University of Wisconsin School of Medicine and Public Health, Milwaukee, Wisconsin

SECTION EDITORS

MASOOD AKHTAR, MD, FACC, FACP, FAHA, MACP
Clinical Professor of Medicine, Aurora Sinai St Luke's Medical Center, University of Wisconsin School of Medicine and Public Health, Milwaukee, Wisconsin

NITISH BADHWAR, MD, MBBS
Assistant Professor of Medicine, Division of Cardiology, Department of Cardiac Electrophysiology, University of California San Francisco, San Francisco, California

BYRON K. LEE, MD
Assistant Professor of Medicine, Department of Cardiology, University of California San Francisco Medical Center, Cardiac Electrophysiology and Arrhythmia Service, San Francisco, California

GREGORY M. MARCUS, MD, MAS, FAAC
Assistant Professor of Medicine, Division of Cardiology, Electrophysiology Section, University of California, San Francisco, San Francisco, California

WILLIAM P. NELSON, MD
Clinical Professor of Medicine, St Joseph Hospital, Denver, Colorado

AUTHORS

MASOOD AKHTAR, MD, FACC, FACP, FAHA, MACP
Clinical Professor of Medicine, Aurora Sinai St Luke's Medical Center, University of Wisconsin School of Medicine and Public Health, Milwaukee, Wisconsin

MICHAEL ARGENZIANO, MD
Associate Professor of Surgery, Division of Cardiothoracic Surgery, Columbia University, New York, New York

RIMA ARNAOUT, MD
Cardiology Fellow, Cardiology Division, University of California, San Francisco, California

NITISH BADHWAR, MD, MBBS
Assistant Professor of Medicine, Division of Cardiology, Department of Cardiac Electrophysiology, University of California San Francisco, San Francisco, California

GAETANO BARBATO, MD
Cardiology Department, Maggiore Hospital, Bologna, Italy

PRASHANT D. BHAVE, MD
Fellow, Department of Cardiology, University of California San Francisco Medical Center, San Francisco, California

VALERIA CARINCI, MD
Cardiology Department, Maggiore Hospital, Bologna, Italy

JOSÈ DIZON, MD
Associate Professor of Medicine, Division of Cardiology, Columbia University, New York, New York

HASAN GARAN, MD
Department of Medicine, Columbia University Medical Center, New York, New York

NORA GOLDSCHLAGER, MD
Professor of Clinical Medicine, Division of Cardiology, Department of Medicine, San Francisco General Hospital, University of California San Francisco, San Francisco, California

JONATHAN C. HSU, MD
Cardiology Fellow, Division of Cardiology, Department of Medicine, University of California, San Francisco, San Francisco, California

COLLEEN JOHNSON, MD, MS
Division of Cardiology, Department of Cardiac Electrophysiology, University of California San Francisco, San Francisco, California

MARK E. JOSEPHSON, MD
Chief, Cardiovascular Division, Beth Israel Deaconess Medical Center, Boston, Massachusetts

DAVID S. KWON, MD, PhD
Cardiac Electrophysiology Fellow, Section of Cardiac Electrophysiology, Division of Cardiology, University of California, San Francisco, San Francisco, California

BYRON K. LEE, MD
Assistant Professor of Medicine, Department of Cardiology, University of California San Francisco Medical Center, Cardiac Electrophysiology and Arrhythmia Service, San Francisco, California

RANDALL J. LEE, MD
Professor of Medicine, Cardiac Electrophysiology, Cardiology Division, University of California San Francisco, San Francisco, California

GREGORY M. MARCUS, MD, MAS, FAAC
Assistant Professor of Medicine, Division of Cardiology, Electrophysiology Section, University of California, San Francisco, San Francisco, California

WILLIAM P. NELSON, MD
Clinical Professor of Medicine, St Joseph Hospital, Denver, Colorado

DUY THAI NGUYEN, MD
Electrophysiology Fellow, Division of Cardiology, Section of Cardiac Electrophysiology, University of California San Francisco, San Francisco, California

MELVIN SCHEINMAN, MD
Professor of Medicine, Division of Cardiology, Cardiac Electrophysiology Section, University of California San Francisco, San Francisco, California

DAVID SINGH, MD
Electrophysiology Fellow, Division of Cardiology, Department of Cardiac Electrophysiology, University of California, San Francisco, California

RONN E. TANEL, MD
Associate Professor Department of Pediatrics, University of California San Francisco School of Medicine; Director, Pediatric Arrhythmia Center, Division of Pediatric Cardiology, University of California San Francisco Children's Hospital, San Francisco, California

ANNE THORSON, MD
Associate Clinical Professor of Medicine, Cardiology Division, University of California, San Francisco, San Francisco, California

ZIAN H. TSENG, MD, MAS
Assistant Professor of Medicine, Section of Cardiac Electrophysiology, Division of Cardiology, Department of Medicine, University of California, San Francisco School of Medicine, San Francisco, California

VASANTH VEDANTHAM, MD, PhD
Clinical Fellow, Cardiac Electrophysiology Section, Cardiology Division, University of California, San Francisco, San Francisco, California

MOHAN N. VISWANATHAN, MD
Assistant Professor of Medicine, Section of Cardiac Electrophysiology, Division of Cardiology, University of Washington School of Medicine, Seattle, Washington

DANIEL Y. WANG, MD
Cardiac Electrophysiology Fellow, Instructor in Clinical Medicine, Department of Medicine, Columbia University Medical Center, New York, New York

SHEPARD D. WEINER, MD
Cardiology Fellow, Department of Medicine, Columbia University Medical Center, New York, New York

WILLIAM WHANG, MD
Assistant Professor of Clinical Medicine, Department of Medicine, Columbia University Medical Center, New York, New York

YANFEI YANG, MD
Division of Cardiology, Cardiac Electrophysiology Section, University of California San Francisco, San Francisco, California

Contents

Foreword xv

RanjanThakur and Andrea Natale

Preface xvii

Melvin Scheinman and Masood Akhtar

Abnormalities of Impulse Formation and Conduction

William P. Nelson, Section Editor

Syncope in Patient with Long-Standing Hypertension, Diabetes, and Mild Aortic Stenosis 151

Mark E. Josephson

This article presents a case study of a patient with long-standing hypertension, diabetes, and mild to moderate aortic stenosis presenting with syncope without premonitory symptoms. Electrophysiology confirmed intra-His block. After placement of a permanent pacemaker, the patient remains free of syncope and her high blood pressure is more readily controlled.

Exercise-Induced Near Syncope 155

Mark E. Josephson

This article provides a case study of a patient with exercised-induced near syncope. Intracardiac electrophysiologic study confirmed an intra-His block and a pacemaker was implanted.

Abnormalities of Impulse Formation and Conduction 159

William P. Nelson

This article examines abnormalities of impulse formation and conduction through the examples of various case studies.

SupraventricularTachycardia

Nitish Badhwar, Section Editor

Introduction to Supraventricular Tachycardia 179

Nitish Badhwar

Paroxysmal supraventricular tachycardia (PSVT) is a clinical syndrome characterized by a rapid tachycardia with an abrupt onset and termination cardiomyopathy. The three most common causes of PSVT are atrioventricular nodal reentrant tachycardia (50%–60%), atrioventricular reentrant tachycardia in patients with Wolff-Parkinson-White syndrome (25%–30%), and atrial tachycardia (10%). Rare causes of PSVT include focal junctional tachycardia, atriofascicular tachycardia, permanent reciprocating junctional tachycardia, and nodoventricular/nodofascicular

distal to the AP recording within the CS, then the AP potential itself at the os. The current case highlights the complexity of the AV connection and the importance of careful mapping of the CS in patients with PJRT.

Supraventricular Tachycardia in a Patient with Repaired Congenital Heart Disease **231**

Ronn E. Tanel

This case illustrates the difficulty in diagnosing atrial tachycardia in a patient who had a Mustard procedure for transposition of great arteries. Identification of atrial arrhythmias, even when they occur at physiologic ventricular rates, is important, because these patients are at risk for thrombus development and symptoms related to periods of a more rapid ventricular response. Another potential concern is that if the heart rate is elevated moderately during an unrecognized arrhythmia, the patient may develop a tachycardia-mediated cardiomyopathy over time. Patients with repaired congenital heart disease who develop postoperative tachyarrhythmias usually are treated aggressively to restore sinus rhythm. This is especially true in those who have residual intracardiac lesions or depressed myocardial function.

Supraventricular Tachycardia and Atrioventricular Block **235**

Duy Thai Nguyen and Nitish Badhwar

The differential diagnosis for a mid- to long-RP supraventricular tachycardia include atrial tachycardia, atypical atrioventricular nodal reentrant tachycardia (AVNRT), and atrioventricular reentrant tachycardia (AVRT) utilizing a slowly conducting concealed accessory pathway. The presence of spontaneous atrioventricular block excludes AVRT. This case reviews pacing maneuvers to distinguish atrial tachycardia from AVNRT. Atypical AVNRT generally demonstrates the presence of a lower common pathway and has its site of earliest retrograde atrial activation near the coronary sinus ostium, which would be the target for ablation.

Changing QRS Morphology in a Patient with Wolff-Parkinson-White Syndrome **239**

Vasanth Vedantham and Zian H. Tseng

A case of Wolff-Parkinson-White syndrome with supraventricular tachycardia is presented in which 2 atrioventricular (AV) reentry circuits are identified. The first circuit used the AV node in the antegrade limb and a left lateral accessory pathway in the retrograde limb. The second circuit used an atriofascicular accessory pathway as the antegrade limb and the left lateral accessory pathway as the retrograde limb. The characteristics of these tachycardias are described, along with diagnostic maneuvers used in the electrophysiology laboratory. Mapping and ablation of both of these accessory pathways is also described. This article is aimed at clinical electrophysiologists interested in management of complex supraventricular tachycardias in the electrophysiology laboratory.

Ventricular Tachycardia

Masood Akhtar, Section Editor

Ventricular Tachycardia **245**

Masood Akhtar

Understanding of ventricular tachycardia has improved greatly in recent years. Still diagnosis has remained challenging. This article presents four cases to illustrate different presentations of this disorder.

Supraventricular Tachycardia After Atrial Fibrillation Ablation **313**

Duy Thai Nguyen, Randall J. Lee, and Zian H. Tseng

Atrial arrhythmias occur commonly after atrial fibrillation (AF) ablation. Initial conservative management with medical therapy and cardioversion is reasonable, particularly in the early period (first 3 months) after ablation, because many of these arrhythmias remit over time. However, definitive therapy with ablation may be required, depending on the clinical circumstances, and should focus on the putative mechanism of tachycardia and its likely location, both of which can be suggested by the initial AF ablation strategy. Response to pacing, entrainment, and electroanatomic activation mapping are useful to confirm the mechanism, define complex circuits, and guide ablation targets.

Supraventricular Tachycardia in Pulmonary Hypertension **317**

Duy Thai Nguyen and Melvin Scheinman

Pulmonary hypertension is a disease with significant morbidity and mortality. It is characterized by right-sided volume and pressure overload, which leads to structural changes and fibrosis in the right atrium, thus predisposing to supraventricular arrhythmias. This article presents a case discussion of supraventricular tachycardia in pulmonary hypertension. A 48-year-old woman, with a history of primary pulmonary hypertension and right heart failure, was admitted with a supraventricular tachycardia, hypotension, and congestive heart failure.

Index **321**

Cardiac Electrophysiology Clinics

FORTHCOMING ISSUES

September 2010

Arrhythmogenic Right Ventricular Cardiomyopathy/Dysplasia
Domenico Corrado, MD, PhD,
Cristina Basso, MD, PhD, and
Gaetano Thiene, MD, *Guest Editors*

December 2010

Advances in Antiarrhythmic Drug Therapy
Peter R. Kowey, MD, and
Gerald V. Naccarelli, MD, *Guest Editors*

March 2011

Basic Science for the Clinical Electrophysiologist
Charles Antzelevitch, PhD, FACC, FAHA, FHRS,
Guest Editor

RECENT ISSUES

March 2010

Epicardial Interventions in Electrophysiology
Kalyanam Shivkumar, MD, PhD, FHRS, and
Noel G. Boyle, MD, PhD, FHRS,
Guest Editors

December 2009

Sudden Cardiac Death
Ranjan K. Thakur, MD, MPH, FHRS, and
Andrea Natale, MD, FACC, FHRS,
Guest Editors

ISSUES OF RELATED INTEREST

Cardiology Clinics November 2009 (Vol. 27, No. 4)
Advances in Cardiac Computed Tomography
Mario J. Garcia, MD, FACC, *Guest Editor*
Available at: http://www.cardiology.theclinics.com/

Heart Failure Clinics January 2010 (Vol. 6, No. 1)
Pharmacogenetics in Heart Failure: How It Will Shape the Future
Dennis M. McNamara, MD, *Guest Editor*
Available at: http://www.heartfailure.theclinics.com/

VISIT THE CLINICS ONLINE!

Access your subscription at:
www.theclinics.com

Foreword

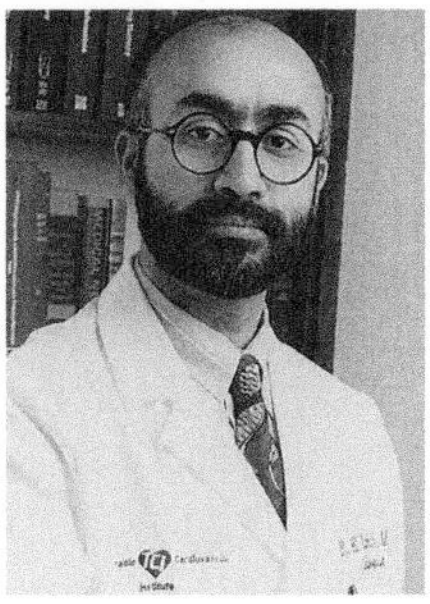

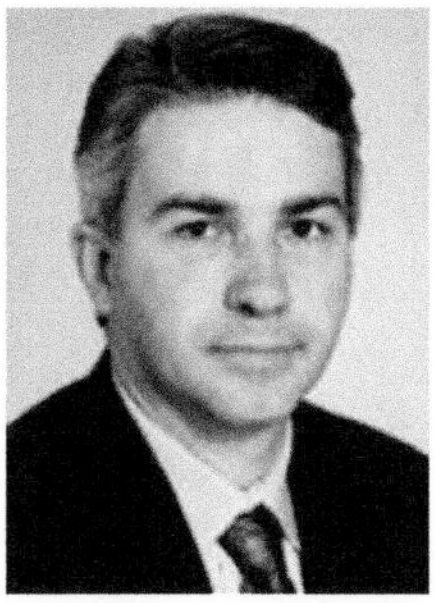

Ranjan Thakur, MD, MPH, FHRS   Andrea Natale, MD, FHRS
Consulting Editors

The practice of electrophysiology requires an understanding of theoretic principles, but beyond that, it needs cognitive application of those principles to solve electrophysiologic puzzles in the laboratory. In that respect, electrophysiology is unique in cardiology and among medical specialties.

Although one can learn the principles by reading a book, learning how and when to invoke those principles for solving problems comes through deliberate practice, getting it wrong at times, and then having someone show you how to get to the answer and by watching others do it. This was our thinking when we invited Dr Melvin Scheinman and Dr Masood Akhtar to edit this issue of *Cardiac Electrophysiology Clinics* devoted to interpretation of complex surface and intracardiac electrocardiographic tracings.

Dr Scheinman and Dr Akhtar are well-known pioneers in cardiac electrophysiology, and many of the principles that we take for granted were, in fact, first elucidated by them. In addition to their enormous contribution to electrophysiology, they are master teachers.

We were delighted when they accepted our invitation to edit this issue. Electrophysiologists at all levels will find this issue useful. Beginners should pore over these pages slowly and repeatedly. Practicing electrophysiologists will gain by reviewing these cases, which will remind them of many things they may have long forgotten. Teachers will find these cases useful for teaching their fellows and staff. The case slides are available in PowerPoint format on the *Cardiac Electrophysiology Clinics* Web site (http://www.cardiacep.theclinics.com/) so they can be downloaded for educational purposes. Dr Scheinman and Dr Akhtar and the contributors have made an excellent effort and we hope that you, the reader, will gain from their wisdom and exposition. We intend to devote an issue of the *Cardiac Electrophysiology Clinics* every few years to a similar endeavor, edited by a master clinician/teacher.

We would like to receive your feedback and critique so that the *Cardiac Electrophysiology Clinics* can continually improve to meet your educational needs.

Ranjan Thakur, MD, MPH, FHRS
Thoracic and Cardiovascular Institute
Michigan State University
405 West Greenlawn, Suite 400
Lansing, MI 48910, USA

Andrea Natale, MD, FHRS
Texas Cardiac Arrhythmia Institute
Center for Atrial Fibrillation at
St David's Medical Center
1015 East 32nd Street, Suite 516
Austin, TX 78705, USA

E-mail addresses:
Thakur@msu.edu (R. Thakur)
Andrea.natale@stdavids.com (A. Natale)

Card Electrophysiol Clin 2 (2010) xv
doi:10.1016/j.ccep.2010.02.008
1877-9182/10/$ – see front matter

Preface

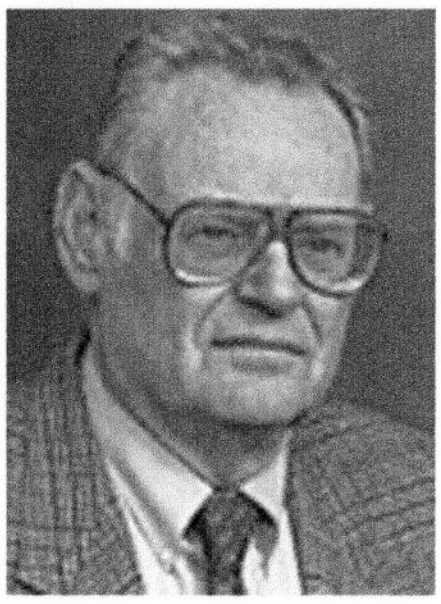

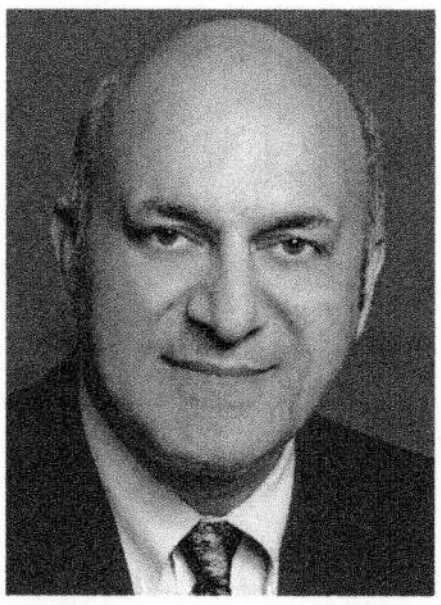

Melvin Scheinman, MD Masood Akhtar, MD, MACP
Guest Editors

We are delighted to launch an educational endeavor that differs from the usual *Cardiac Electrophysiology Clinics* format. This issue is devoted to analyses of cardiac arrhythmias entirely using a case-based format. We have always thought that a case-based approach is a unique teaching technique, forcing readers to think along with the experts. Unfortunately, it has become difficult for arrhythmia journals to publish all the excellent case reports submitted. It was, therefore, felt that this issue of *Cardiac Electrophysiology Clinics* would provide a venue for readers to enjoy and learn from case vignettes from the masters.

This issue is designed for clinicians interested in cardiac rhythm analyses and for cardiac electrophysiology specialists. We have tried to collect case gems that span the gamut of arrhythmia experience. This issue is especially valuable for cardiology trainees reviewing material for board examinations.

We are greatly indebted to some of the most eminent authorities in the field of arrhythmias for their contributions to this issue. Dr William Nelson is a disciple of the Pick-Langendorf school and provided the introductory surface tracings together with their elegant analyses. We acknowledge the important contribution of Dr Mark Josephson. We are particularly indebted to colleagues at the University of California, San Francisco, who worked very hard as section editors to collate and integrate these cases. We sincerely hope that you enjoy this issue. Please let us know if you think this is a worthwhile approach.

Melvin Scheinman, MD
Electrophysiology Service
500 Parnassus Avenue
Suite 433, San Francisco
CA 94143-1354, USA

Masood Akhtar, MD, MACP
Aurora Sinai Medical Center
960 North 12th Street
Milwaukee, WI 52333, USA

E-mail addresses:
scheinman@medicine.ucsf.edu (M. Scheinman)
llandis@hrtcare.com (M. Akhtar)

Card Electrophysiol Clin 2 (2010) xvii
doi:10.1016/j.ccep.2010.02.007
1877-9182/10/$ – see front matter

Syncope in Patient with Long-Standing Hypertension, Diabetes, and Mild Aortic Stenosis

Mark E. Josephson, MD

KEYWORDS

• Syncope • Intra-His block • Hypertension

An 86-year-old Russian-speaking woman with long-standing hypertension, diabetes, and mild to moderate aortic stenosis presented with syncope without premonitory symptoms. She had no symptoms of congestive heart failure or chest pain. She had a prior episode of syncope the preceding year that was believed by her primary care physician to be vasovagal and was not specifically treated. She also had a history of atrial fibrillation that was intermittent, occurring one to two times per year, but no known sinus node.

Two weeks before the present syncopal episode she felt weak and tired. She was sent to the Outpatient Arrhythmia Clinic at the Beth Israel Deaconess Medical Center for evaluation. On physical examination she was an elderly woman, in no acute distress, resting comfortably. Her blood pressure was 180/65, her heart rate was 35 and regular, and respirations were 14 unlabored. Her physical examination was significant only for elevated jugular venous pressure with intermittent cannon a waves, a murmur of aortic stenosis, some mild edema, and diminished peripheral pulses. Her electrocardiogram is shown in **Fig. 1**.

Carefully analysis of the tracing demonstrates sinus rhythm at about 70 beats per minute with no relationship to the QRS complexes, which have a right bundle branch block, left anterior hemiblock morphology. Complete atrioventricular (AV) block is present. Of note, the P-P intervals surrounding the QRS seem to be shorter than the PR intervals between the QRS. This phenomenon is called "ventriculoaphasic effect." It is thought to be caused by baroreceptor responsiveness in the aorta to each of the conducted QRS complexes, which produces a systolic pressure wave that increases vagal tone to slow the next sinus cycle. Experimentally, this has been abolished with atropine. The question that arises is whether or not the escape rhythm is arising from the posterior fascicle or whether it is arising in the AV junction itself. An electrocardiogram taken 6 years previously is shown in **Fig. 2**. Is this of any help?

This tracing demonstrates normal sinus rhythm at a rate of approximately 60 beats per minute with a normal PR interval of 190 milliseconds. Of note, left anterior hemiblock is present and the QRS is on the high side at 102 milliseconds. Left ventricular hypertrophy is probably also present. Because this was taken 6 years previously it is of no help in answering the question of whether the rhythm shown in **Fig. 1** is a fascicular rhythm or junctional rhythm. More recent electrocardiograms are necessary to make a more definitive statement.

What is the next step? Specifically, one should ask what medication she was taking, because medications that are commonly used for hypertension and atrial fibrillation could affect AV

Cardiovascular Division, Beth Israel Deaconess Medical Center, 185 Pilgrim Road, West Baker 4, Boston, MA 02215, USA
E-mail address: mjoseph2@bidmc.harvard.edu

Card Electrophysiol Clin 2 (2010) 151–153
doi:10.1016/j.ccep.2010.02.002
1877-9182/10/$ – see front matter

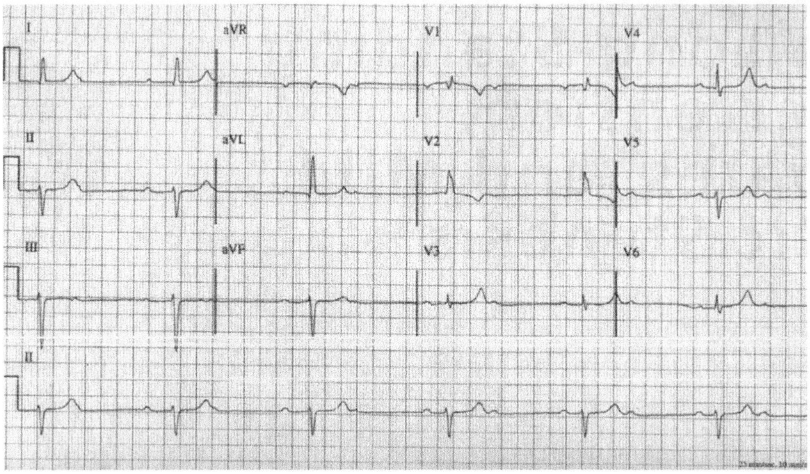

Fig. 1. What is the rhythm?

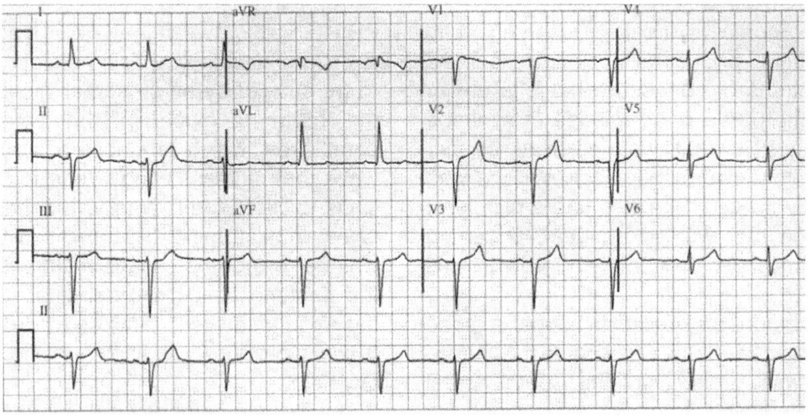

Fig. 2. Electrocardiogram of the same patient shown in **Fig. 1,** taken 6 years earlier.

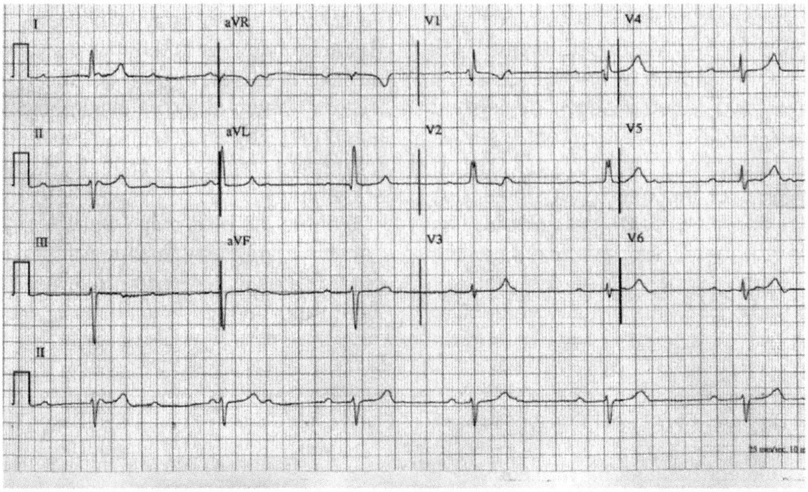

Fig. 3. Where is the site of the block? Where is escape rhythm originating? Why is fourth QRS early?

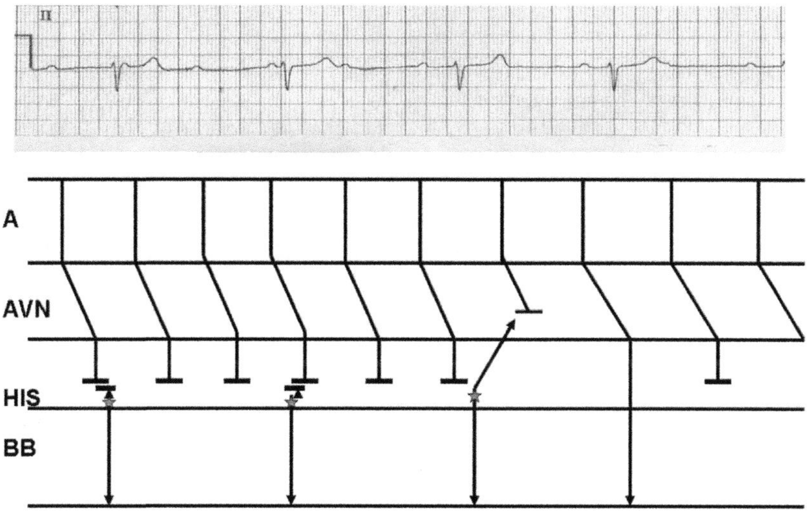

Fig. 4. This schematic drawing shows the reason for the early QRS.

conduction. Indeed, she had been on 50 mg of Toprol, an angiotensin-converting enzyme inhibitor, and hydrochlorothiazide.

During her visit a continuous traveling electrocardiogram was taken. **Fig. 3** demonstrates an electrocardiogram taken at the end of her physical examination. There are three questions that can be asked of this tracing, the answers of which provide important diagnostic information: (1) Where is the site of block? (2) Where is the escape rhythm originating? (3) Why is the fourth QRS early? First, unlike **Fig. 1**, this tracing is slightly irregular. The first three complexes occur at the same rate, but the fourth complex is slightly early. This means that during this tracing complete heart block is not present. The early QRS complex has an identical QRS to all the other escape complexes, suggesting that this rhythm originates in the His bundle. This slow rate suggests that it is in the distal His bundle. The reason for the early QRS is shown in the schema (**Fig. 4**). I believe the block is within the His bundle and the escape is in the distal His bundle. If the block was in the node and there was a distal His escape no retrograde conduction producing subsequent facilitation of conduction could be possible. With the block being within the His bundle itself, however, the third QRS penetrates the AV node and the P wave, which falls within the T wave blocks in the node. This provides time for the site of block within the His bundle to recover excitability and allows the subsequent P wave to conduct with the PR interval with 245 milliseconds. It should be noted that block in the His Purkinje system can be associated with retrograde conduction to the node and sometimes to the atrium.[1–3] This is never the case when block is in the AV node. This is clinically important because placement of a VVI pacemaker in some of these patients produces VA conduction and a "pacemaker syndrome."

The patient was admitted for work-up for a permanent pacemaker, which was accomplished without complication. The electrophysiologist confirmed intra-His block. No abnormalities of sinus node function were observed and no tachyarrhythmias were induced during an electrophysiologic study at the time of pacemaker implantation. The patient remains free of syncope and her high blood pressure is more readily controlled.

REFERENCES

1. Josephson ME. Atrioventricular conduction. In: Clinical cardiac electrophysiology: techniques and interpretations. 4th edition. Philadelhia: Wolters Kluwer/Lippincott Williams and Wilkins; 2008. p. 93–113.
2. Zimetbaum PJ, Josephson ME. Bradycardias. In: Practical clinical electrophysiology. Philadelhia: Wolters Kluwer/Lippincott Williams and Wilkins; 2009. p. 163–78.
3. Wellens HJJ, Conover M. Bradyarrhythmias. In: The ECG in emergency decision making. 2nd edition. Philadelhia: Saunders Elsevier; 2006.

Exercise-Induced Near Syncope

Mark E. Josephson, MD

KEYWORDS

- Atrioventricular block • His bundle
- Exercise-induced near syncope

The patient is a 29-year-old man with a history of exercise-induced near syncope. He is the product of a normal pregnancy and was not known to have any cardiovascular abnormalities as a child. He has no family history of hypertrophic cardiomyopathy, sudden cardiac death, or electrocardiographic abnormalities consistent with long QT syndrome or Brugada syndrome. All of his symptoms were exertional and unrelated to use of alcohol, illicit drugs, or dehydration.[1–4]

He went to his primary care physician and was found to be normotensive with a heart rate of 70, and normal respirations. He had clear lungs, and cardiac examination revealed no murmurs, rubs, or gallops. He had no arthritis, organomegaly, or rashes. Chest radiograph was normal. His electrocardiogram (ECG) is shown in **Fig. 1**. His ECG at that time revealed normal sinus rhythm at a rate of 65 with normal P waves, normal PR interval, normal QRS interval, and normal QT interval. He had no ST elevation in his precordial leads. His QT interval was neither short nor long.

The differential diagnosis by his primary care physician included (1) exercise-induced supraventricular tachycardia, (2) exercise-induced ventricular tachycardia from the right ventricular outflow tract, (3) catechoaminergic polymorphic ventricular tachycardia, (4) paroxysmal atrioventricular (AV) block, or (5) sinus node dysfunction or (6) exercise-induced AV block. A Lyme titer was sent and came back negative. Laboratory tests for vasculitis and rheumatoid arthritis were negative. His chest and spine radiographs were normal and there was no mediastinal or hilar adenopathy or pulmonary nodules or evidence of ankylosing spondylitis. An angiotensin-converting enzyme level was also taken to rule out sarcoidosis (it was negative). An echocardiogram was done and there was no evidence of hypertrophy (septal or otherwise) and there was no evidence of abnormal right ventricular function. An MRI was also done with no delayed enhancement and normal ventricular function.

He was then referred to the electrophysiology group for further evaluation. Physical examination by the electrophysiologist was also normal. In addition to what was observed previously, carotid pressure produced sinus slowing but no evidence of paroxysmal or bradycardic-dependent block. The most important and obvious test that should be done in such an individual is an exercise test, not an electrophysiology study. Because all his symptoms were related to exercise, the most direct way to demonstrate what is causing his symptoms is to have him exercise. This is important for any exercise-induced tachyarrhythmia or AV block. The failure to produce bradycardic-induced block following carotid sinus pressure, despite a pause of 2.5 seconds, was reassuring but not necessarily proof that there was no paroxysmal AV block. A tilt test was not done because his symptoms were during exercise and not just following exercise. Moreover, there were no other episodes of syncope that occurred under different circumstances known to produce vagal, vasodepressor, or mixed neurocardiac syncope.

Cardiovascular Division, Beth Israel Deaconess Medical Center, 185 Pilgrim Road, West Baker 4, Boston, MA 02215, USA
E-mail address: mjoseph2@bidmc.harvard.edu

Card Electrophysiol Clin 2 (2010) 155–157
doi:10.1016/j.ccep.2010.02.004
1877-9182/10/$ – see front matter

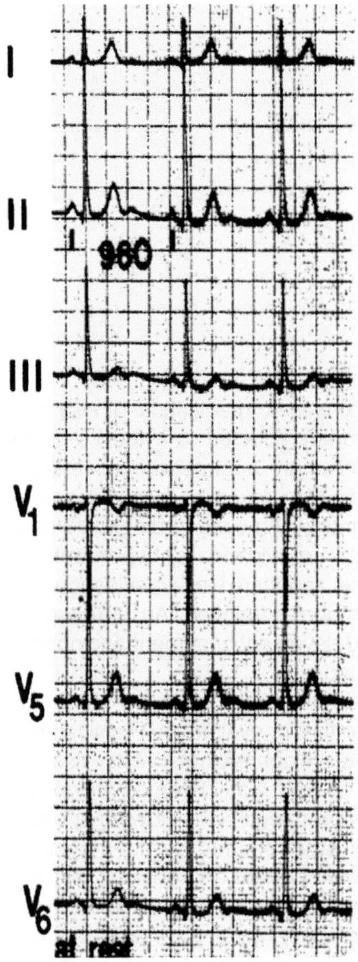

Fig. 1. ECG at the onset of exercise (first 3 minutes).

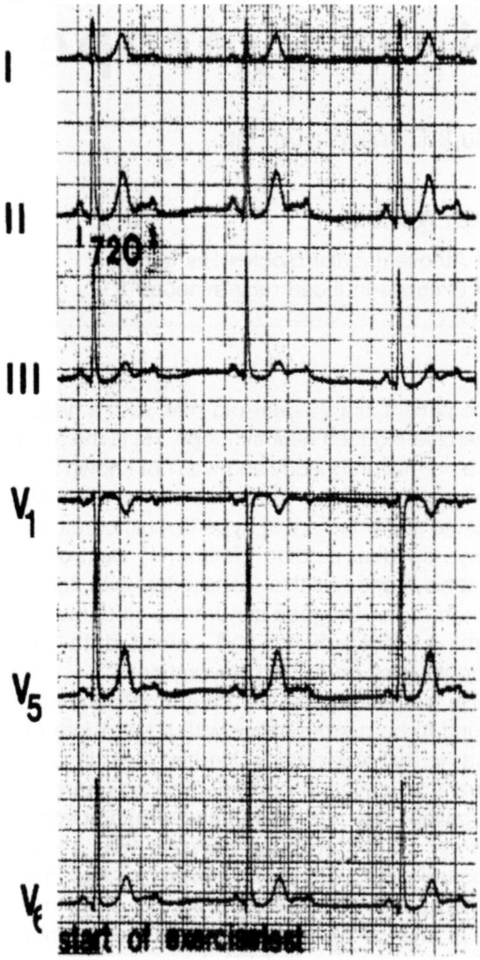

Fig. 2. Continuation of exercise resulted in near syncope during the ECG.

As such he was sent for an exercise test. An ECG at the onset of exercise (first 3 minutes) is shown in **Fig. 2**. Here his sinus rhythm has accelerated to approximately 80 beats a minute and two to one AV block has appeared. His PR interval of his conducted complexes remains short. One also notes that the PP intervals surrounding the QRS were shorter than those in between the QRS demonstrating the so-called "ventriculophasic effect." It is a normal finding, particularly in healthy people with a normal baroreceptor response. The appearance of block on exercise generally points to a disease of the His-Purkinje system. Similarly, a short PR of conducted beats favors subnodal conduction problems. In view of the fact that his QRS was normal it was assumed that the lesion in this individual was in the His bundle. Continuation of exercise resulted in near syncope during the ECG shown in **Fig. 3**. Here, at 9 minutes of exercise, with a sinus rate of 150 beats a minute, three to one AV block is observed. The chronotropic insufficiency at this level of exercise resulted in hypotension and near syncope. The exercise test was stopped and as his sinus rate slowed to baseline, within 5 minutes, one to one conduction appeared.

It was the contention of the electrophysiologist that this was indeed rate-dependent infranodal block. The cause of such block is often idiopathic but can be related to granulomas disease in the His bundle, such as sarcoidosis; valve calcification in elderly people; or as a complication of mitral or aortic valve disease with extension of calcification into the His bundle. Anterior infarction or inferior infarction involving the His bundle has been noted, but neither was seen in this patient. Intracardiac electrophysiologic study confirmed an intra-His block and a pacemaker

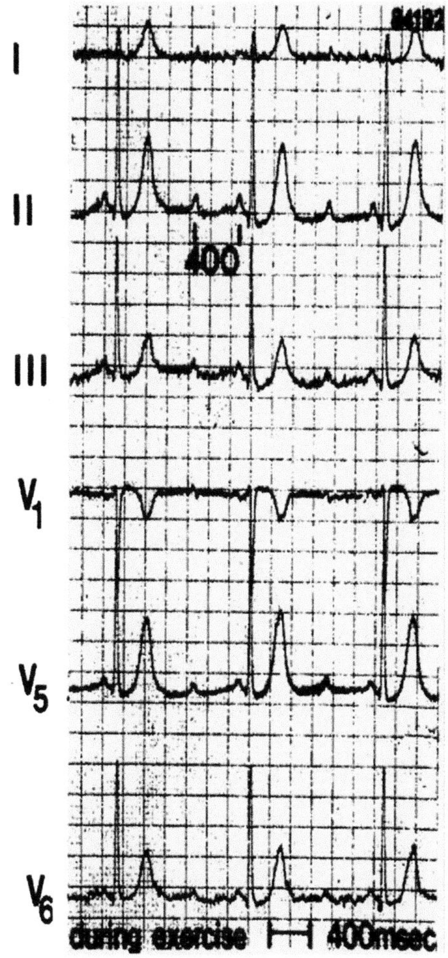

Fig. 3. The patient's ECG on presentation.

was implanted. In this case the pacemaker was a dual-chamber pacemaker, first to maintain AV synchrony during exercise and second to prevent pacemaker syndrome, which not infrequently can occur when infranodal AV block is present. This results because of the potential for VA conduction in perhaps half of all patients. This patient has done remarkably well and complete AV block was observed in his first year of follow-up.

In evaluating AV block it is important to know whether it occurs with enhanced sympathetic tone or withdrawal of vagal tone. In such instances block is mostly always infranodal. Slowing down the sinus rate with carotid sinus pressure may even produce one to one conduction. This is in contradistinction to block in the AV node where carotid sinus pressure makes conduction worse and vagal withdrawal and enhanced sympathetic tone improves conduction.

REFERENCES

1. Josephson ME. Atrioventricular conduction. In: Clinical cardiac electrophysiology: techniques and interpretations. 4th edition. Philadelphia: Wolters Kluwer/ Lippincott Williams and Wilkins; 2008. Chapter 4.
2. Zimetbaum PJ, Josephson ME. Bradycardias. In: Practical clinical electrophysiology. Philadelphia: Wolters Kluwer/Lippincott Williams and Wilkins; 2009.
3. Lee S, Wellens HJJ, Josephson ME. Paroxysmal atrioventricular block. Heart Rhythm 2009;6:1229–34.
4. Wellens HJJ, Conover M. Bradyarrhythmias. In: The ECG in emergency decision making. 2nd edition. Philadelphia: Saunders Elsevier; 2006.

Abnormalities of Impulse Formation and Conduction

William P. Nelson, MD

KEYWORDS

- Impulse formation • Electrocardiography • Tracing
- Conduction

A first approach to electrocardiogram (EKG) interpretation can be provided by observations available at a glance. Are there regular R-R cycles? Are P waves present with normal PR intervals? Is the frontal plane axis normal? Are significant "Q waves" absent? Is there appropriate precordial R wave development and QRS transition? If all the observations are present, then the tracing is normal, a conclusion that requires only a few seconds. The commandments of electrocardiography include the following:

1. Be mindful of the mischievous machine. In bygone days, the problem was the electrocardiograph itself, requiring attention to recording stylus heat and pressure. Today, it is computer interpretation of EKGs. Computer errors are frequent and can be disastrous to the unwary (both patient and doctor).
2. Beware the treacherous technician. The possibilities for technician errors are numerous. Reflect on this: if there are four extremity leads and a single precordial lead, the number of different lead combinations is 120, only one of which is correct.
3. "Thou shalt not interpret the EKG without reference to prior tracings." It is essential that previous tracings be included in the interpretation of the current EKG. Seeming minor differences in two tracings may indicate a significant new abnormality.
4. Assiduously avoid rhythm strips. Insist on 12-lead tracings with three rhythm strips at the bottom. Single leads may be misleading, as is apparent in the examples in **Fig. 1**. In **Fig. 1**A, atrial flutter is evident in lead II but not apparent in the simultaneous V_1. In **Fig. 1**B, the opposite is seen. There is no such thing as the best lead for a rhythm strip.
5. Learn to use ladder diagrams. Simple arrhythmias are easily analyzed and are obvious at first glance (eg, atrial or ventricular premature beats). Complex arrhythmias require a logical step-wise approach, which can be provided by using a ladder diagram. Plot obvious events (P-QRS) and determine their relationship.

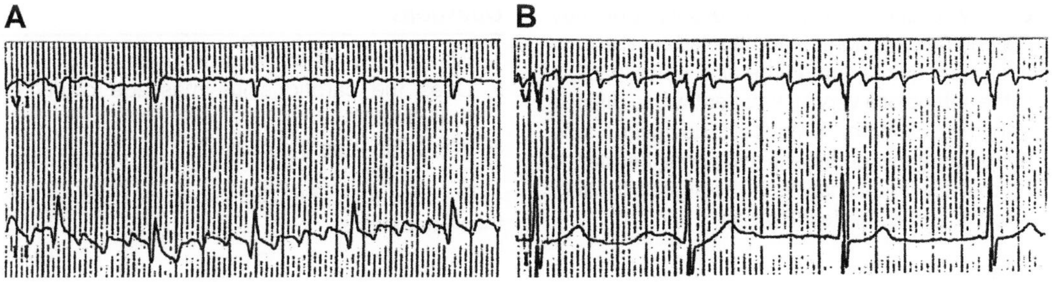

Fig. 1. (*A*) Atrial flutter apparent in lead II is not seen in V1. (*B*) Atrial flutter evident in V1 is not seen in lead II.

St Joseph Hospital, 1835 Franklin Street, Denver, CO 80218, USA
E-mail address: wpan747@comcast.net

Card Electrophysiol Clin 2 (2010) 159–177
doi:10.1016/j.ccep.2010.02.001

cardiacEP.theclinics.com

Box 1
The possibilities

Irregular narrow complex tachycardias
Atrial fibrillation
Atrial flutter with variable AV conduction
Multifocal atrial tachycardia

Regular narrow complex tachycardias
Sinus tachycardia
A-V nodal reentrant tachycardia
A-V reentrant tachycardia using an accessory pathway (orthodromic tachycardia)
Primary atrial tachycardia
Junctional tachycardia

Irregular wide QRS tachycardias
Atrial fibrillation with bundle branch block
Atrial fibrillation with an accessory pathway

Regular wide QRS tachycardias
Supraventricular tachycardia with bundle branch block
Antidromic tachycardia using an accessory pathway
Ventricular tachycardia

Early beats
Atrial ventricular or junctional premature beats
Capture beats during A-V dissociation
Reciprocal beats

Pauses in the rhythm
Atrial premature contractions conducted or nonconducted
Ventricular premature beats with or without retrograde conduction
Type 1 or 2 A-V block
Sinoatrial exit block
Concealed junctional extrasystoles

Usually, calipers are not necessary, but they may be helpful. Completing the ladder diagram analysis requires some time and is not feasible in the setting of a very sick patient with a difficult arrhythmia. With practice, however, one becomes more confident and more frequently correct in a quick analysis in the acute situation.

6. Know the possibilities (**Box 1**).

CASE 1

A 62-year-old man seen postoperatively after abdominal aortic aneurysm resection had intraoperative atrial fibrillation; he was given intravenous digoxin (**Fig. 2**A).

Questions

1. What might the tachycardia represent?
2. Does the carotid sinus massage clarify the arrhythmia?
3. What might be the cause?

The legend to **Fig. 2**B provides discussion of these questions.

CASE 2

The patient is a 77-year-old woman (**Fig. 3**). The computer interpretation was "sinus rhythm with premature atrial contraction and one fusion beat and probably lateral region infarction—age indeterminate."

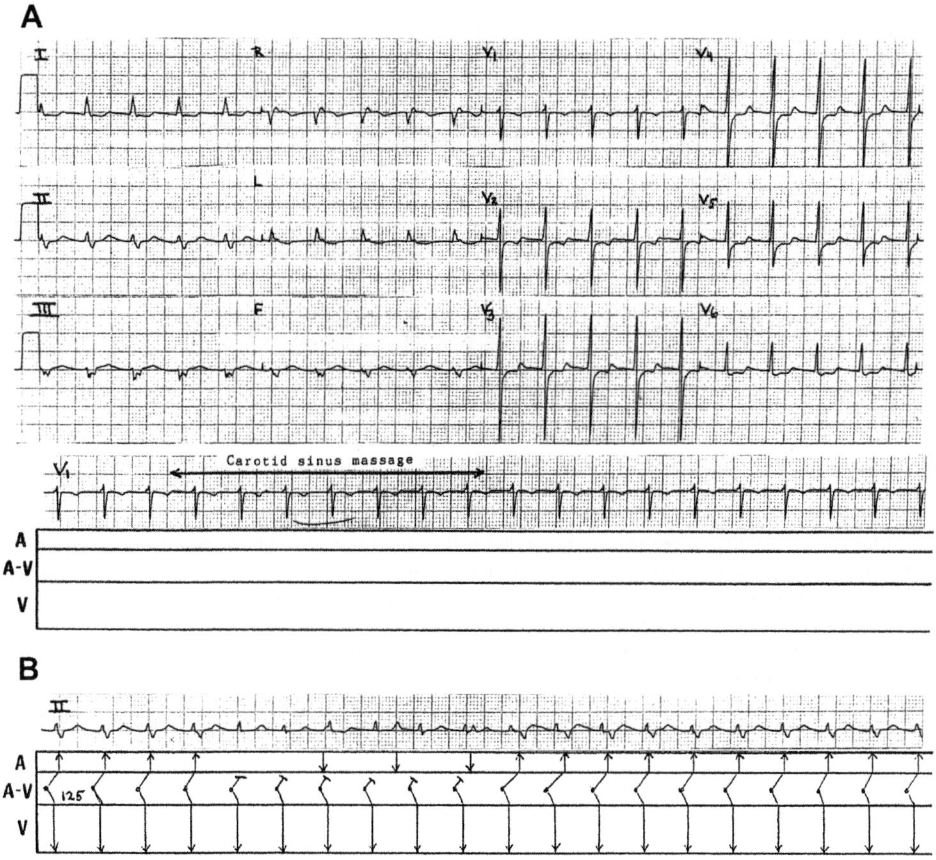

Fig. 2. (*A*) Tracing from a 62-year-old man with intraoperative atrial fibrillation. (*B*) The 12-lead tracing shows a supraventricular tachycardia at 125 per minute, with no P waves evident in front of the QRS complexes. There is an axis of 0 degrees and worrisome ST-T changes. Carotid sinus massage (CSM) clarifies the arrhythmic mechanism, the vagotonic effect of CSM results in a change in QRS morphology and transiently surfaces P waves (*upper arrows*), but does not convert the arrhythmia. The first four complexes are caused by the discharge of a junctional focus with retrograde atrial activation. The apparent S wave in lead II is an inverted P wave. CSM prevents the retrograde conduction but does not alter the accelerated focus. At the end of the CSM, the junctional focus once again conducts retrograde. Note the delay in retrograde conduction (*lower arrows*) as the vagal influence wanes. Clinical correlation: during surgery, the patient developed atrial fibrillation and was given repetitive doses of intravenous digoxin. When the drug was withheld, the arrhythmia disappeared.

Questions

1. What correction would you make?
2. What additional observations would you provide?
3. What do the wide QRS complexes represent?
4. Is there evidence of myocardial Infarction? How might you clarify?

CASE 3

The patient is an 85-year-old man (**Fig. 4**).

Questions

1. What do the irregular, multiformat P waves indicate?
2. What are the implications of the "Shamroth pattern"?

CASE 4

The patient is a 50-year-old man seen after cardiac surgery (**Fig. 5**).

Questions

1. What two pacing sites are seen?
2. Does this represent AV dissociation by the "default" of the sinus node?
3. What "turns off" the auxiliary pacemaker?

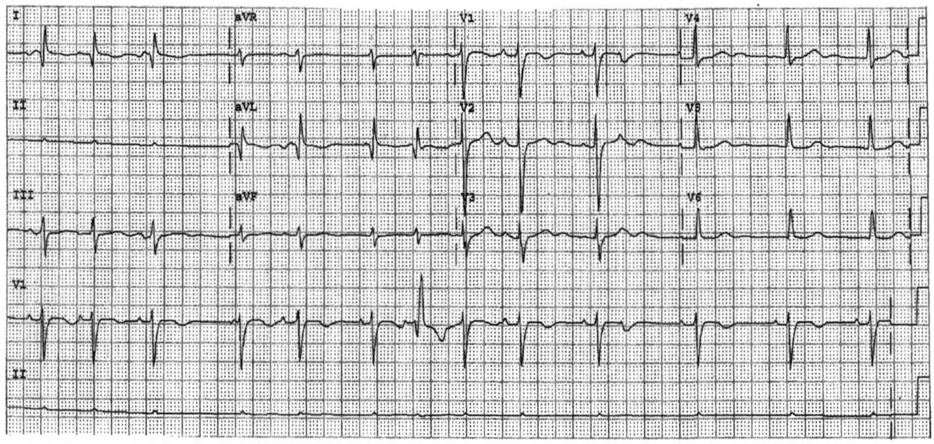

Fig. 3. Tracing from a 77-year-old woman. The rhythm is sinus in origin with several atrial premature contractions (APCs), one of which is aberrantly conducted with the morphology of right bundle branch block (RBBB), which was misdiagnosed by the computer as a fusion beat. Before concluding the interpretation as "abnormal EKG," always consider the possibility of technician error. Note that lead II is virtually a straight line. This bipolar lead connects the right arm and left leg, reflecting the electrical potential recorded from that vantage point. In this tracing, the right arm electrode has been placed on the right ankle and lead II is recording the potential across the ankles (where there is none). The rearrangement also inverts the P waves in lead I and completely changes the QRS morphology in the frontal plane. The interpretation should read "technically poor tracing, unsuitable for interpretation. Please repeat."

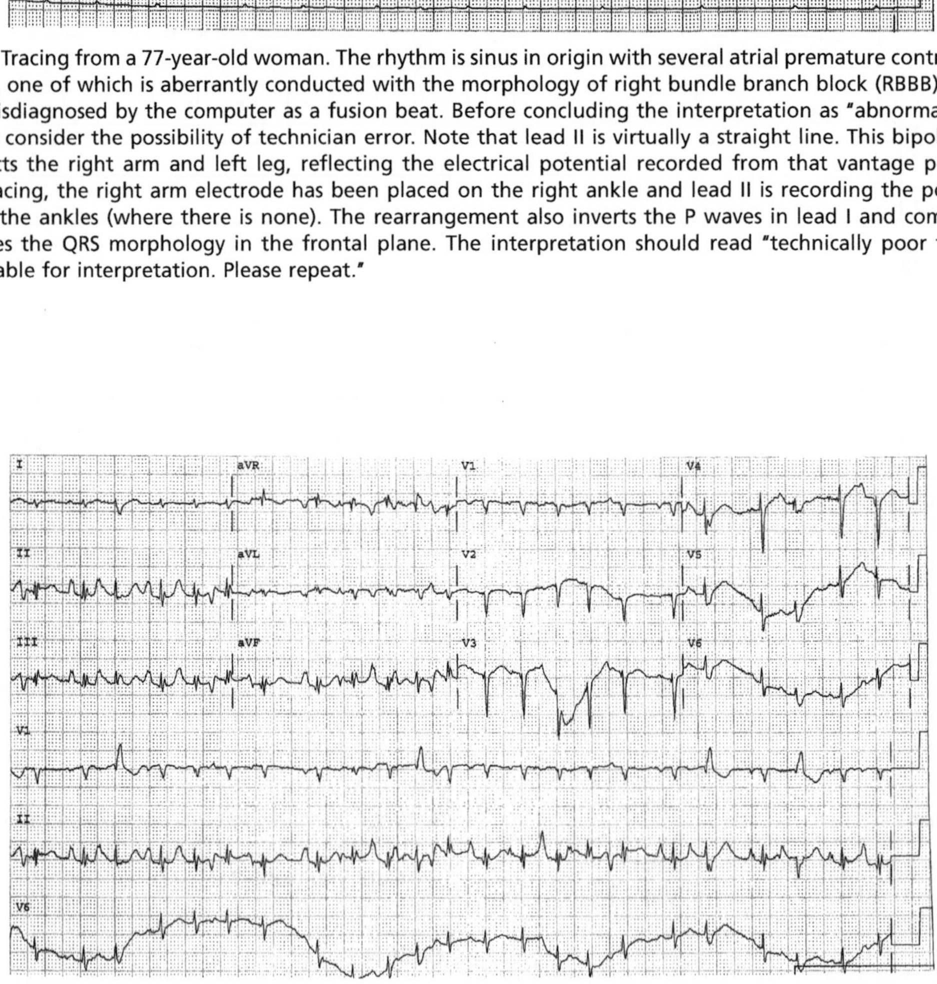

Fig. 4. Tracing from an 85-year-old man. The late Dr Leo Shamroth pointed out that if the P-QRS-T were all reasonably isoelectric in lead I, the patient had advanced chronic obstructive pulmonary disease. The multiple and variable APCs identify multifocal atrial tachycardia, most often seen in the setting of serious lung disease. The wide-QRS complexes are not ventricular premature beats but are aberrantly conducted beats. Note that they are preceded by P waves and show typical RBBB morphology, supporting their atrial origin. The absence of initial R waves in leads V_1 to V_3 is consistent with anterior infarction. With hyperinflation, however, the heart descends with the low-lying diaphragms. The "normal" precordial electrode position may be "too high" and lower lead position should be used. (A "precordial map" would be precordial leads 1 to 2 and three interspaces below the normal location). If additional waves are recorded in these leads, the diagnosis of anterior infarction is canceled.

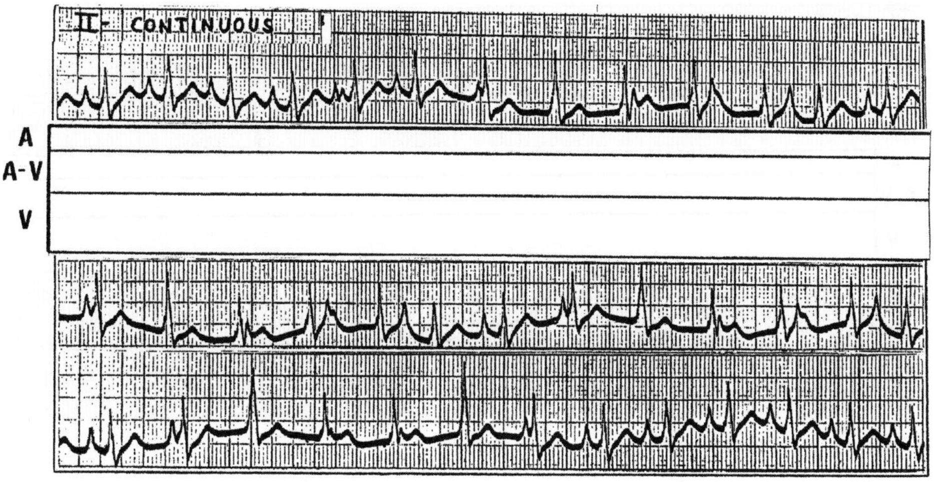

Fig. 5. Tracing from a 50-year-old man.

The legend to **Fig. 6** provides discussion of these questions.

CASE 5

Which of the following statements about **Fig. 7** are correct?

1. There is a sinus discharge rate of approximately 70 per minute with frequent atrial and ventricular complexes.
2. There is a stable atrial tachycardia of approximately 130 per minute with variable second-degree A-V block.

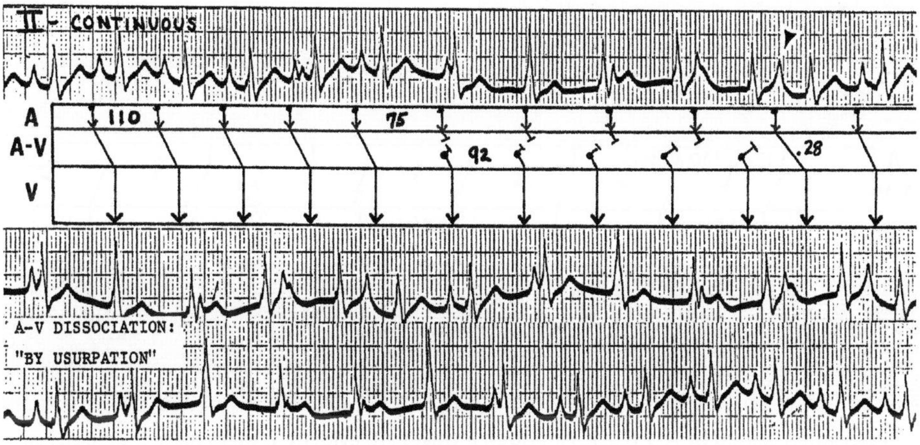

Fig. 6. This tracing is an example of AV dissection caused by a usurping junctional pacemaker. Sinus impulse (*arrowhead*). There is variability in the sinus rate, and whenever it slows to the critical degree, an "enhanced" pacemaker at a rate of 92 per minute appears in the A-V junction and activates the ventricles. The slower sinus P waves gradually march through the QRS complex, and when they reach an appropriate time in the refractory period of the preceding beat, the sinus impulse (*arrowhead*) is conducted (with a somewhat longer PR interval of 0.28 seconds). The successful penetration of the sinus impulse momentarily extinguishes the forming impulse in the A-V junction and allows the sinus pacemaker temporarily to regain control of ventricular activation. Subsequent sinus slowing, however, permits the junctional focus to reappear with the P waves "leapfrogging" the QRS and T until the A-V junction is responsive, permitting another "capture beat." This phenomenon is repetitively seen in the second and third strips. Notice the interesting coincidental effect of the P waves merging with the QRS complexes, adding to their height or somewhat changing their morphology. In this patient, the accelerated junctional focus was caused by digitalis intoxication, and the correct interpretation is important. When the drug was stopped, sinus activity continued, and the enhanced junctional pacemaker disappeared.

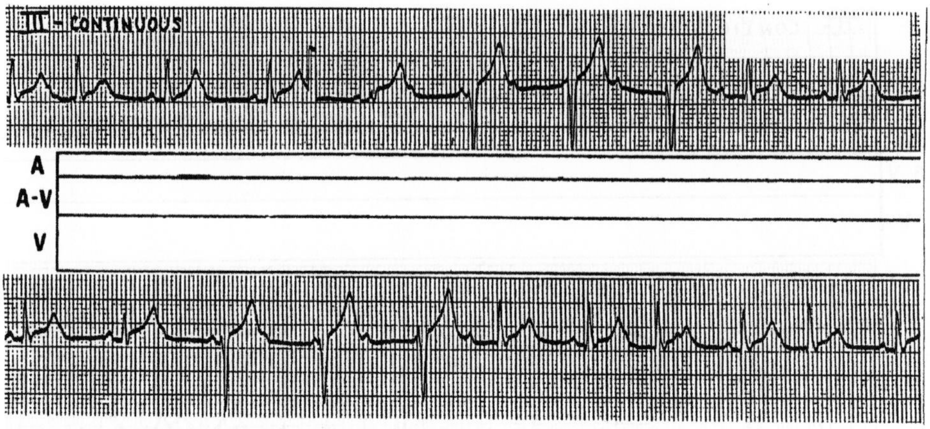

Fig. 7. See text for a list of statements about this tracing.

3. AV block promotes the appearance of a subsidiary pacemaker, which emerges with a discharge rate of 88 per minute. This is AV dissociation caused by AV block.
4. The changed QRS morphology, caused by the discharge of the ectopic pacemaker, indicates that it arises below the level of the bundle of His and is ventricular in origin.
5. The competition of penetrating atrial impulse and ventricular ectopic focus results in fusion beats.

The legend to **Fig. 8** provides discussion of these questions.

CASE 6

The tracing in **Fig. 9** is from a 70-year-old man with arteriosclerotic heart disease, chronic obstructive pulmonary disease, and chronic renal disease.

Question

What is going on in the tracing?

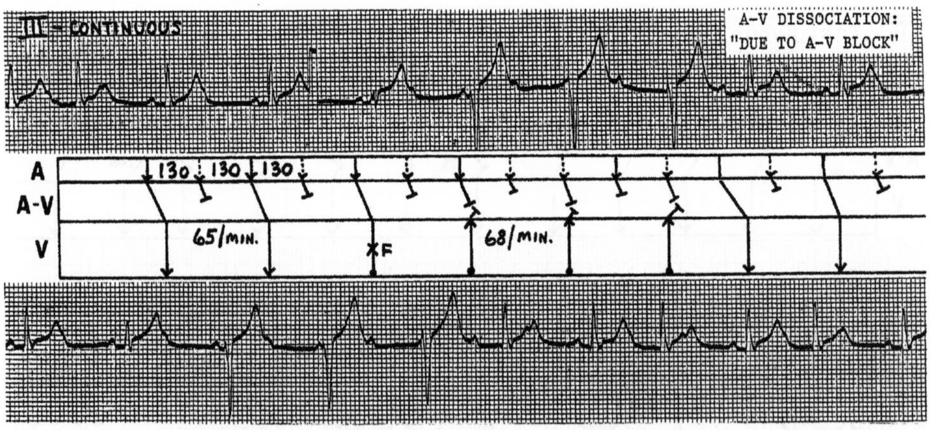

Fig. 8. A-V dissociation caused by A-V block. Although P waves are evident, it takes more than a casual glance to determine that the true atrial rate is 130 per minute, and that initially the atrial stimuli are conducted 2:1 to the ventricle. The effective rate is 65 per minute. Lurking in the ventricle is an ectopic pacemaker with a firing rate of 68 per minute. A little reflection should make it obvious who wins this duel. The ventricular focus assumes command with a fusion complex (F), indicating the participation of both atrial and ventricular impulses in cardiac excitation. The ventricular focus remains in charge for the next three beats, then the dissociated P wave finds a critical time in refractory period established by the ventricular focus and "captures" the ventricle. This phenomenon is repeated in the bottom strip. Of interest, this strip ends with an interlude of 3:2 Wenckebach A-V block. There are several abnormalities and considerations to emphasize in this EKG: (1) it is evident that some degree of AV block must be present or all of the atrial stimuli would be conducted; (2) the rate of the ventricular focus (68 per minute) is certainly abnormal and it must be an accelerated discharge site; and (3) the fusion complex proves that the ectopic pacemaker is arising in the ventricle. AV block sets the stage where an accelerated ventricular focus can surface to cause AV dissociation. If the ladder diagram is completed, it should be evident that all statements are correct except for the first.

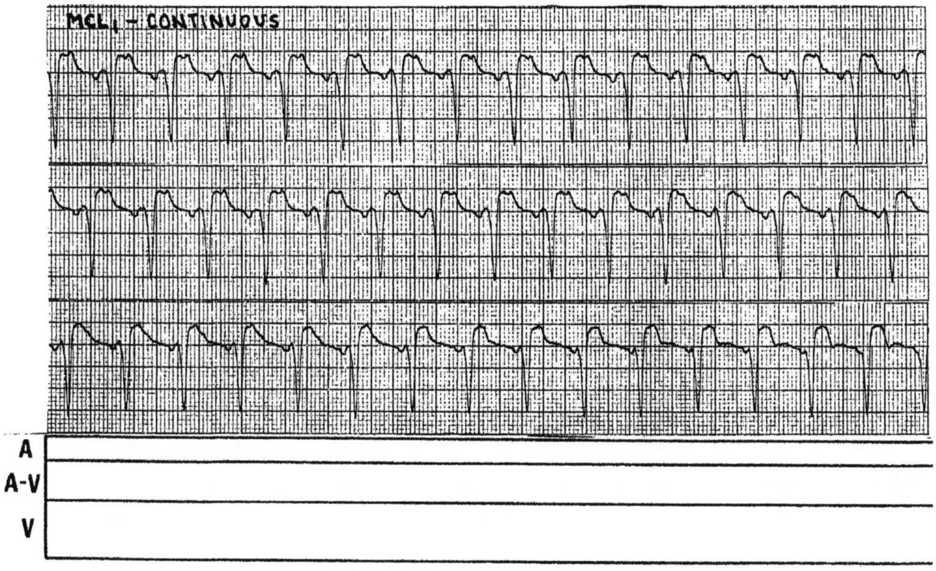

Fig. 9. Tracing from a 70-year-old man with arteriosclerotic heart disease, chronic obstructive pulmonary disease, and chronic renal disease.

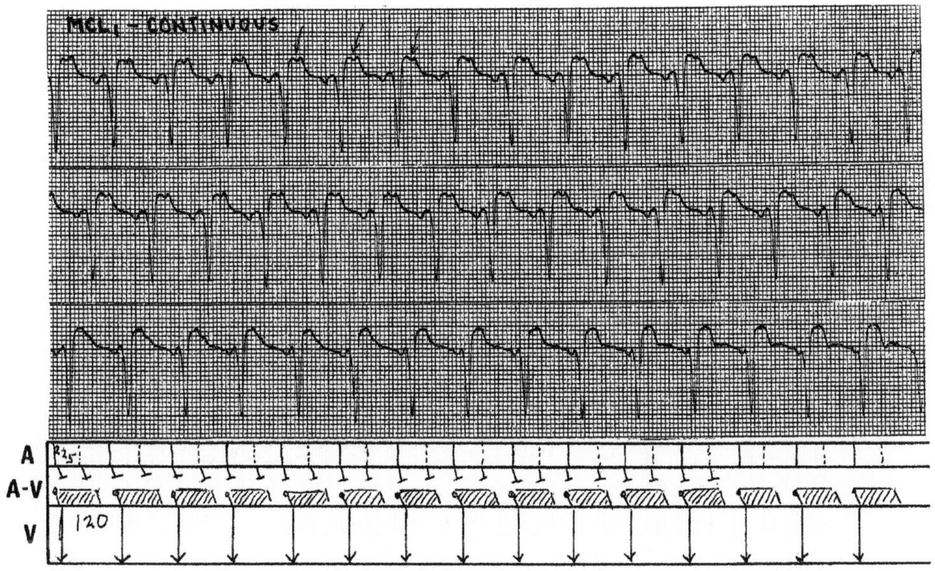

Fig. 10. Tracing from **Fig. 9** is shown with completed ladder diagram. P wave hiding in the ST segment (*arrows*). In bygone days, the mainstay of therapy for congestive heart failure was digoxin, and the occurrence of digitalis toxicity was common. Virtually every imaginable arrhythmia could be seen. In this example, the rhythm seems to be sinus tachycardia at 120 per minute, but if one looks closely there is another P wave hiding in the ST segment (*arrows*). Given only the top tracing, this is an example of atrial tachycardia (atrial flutter) at 240 per minute with 2:1 A-V conduction. The second and third strips, however, prove that this interpretation is incorrect. The obvious P wave and R-R cycles remain regular, but the PR interval gradually shortens. Ultimately, it becomes evident that the P waves are not conducted and that the P waves and QRS complexes are dissociated. An accelerated junctional focus at 120 per minute is in command. The rhythm represents a combination of some A-V "block," accompanied by a usurping ectopic focus. The status of the A-V bridge cannot be determined because, as diagrammed, the discharge of the junctional focus repetitively sets up a refractory wake that prevents transmission of the atrial stimuli. Digoxin dose in this man was increased because of progressive heart failure. This arrhythmia correlated with a plasma "dig." level of 4.8.

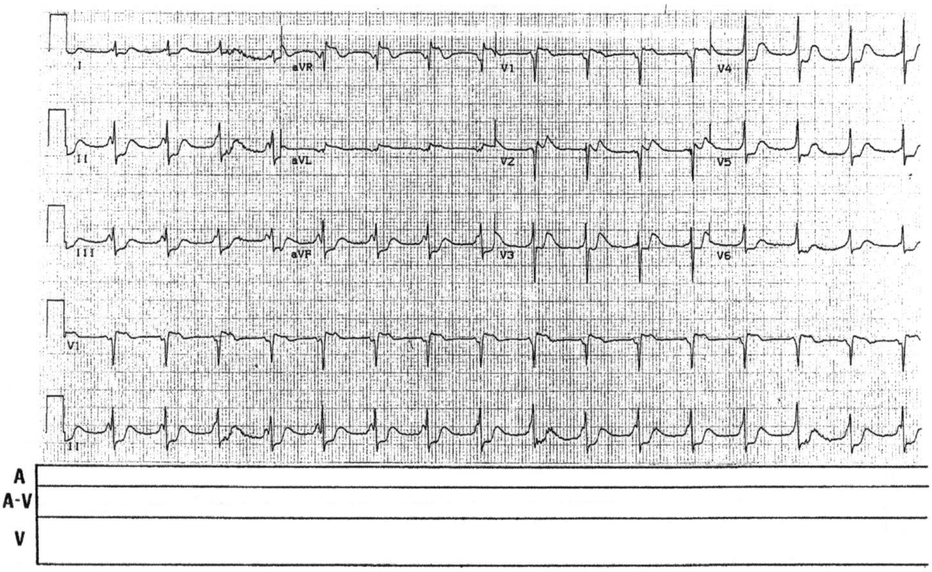

Fig. 11. Tracing from a 37-year-old man with drug overdose.

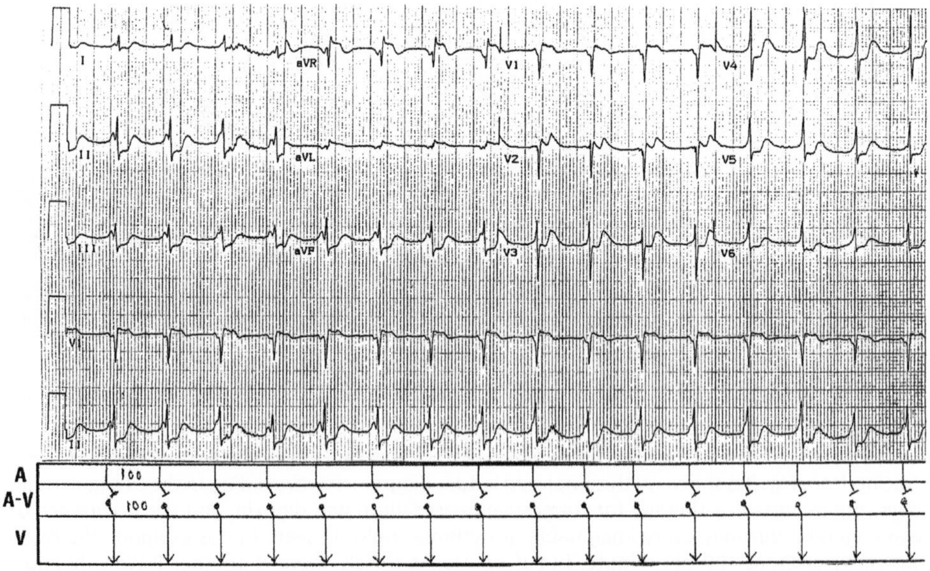

Fig. 12. Tracing in **Fig. 11** is shown with completed ladder diagram. Over the course of several days, this young man repetitively smoked "crack" cocaine. The resulting high prevented sleep, so he attempted to "come down" by taking a large dose of morphine. He quickly slipped into the arms of Morpheus, and it was not until he stopped breathing that his friend became concerned and called emergency medical services. He was intubated in the field but was "brain-dead" on arrival at the hospital. The ladder diagram depicts his rhythm disturbance. An accelerated junctional focus is competing with sinus rhythm. The rates of the two are virtually identical, and the rhythm represents so-called "isochronic" A-V dissociation. It should be obvious that the P waves are so closely related to the QRS complexes that they cannot be conducted. Similarly, because the atrial events are so aligned, no conclusion can be made about AV block.

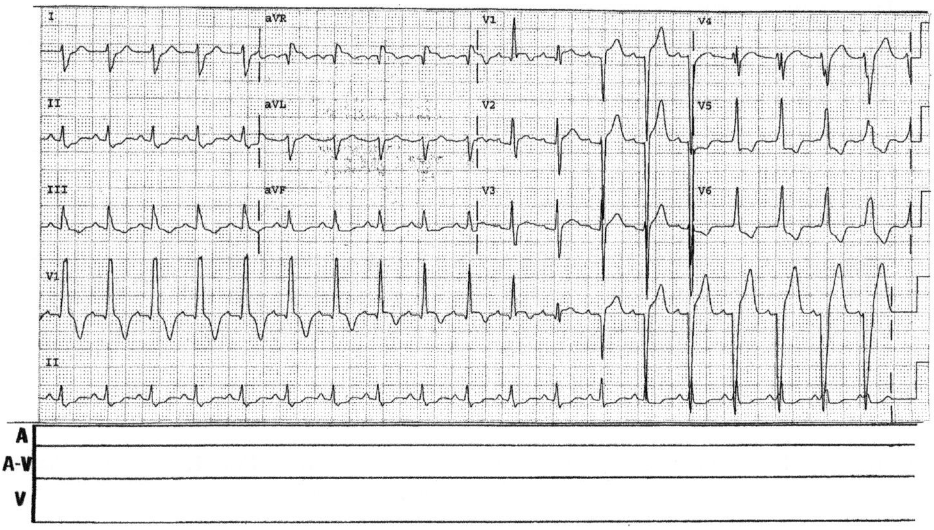

Fig. 13. Tracing from 52-year-old man.

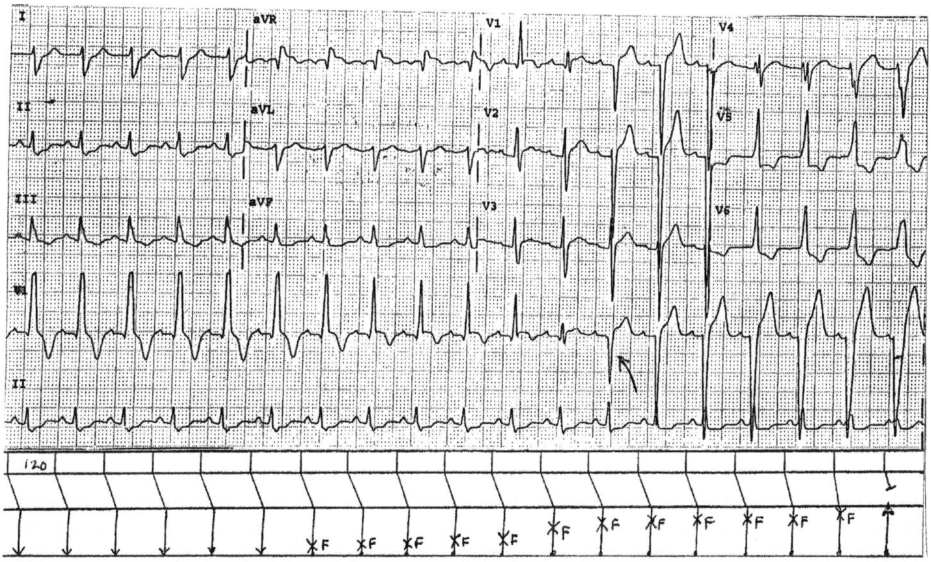

Fig. 14. Tracing from **Fig. 13** with completed ladder diagram. Normal QRS complex (*arrow*). The tracing starts with a sinus tachycardia at 120 per minute with a wide QRS. The morphology and frontal plane axis indicate that this is caused by bifascicular block: RBBB plus left posterior fascicular block. It ends with an accelerated ventricular focus with left bundle branch block (LBBB) morphology at a very similar rate. The configuration during this rhythm suggests that the ectopic site is probably in the right ventricle. When its discharge is coincident with the arrival of the sinus impulses, ventricular fusion beats result. In the middle portion of the tracing, a number (12) of these are present. Their changing configuration demonstrates the variable participation of the conducted and ectopic stimuli. Of particular interest, when the RV focus discharges at "just the right time," it cancels the RBBB, and a normal QRS complex results (*arrow*). The next day the accelerated ventricular focus was gone and only the bifascicular block remained.

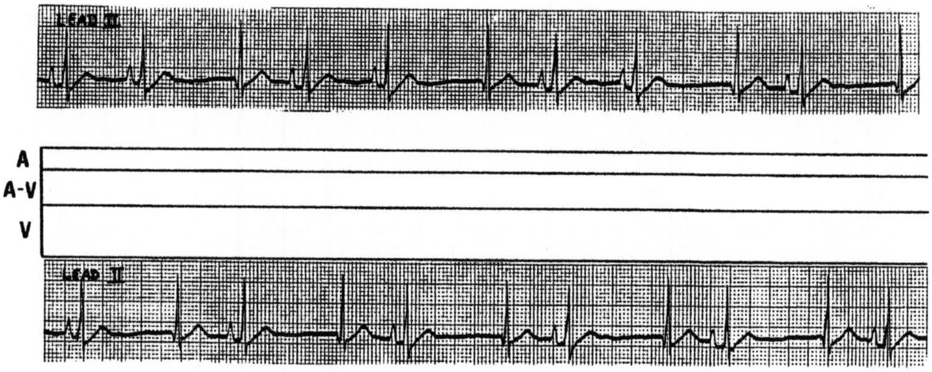

Fig. 15. Tracing from a 40-year-old man with chronic cor pulmonale and right heart failure.

The legend to **Fig. 10** provides discussion of this question.

CASE 7

The patient is a 37-year-old man with drug overdose (**Fig. 11**).

Questions

1. The relationship of the P waves and QRS complexes is stable. Are they cause and effect?
2. Do you agree with the following statement: if no P waves are conducted, there is complete AV block?

The legend to **Fig. 12** provides discussion of these questions.

CASE 8

The patient is a 52-year-old man (**Fig. 13**).

Questions

1. Does this wide-QRS rhythm show right or left bundle branch block?
2. Are there fusion complexes present, and if so, how many?
3. Why is there a narrow complex recorded?

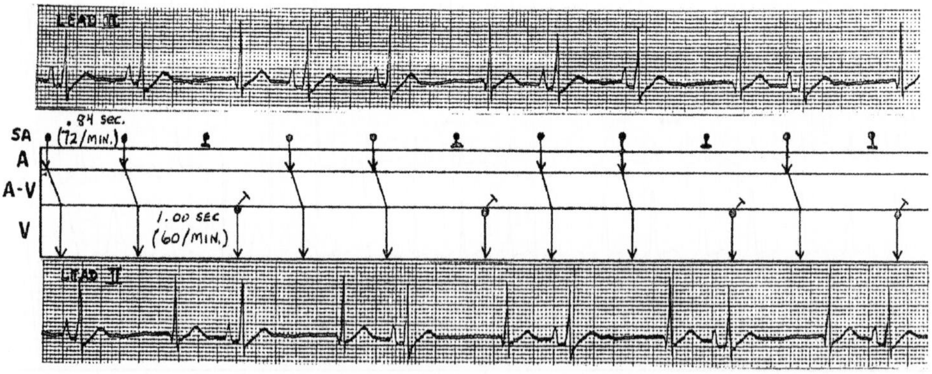

Fig. 16. Tracing from **Fig. 15** with a completed ladder diagram. A quick glance indicates that there are "missing P waves." If one measures the manifest P-P interval (0.84 seconds), it is clear that the missing P waves do not alter the basic sinus node cycle. As diagrammed in the top strip, this is an example of a sinoatrial (SA) exit block. Every third potential SA impulse is not transmitted to the atria. An escape pacemaker surfaces at a rate of 60 per minute to continue cardiac activation. Note that it is slightly different in morphology from the sinus-conducted beats, suggesting that it might arise just below the bundle of His, so-called "fascicular rhythm." In the bottom strip, SA exit block occurs every other impulse, leading to "doublets" consisting of escape pacemaker, followed by a sinus impulse, an example of "escape-capture bigemini." Block of SA impulses can be envisioned similar to "degrees" of A-V block and can classify disturbed transmission into first-, second-, and third-degree SA block. First-degree exit block cannot be identified on the surface EKG because one cannot determine the timing of SA nodal discharge. Similarly, third-degree SA block could not be identified, because there are no P waves present. Second-degree SA block can be likened to type I or II A-V block in the top strip in the present tracing, the P-P cycle remains regular, and the "missing P waves" occur without the alert of changing P-P intervals. This is an example of the type II SA exit block.

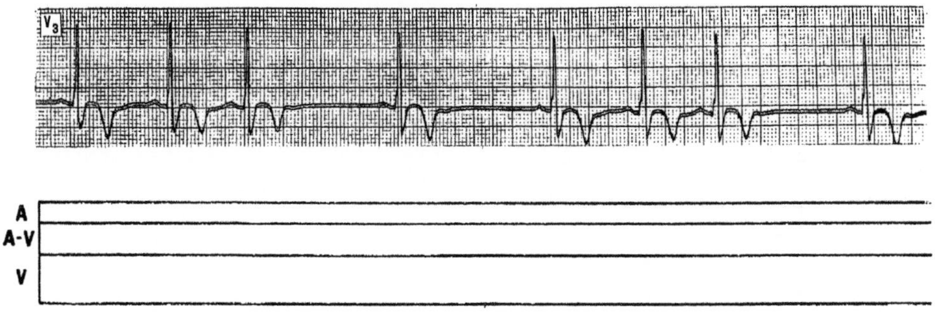

Fig. 17. See text for questions about this tracing.

The legend to **Fig. 14** provides discussion of these questions.

CASE 9

The patient is a 40-year-old man with chronic cor pulmonale and right heart failure (**Fig. 15**). Treatment was with diuretics and digitalis.

Questions

1. What is the cause of the pause?
2. Is the rhythm abnormality caused by disturbed impulse formation or conduction?
3. With what does the pause terminate?
4. In the bottom strip, what is "escape capture bigemini"?
5. What might be the cause and the treatment?

The legend to **Fig. 16** provides discussion of these questions.

CASE 10

See the tracing in **Fig. 17**.

Questions

1. What is the cause of the irregularity of the R-R and P-P intervals?
2. Is this a disturbance of impulse formation or conduction?
3. Is this an example of "sinus arrest"?

The legend to **Fig. 18** provides discussion of these questions.

CASE 11

The patient is a 40-year-old woman who was seen in the emergency department (**Fig. 19**).

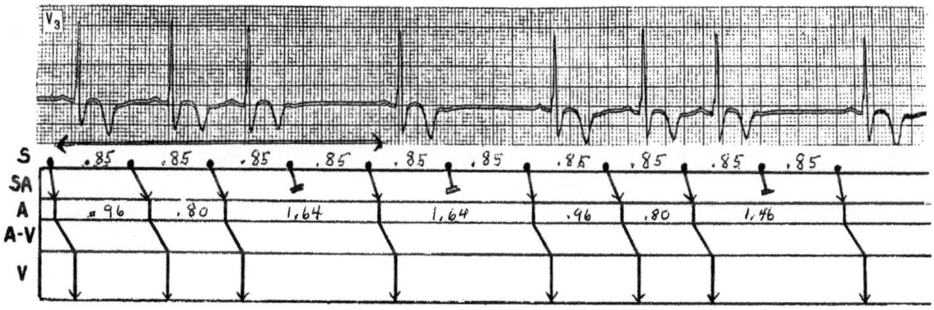

Fig. 18. Type I sinoatrial exit block. Note the grouping of the P waves and QRS complexes and the obvious "missing P waves". This is an example of type 1 SA exit block, a disturbance of impulse conduction. The ladder diagram provides a depiction of the presumed events. There is gradual prolongation in passage of the sinus node signal to the atrial myocardium until a "drop beat" occurs. Note the shortening of the P-P cycle before the drop beat. This is analogous to Wenckebach AV block in which shortening of the R-R interval occurs because of a decreasing amount of prolongation of the PR interval. The measured P wave intervals are 0.96 + 0.80 + 1.64 = 3.40 seconds. Presuming that there is SA discharge during the pause, there are four cycles present between the arrowheads. The calculated rate of the SA node is 3.40 – 4 = 0.85, a rate of 70 per minute. This arrhythmia could be caused by drugs that depress the sinus and AV nodes or by "ischemic disease."

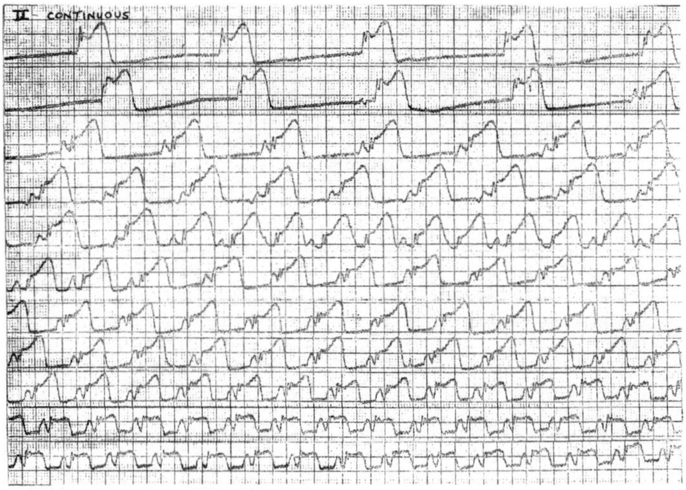

Fig. 19. Tracing from a 40-year-old woman. The marked ST segment elevation in this lengthy rhythm strip anticipates an acute inferior infarction. Receptors in the inferior aspect of the ventricular septum can prompt a powerful parasympathetic response, the Bezold-Jarisch reflex. It results in a vagatonic suppression of sinus node formation or A-V nodal conduction. In addition, the reflex results in peripheral vasodilation. The effect is bradycardia and hypotension, a life-threatening combination. The immediate therapy is the administration of intravenous atropine. In the example, the rhythm begins with a junctional focus at 30 per minute. Note the prompt and dramatic effect of 1 mg of atropine. The P waves reappear, the rate increases, and the magnitude of the injury current decreases.

Questions

1. If a 12-lead tracing was available, instead of only this rhythm strip, what would one expect it to show?
2. The rhythm is irregular with significant pauses. What are they caused by?
3. What is the Bezold-Jarisch reflex? When does it appear and what are the consequences?
4. What treatment would you recommend?

The legend to **Fig. 19** provides a discussion of these questions.

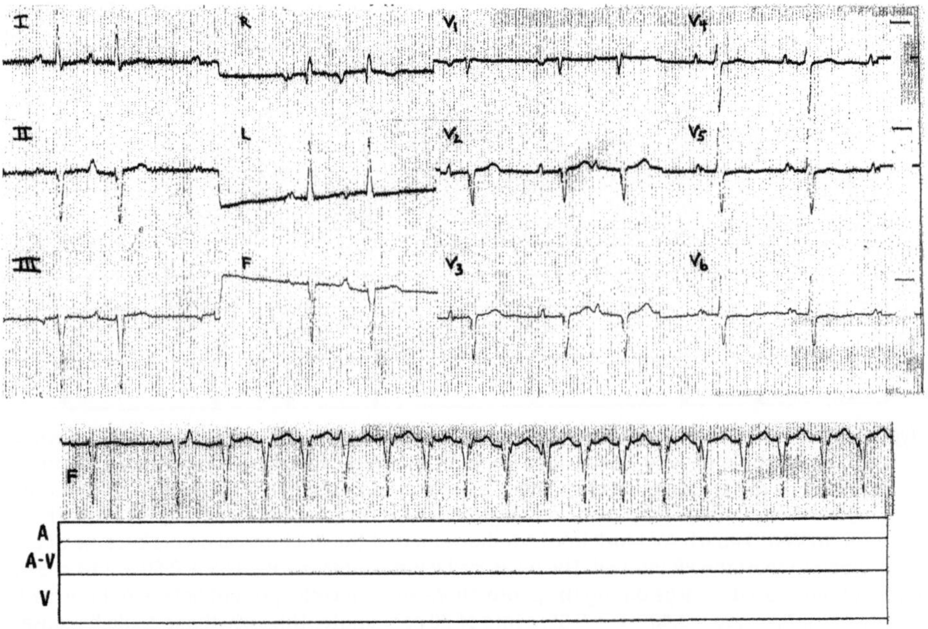

Fig. 20. Tracing from a 75-year-old man complaining that his heart was racing and he felt dizzy.

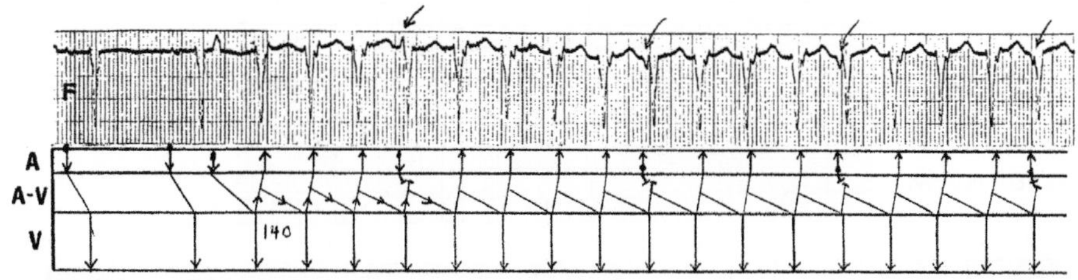

Fig. 21. Tracing from **Fig. 20** with completed ladder diagram. The 12-lead EKG is straightforward: there is normal sinus rhythm with frequent APCs. Sinus impulses are conducted with a long PR interval and there is left axis deviation of –70 degrees consistent with left anterior fascicular block. Evidence of a prior anterior myocardial infarction is present. Sinus P waves are abnormal in morphology consistent with bilateral abnormality. The obvious point of interest is the salvo of supraventricular tachycardia. The evident atrial premature impulse is conducted with a long PR interval and initiates an AV nodal reentrant tachycardia, with the retrograde P wave distorting the terminal part of the QRS complex. This is typical AV nodal reentry using a slow pathway for anterograde conduction and a fast conducting limb for retrograde passage. A point of particular interest is the beats marked with the arrows. Note that these show an abnormality of the initial portion of the QRS complex with loss of the retrograde P wave distorting the terminal part of the QRS. The ladder diagram depicts what is happening. There are four atrial premature stimuli, which depolarize the atria but do not interrupt the tachycardia. This tracing is an electrophysiologist's dream. The APCs prove that the atria are not an essential part of the reentrant circuit. This indicates that the arrhythmia must be AV nodal in location and cannot be caused by reentry using an accessory pathway because the retrograde impulse requires atrial participation to complete the reentrant loop.

CASE 12

The patient is a 75-year-old man complaining of heart racing and dizziness (**Fig. 20**).

Questions

1. Several observations can be made in this tracing. Can you identify five of them?
2. What is the arrhythmia an example of? Is it completely typical?

The legend to **Fig. 21** provides a discussion of these questions.

CASE 13

The patient is an 81-year-old man with previous inferior wall infarction. The rhythm strip of the V_1 (**Fig. 22**) shows an unusual phenomenon.

Questions

1. What do the differing QRS morphologies represent?
2. What does this phenomenon represent?
3. Why are there normal beats?
4. Does the increasing T-wave abnormality indicate progressive "ischemia"?

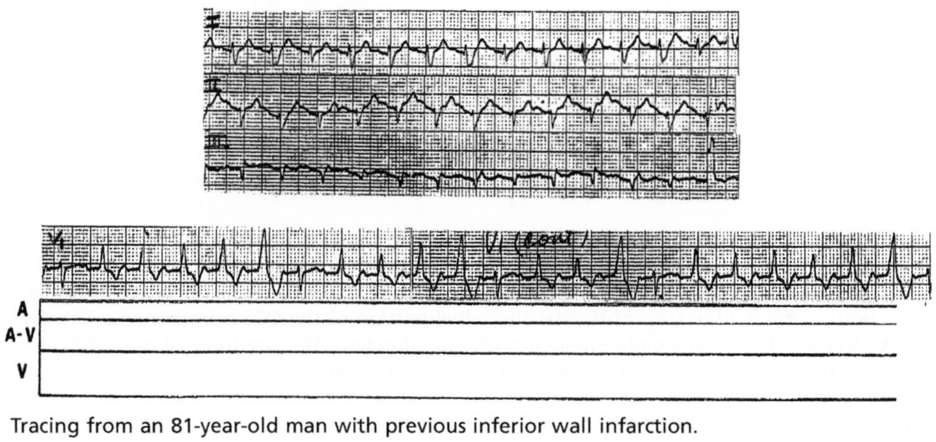

Fig. 22. Tracing from an 81-year-old man with previous inferior wall infarction.

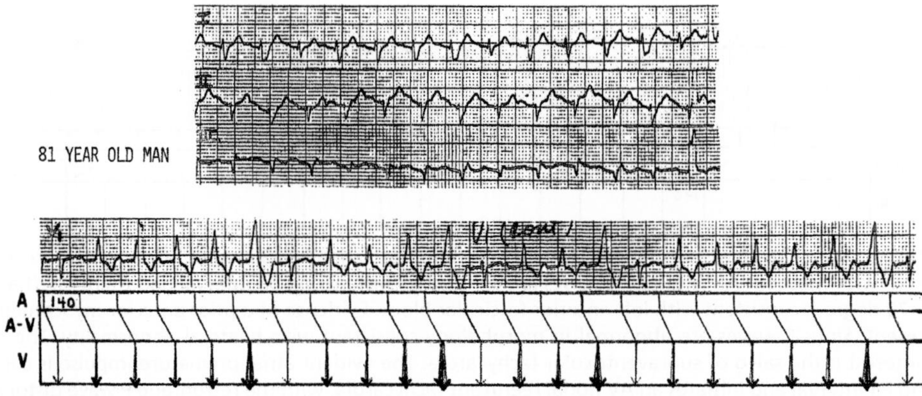

Fig. 23. Ladder diagram for the tracing in **Fig. 22**. This elderly gentleman has had a previous inferior wall infarction. The obvious point of interest is the changing QRS morphology, which in lead V_1 seems to represent varying degrees of RBBB. Intermittently, there is a single normal QRS with subsequent beats showing gradual and progressive QRS delay until "complete RBBB" develops. The subsequent beat is normally conducted once again, and the sequence repeats itself several times. This is an example of an usual abnormality: Wenckebach (type 1) delay in RBB conduction and the phenomenon of Wenckebach block of a bundle branch is an obvious extension of Wenckebach A-V block. It seems to be caused by gradual conduction delay in the affected bundle resulting in increased degrees of QRS prolongation, culminating in complete RBBB. The interlude during which the right bundle is "not used" permits a longer recovery time, and the next sinus impulse is able to traverse the right bundle in normal fashion. The repetitive occurrence helps to ensure that is not accidental. The changing T waves parallel the "amount" of depolarization abnormality.

The legend to **Fig. 23** provides discussion of these questions.

CASE 14

The patient is a 77-year-old man. The rhythm strip shows a peculiar alternation in the QRS morphology (**Fig. 24**).

Questions

Which of the following is the cause of the alternation in QRS morphology?

1. Intermittent bifascicular block?
2. Ventricular bigemini?
3. Atrial bigemini with alternating aberration?

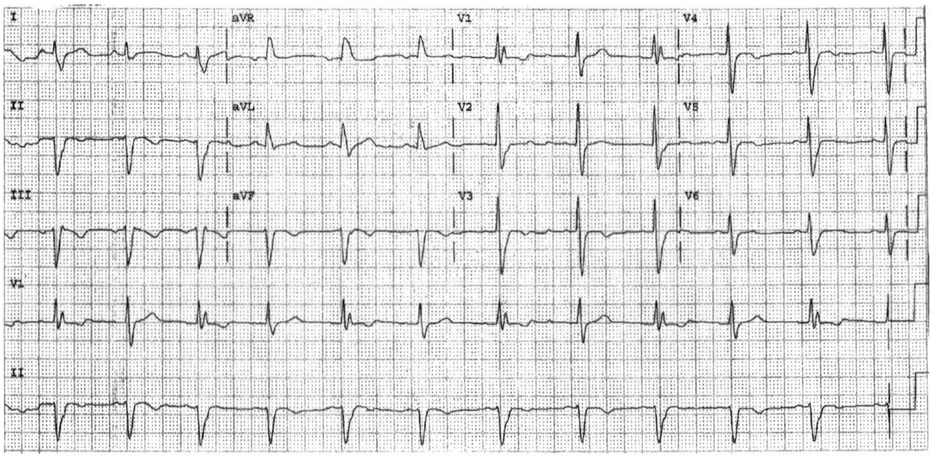

Fig. 24. Tracing from a 77-year-old man with an alternation in the QRS morphology. There is a regular sinus rhythm at 70 per minute and all atrial impulses are conducted with a constant PR interval. The QRS complexes show left axis deviation consistent with left anterior fascicular block, but there is an alternating duration and morphology. Note in the rhythm strip of V_1 that the initial portion of the QRS is unchanged. The prominent R waves in V_1-V_2-V_3 point to an aged undetermined posterior infarction. The late forces show RBBB in every other beat. When a stimulus does conduct over the RBBB, it is rendered refractory, and if its recovery time is prolonged, the next impulse is conducted with RBBB. The "peculiar alternation" is caused by the combination of left anterior fascicular block and alternating RBBB.

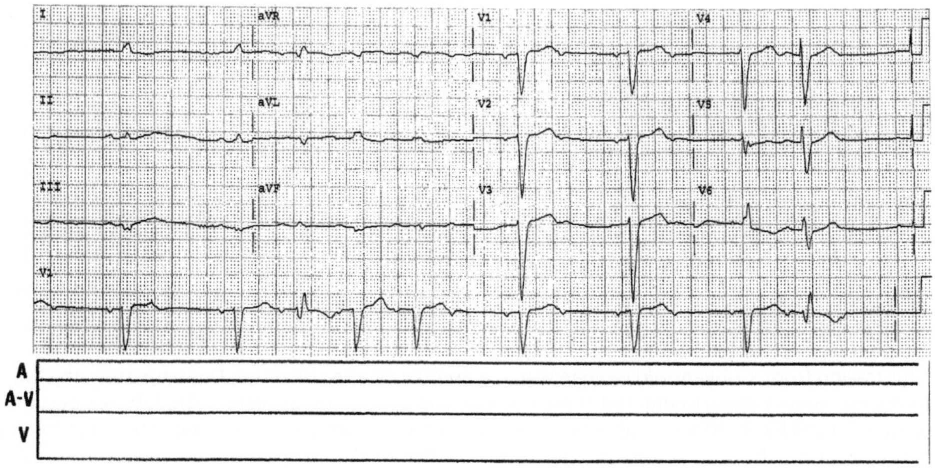

Fig. 25. Tracing from a 70-year-old man.

4. Rate-related bundle branch block?

CASE 15

The patient is a 70-year-old man (**Fig. 25**).

Questions

1. Is there any irregularity in the atrial rhythm?
2. What is causing the pauses in the rhythm?
3. What is "postextrasystolic sinus node suppression"?
4. What is "bilateral bundle branch block"?

The legend to **Fig. 26** provides discussion of these questions.

CASE 16

The patient is a 74-year-old woman complaining of marked weakness. A number of abnormalities are present (**Fig. 27**).

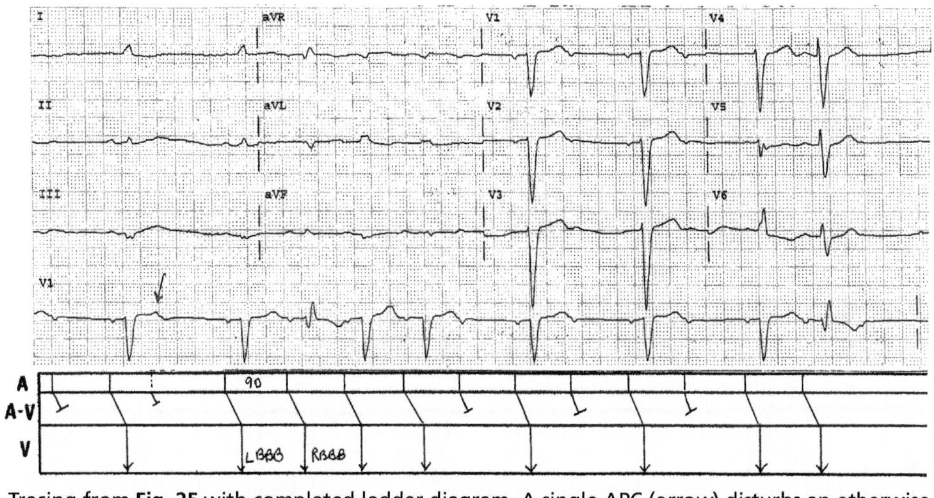

Fig. 26. Tracing from **Fig. 25** with completed ladder diagram. A single APC (*arrow*) disturbs an otherwise regular sinus rhythm at 90 per minute. The APC depolarizes the sinus node and forces it to "reset." The original sinus P-P cycle does not immediately return, reflecting "post-extrasystolic sinus node suppression." Subsequently, the atrial impulses are transmitted in peculiar fashion. Some are not conducted; some are conducted with LBBB morphology and some with RBBB pattern. The varying bundle branch conduction has been termed "bilateral bundle branch block." It signals the imminent demise of the intraventricular pathways and justifies insertion of an electronic pacemaker.

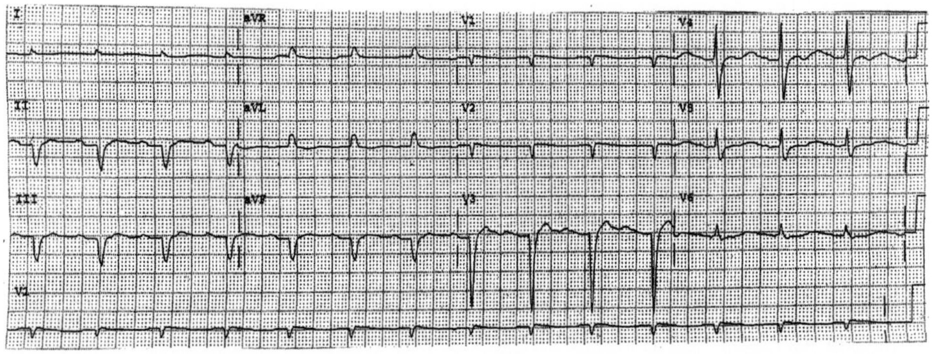

Fig. 27. This tracing from a 74-year-old woman shows a number of abnormalities. Unfortunately, this was a single EKG from the emergency department and there is no clinical correlation available. The left axis deviation in the frontal plane is caused by an inferior wall infarct, and the lack of R waves in V_1 to V_3 indicates an anterior myocardial infarction. Noteworthy observations are the short Q to the onset and apex of the T wave and very prominent U waves, the combination consistent with hypercalcemia, and hypokalemia. Recall that cellular "excitability" reflects the difference between the resting membrane potential = (–) 90 mV and the threshold potential = (–) 60 mV. The normal excitability is $\pm$30 mV. Hypokalemia increases the resting membrane potential (eg, to 100 mV) and hypercalcemia decreases threshold level (eg, to –50mV). With the combined electrolyte derangement, the stimulus now required to reach the threshold is 50 mV, with resultant profound weakness.

Questions

1. What is causing the left axis deviation?
2. Is the precordial R wave development appropriate?
3. Is there evidence of ion sufficiency or deficiency?
4. Is the "excitability requirement" normal?

CASE 17

The patient is a 77-year-old woman.

Questions

Which of the following problems does her tracing (**Fig. 28**) suggest:

1. Diabetes
2. Chronic renal failure
3. Pancreatitis
4. All of the above.

The legend to **Fig. 28** provides discussion of this question.

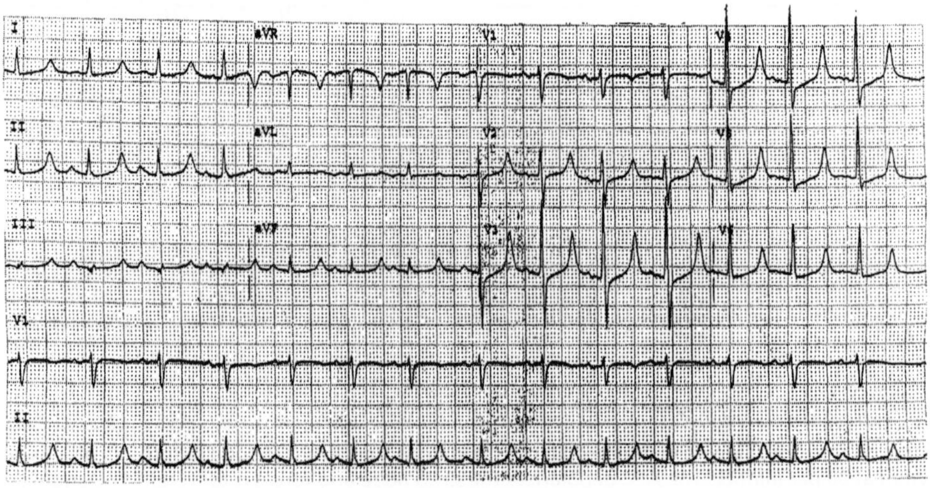

Fig. 28. This tracing is from a 77-year-old woman. The prolonged Q to the onset and apex of the T wave indicates hypocalcemia, and tall, narrow-based T waves hyperkalemia. All three of the suggested problems were present. The patient's pancreatitis caused the release of lipase and the resulting free fatty acids were "saponified" by calcium, resulting in a decreased calcium level of 7.2 mg/dL. Diabetic ketoacidosis and chronic renal failure combined to increase the potassium to 8.2 mEq/L.

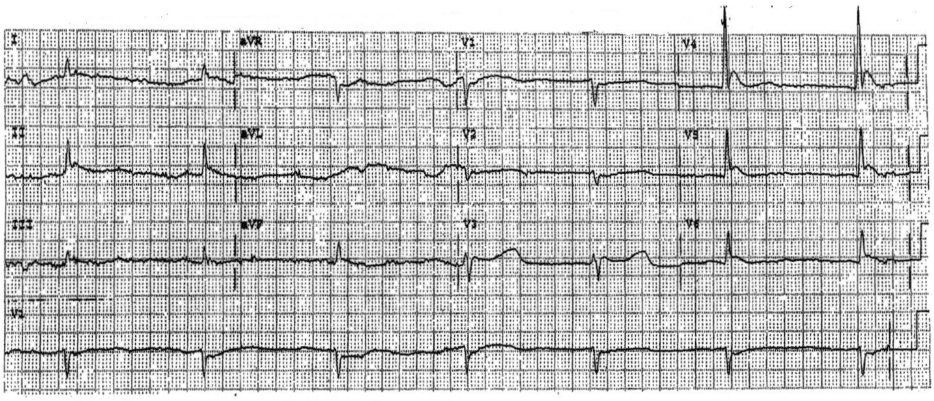

Fig. 29. Tracing from a 52-year-old woman "found down."

CASE 18

The patient is a 52-year-old woman "found down" (**Fig. 29**). The computer interpretation was atrial fibrillation with rapid ventricular response of 121 (now present), indeterminate QRS axis, nonspecific intraventricular conduction delay (now present), low voltage in frontal leads (now present), and anterolateral region infarct, age indeterminate (now present).

Questions

1. Do you agree with the computer's interpretation?
2. What is this patient's problem?
3. What eponymic term has been applied to this EKG pattern?

The legend to **Fig. 30** provides discussion of these questions.

CASE 19

The patient is an 82-year-old woman seen in the emergency department with chest pain (**Fig. 31**). The computer interpretation was "No further analysis attempted for this ECG—not enough leads could be measured, atrial fibrillation with V

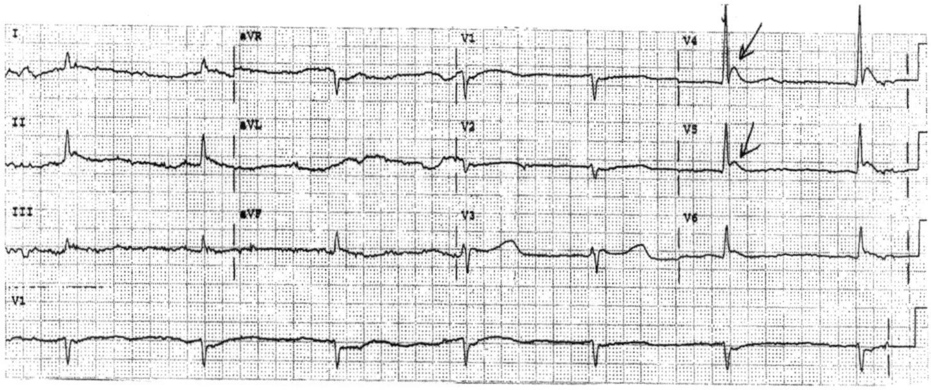

Fig. 30. Arrows show Osborne waves. This EKG pattern was first described in 1953 by Dr J. J. Osborn. Osborn was a cardiac surgeon investigating the application of induced hypothermia to increase the time that the heart could be stepped for correction of defects. He noted that as body temperature decreased, the EKG developed a late contribution to the QRS complex. This has become known as the "Osborne wave." In this tracing, none of the computer diagnoses is correct. This tragic woman was an alcoholic "street person" who apparently passed out in an isolated area on a cold Colorado day. When found and brought to the emergency department her rectal temperature was 75°F. Note the sinus bradycardia, the shiver artifact, and the "Osborn Waves" (*arrows*), particularly in leads V_4 to V_6. A picturesque term that has been applied is "hypothermic humps."

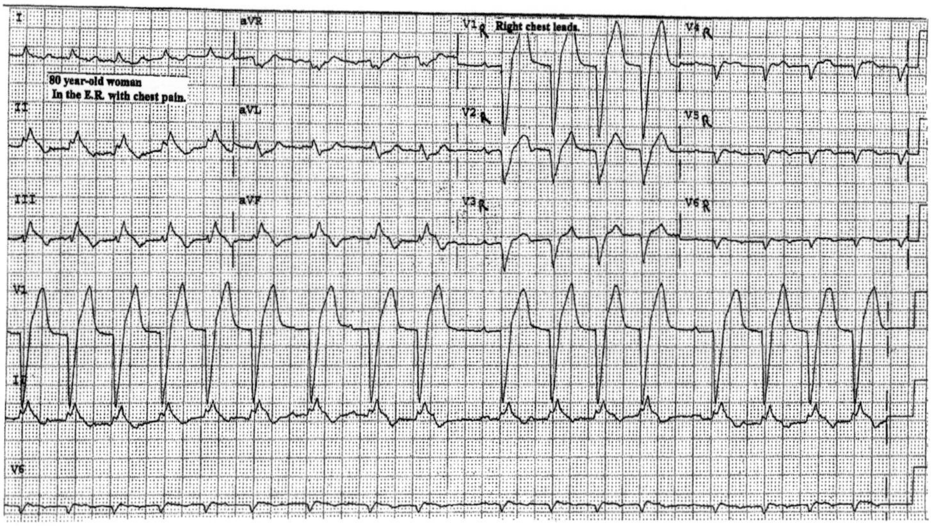

Fig. 31. Tracing from an 80-year-old woman seen in the emergency department.

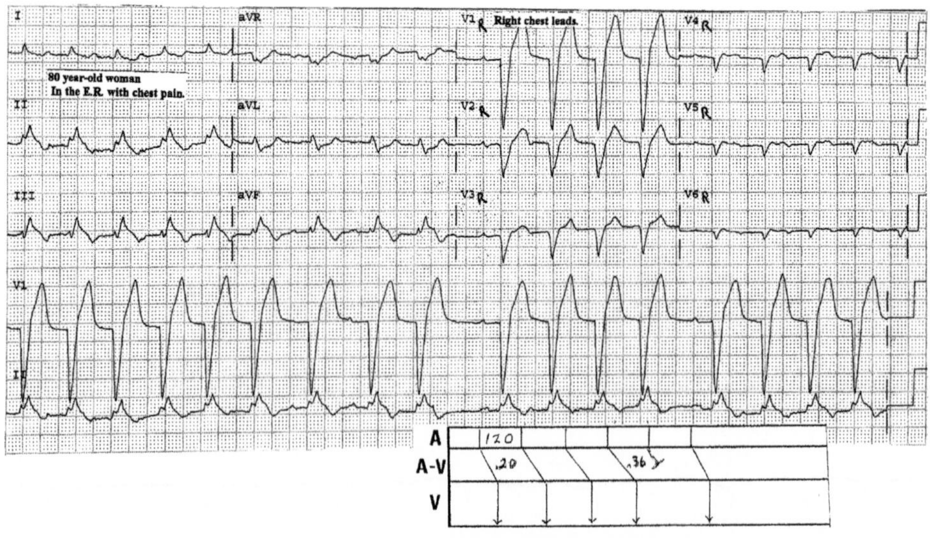

Fig. 32. Tracing from **Fig. 31** shown with completed ladder diagram. The computer interpretation represents a cowardly surrender. Numerous abnormalities are encountered. P waves are present in the rhythm strip of lead II with an atrial rate of 120 per minute. As depicted in the ladder diagram, after the "break" the PR intervals quickly prolong, ending in 5:4 Wenckebach A-V block. The ventricular activation shows LBBB. A validated criterion to diagnose acute myocardial infarction despite LBBB is "ST segment elevation concordant with the QRS complex." This is present in leads II, III, and aVF and is consistent with acute inferior infarction. The presence of 1-mm ST segment elevation, present in the right chest leads V_4R, V_5R, or V_6R, identifies right ventricular involvement in the inferior infarction and indicates a proximal lesion in the right coronary artery.

response of 99 (now absent), and LBBB (now absent)."

Questions

1. Do you agree with the computer?
2. Can you diagnose myocardial infarction in the presence LBBB?
3. Do the right chest leads provide additional information?
4. What causes the pauses?

The legend to **Fig. 32** provides discussion of these questions.

Introduction to Supraventricular Tachycardia

Nitish Badhwar, MD

KEYWORDS

- Supraventricular tachycardia
- Atrioventricular nodal reentrant tachycardia
- Atrioventricular reentrant tachycardia
- Atrial tachycardia

Paroxysmal supraventricular tachycardia (PSVT) is a clinical syndrome characterized by a rapid tachycardia with an abrupt onset and termination. These arrhythmias are frequently encountered in otherwise healthy patients without structural heart disease. Symptoms vary from palpitations and dyspnea to tachycardia-induced cardiomyopathy. The three most common causes of PSVT are atrioventricular nodal reentrant tachycardia (AVNRT) (50%–60%), atrioventricular reentrant tachycardia (AVRT) in patients with Wolff-Parkinson-White syndrome (25%–30%), and atrial tachycardia (10%). Rare causes of PSVT include focal junctional tachycardia, atriofascicular tachycardia, permanent reciprocating junctional tachycardia, and nodoventricular/nodofascicular tachycardia. This section, based on challenging PSVT cases, is a guide for clinicians dealing with diagnostic or therapeutic dilemmas in the electrophysiology laboratory.

Surface electrocardiogram offers some useful clues to the diagnosis of PSVT. Typical AVNRT is the most likely diagnosis if there is a short RP tachycardia with RP of less than 70 ms. The main differential diagnoses of a short RP tachycardia but with RP greater than 70 ms include AVRT, AVNRT, and atrial tachycardia. The main differential diagnoses of a long RP tachycardia include atrial tachycardia, atypical AVNRT, and permanent reciprocating junctional tachycardia. If the tachycardia is associated with atrioventricular (AV) dissociation, the diagnosis of AVRT is excluded. If there are more atrial complexes than ventricular complexes, the more likely diagnosis is atrial tachycardia with AV block, although AVNRT with lower common pathway block is also possible. Narrow complex supraventricular tachycardia with ventriculoatrial (VA) block can be seen with AVNRT, junctional tachycardia, and nodoventricular/nodofascicular tachycardia.

Baseline findings in the electrophysiology laboratory that show lack of VA conduction despite the use of isoproterenol argue against AVRT as the supraventricular tachycardia mechanism. Supraventricular tachycardia initiation dependent on a critical atrial-His (AH) interval favors AVNRT, though atrial tachycardia and AVRT are not completely excluded. Spontaneous termination of supraventricular tachycardia with an atrial depolarization argues against atrial tachycardia as the mechanism as does termination with VA block during ventricular pacing. A septal VA interval of less than 70 ms rules out orthodromic AVRT as the mechanism of supraventricular tachycardia.[1] Short VA intervals are not typically seen in atrial tachycardia.

It is important from an ablation standpoint to confirm the participation of an accessory pathway participation in AVRT. This can be established by the presence of any of the following four criteria:

Tachycardia termination obtained with a ventricular stimulus delivered during His refractoriness and without atrial depolarization

Division of Cardiology, Section of Cardiac Electrophysiology, University of California, San Francisco, 500 Parnassus Avenue, Box 1354, San Francisco, CA 94143-1354, USA
E-mail address: badhwar@medicine.ucsf.edu

Card Electrophysiol Clin 2 (2010) 179–181
doi:10.1016/j.ccep.2010.01.001
1877-9182/10/$ – see front matter

Delay in the next atrial depolarization when a ventricular stimulus is delivered during His refractoriness

Increase in VA interval with ipsilateral bundle branch block during tachycardia[2]

An increase in His-ventricular interval results in an increase in His-to-atrial (HA) interval during tachycardia. It is important to note that the HA interval is fixed during AVNRT, but may wobble at the initiation of tachycardia.

Differentiation of atypical AVNRT from orthodromic AVRT using a septal pathway can be a diagnostic dilemma and often requires different pacing maneuvers. Martinez-Alday and colleagues[3] measured the VA interval with differential pacing from the right ventricular apex (RVA) and right ventricular posterobasal region (RVB) during sinus rhythm. VA timing during RVA pacing was more than VA timing during RVB pacing (always >10 ms) with posteroseptal AP conduction. VA timing during RVA pacing was less than or equal to VA timing during RVB pacing with normal AV nodal conduction. Para-Hisian pacing during sinus rhythm and para-Hisian entrainment during tachycardia have also been shown to have diagnostic value in differentiating AVNRT from orthodromic AVRT using a septal accessory pathway.[4,5] In another study, data from right ventricular apex pacing that leads to entrainment of tachycardia was used to differentiate atypical AVRT from septal AVNRT.[6] The investigators measured the VA interval and tachycardia cycle length (TCL) just before the initiation of right ventricular pacing, the interval between the last pacing stimulus and the last entrained atrial depolarization (stimulus-atrial [SA] interval), and the postpacing interval (PPI) at the right ventricular apex. Atypical AVNRT was associated with an SA-VA interval of greater than 85 ms and a PPI-TCL interval of greater than 115 ms. In contrast, orthodromic AVRT using a septal pathway was associated with a SA-VA interval of less than 85 ms and a PPI-TCL interval of less than 115 ms. Miller and colleagues[7] have shown that the change in HA intervals measured during supraventricular tachycardia (HA_{svt}) as well as ventricular pacing at the same tachycardia rate (HA_{pace}) can be used to differentiate AVNRT from orthodromic AVRT using a septal accessory pathway. They concluded that ΔHA ($HA_{pace} - HA_{svt}$) greater than −10 ms reliably differentiates AVNRT (ΔHA >0 ms) from orthodromic AVRT using a septal accessory pathway (ΔHA <−27 ms) without overlap. This technique is limited by technical problems in recording the retrograde His during ventricular pacing. Finally, delivery of late ventricular extrastimulus (preferably from the right ventricular summit) at the time of His refractoriness during tachycardia is a very useful diagnostic maneuver. This is diagnostic of AVRT if it pulls in the atrial signal with the same activation sequence and resets of tachycardia, pushes out the atrial signal, or terminates tachycardia with VA block.

Focal atrial tachycardia is an important differential diagnosis in long RP tachycardia. Atrial tachycardia is the most likely mechanism when an atrial-atrial-ventricular, or "A-A-V," response is seen upon cessation of entrainment ventricular pacing during supraventricular tachycardia, especially when the atrial activation sequence during ventricular pacing differs from that during tachycardia.[8] Man and colleagues[9] found that atrial tachycardia or AVRT consistently showed an AH interval that was similar (ΔAH <20 ms) to the AH interval with right atrial pacing at TCL in a patient with a long RP tachycardia. Atypical AVNRT was always associated with a shorter AH interval (ΔAH >20 ms) than the AH during right atrial pacing at TCL.

Demonstration of VA linking is another diagnostic maneuver that differentiates atrial tachycardia from AVNRT or AVRT. Atrial overdrive pacing during supraventricular tachycardia is performed from different sites in the atrium. The VA interval of the return beat after atrial overdrive pacing will be similar to the VA interval during tachycardia, thus linking the ventricle and atrium and favoring a diagnosis of AVNRT or AVRT.[10]

REFERENCES

1. Knight BP, Ebinger M, Oral H, et al. Diagnostic value of tachycardia features and pacing maneuvers during paroxysmal supraventricular tachycardia. J Am Coll Cardiol 2000;36(2):574–82.
2. Kerr CR, Gallagher JJ, German LD. Changes in ventriculoatrial intervals with bundle branch block aberration during reciprocating tachycardia in patients with accessory atrioventricular pathways. Circulation 1982;66(1):196–201.
3. Martinez-Alday JD, Almendral J, Arenal A, et al. Identification of concealed posteroseptal Kent pathways by comparison of ventriculoatrial intervals from apical and posterobasal right ventricular sites. Circulation 1994;89(3):1060–7.
4. Hirao K, Otomo K, Wang X, et al. Para-Hisian pacing. A new method for differentiating retrograde conduction over an accessory AV pathway from conduction over the AV node. Circulation 1996;94(5):1027–35.
5. Reddy VY, Jongnarangsin K, Albert CM, et al. Para-Hisian entrainment: a novel pacing maneuver to

differentiate orthodromic atrioventricular reentrant tachycardia from atrioventricular nodal reentrant tachycardia. J Cardiovasc Electrophysiol 2003; 14(12):1321–8.
6. Michaud GF, Tada H, Chough S, et al. Differentiation of atypical atrioventricular node re-entrant tachycardia from orthodromic reciprocating tachycardia using a septal accessory pathway by the response to ventricular pacing. J Am Coll Cardiol 2001;38(4):1163–7.
7. Miller JM, Rosenthal ME, Gottlieb CD, et al. Usefulness of the delta HA interval to accurately distinguish atrioventricular nodal reentry from orthodromic septal bypass tract tachycardias. Am J Cardiol 1991;68(10):1037–44.
8. Knight BP, Zivin A, Souza J, et al. A technique for the rapid diagnosis of atrial tachycardia in the electrophysiology laboratory. J Am Coll Cardiol 1999; 33(3):775–81.
9. Man KC, Niebauer M, Daoud E, et al. Comparison of atrial-His intervals during tachycardia and atrial pacing in patients with long RP tachycardia. J Cardiovasc Electrophysiol 1995;6(9):700–10.
10. Sarkozy A, Richter S, Chierchia G-B, et al. A novel pacing manoeuvre to diagnose atrial tachycardia. Europace 2008;10(4):459–66.

Bypass Tract in Patient with Palpitations

Mark E. Josephson, MD

KEYWORDS

- Bypass tract • Palpitations
- Wolff-Parkinson-White syndrome

The patient is a 29-year-old man with a 15-year history of palpitations. He was the product of a normal pregnancy and was completely healthy during his adolescence. He had no family history of sudden cardiac death, atrial fibrillation, or any other atrial arrhythmia. Both parents are alive and well and three siblings have no arrhythmias.

The episodes of palpitations could occur at rest or exercise. Occasionally, they would be precipitated by an earlier beat producing a thump in his chest associated with pulsation in his neck and shortness of breath. His palpitations were always regular and he never had any syncope. He was referred for evaluation.

His physical examination was entirely normal and his electrocardiogram (ECG) is shown in **Fig. 1**. A wide QRS is present with a slurred upstroke suggesting a delta wave. The P wave is normal in morphology and is completed before the beginning of the delta wave. Where does the ECG suggest the bypass tract is located?

To find the location of the bypass tract one needs to assess the first 40-millisecond vector of the delta wave.[1] This is best done if there is maximum pre-excitation. Maximum pre-excitation is rather unlikely, however, in view of the completion of the P wave before any delta wave, because this should allow some component of propagation over the normal conducting system unless there is a primary abnormality in the normal conducting system. The delta wave in leads 2, 3, and F are positive, suggesting the superiorly located bypass tract. The delta wave in lead 1 also looks somewhat positive. This might lead one to suggest a right-sided pathway except when one looks at AVL where the initial vector is isoelectric to negative, suggesting a left-sided bypass tract. Moreover, the delta waves are positive across the precordium, further suggesting a left-sided pathway is present. Nonetheless, the somewhat confusing pattern seen in sinus rhythm should raise the suspicion that more than one bypass tract might be present. Because the presence of the bypass tract does not necessarily mean that the tachycardia that caused palpitations was related to the bypass tract, an electrophysiology study was recommended.

During placement of the catheters a tachycardia was initiated. The 12-lead ECG of that tachycardia is shown in **Fig. 2**. The tachycardia has a slightly wide QRS with the right bundle branch block pattern and no delta wave is seen. During a supraventricular tachycardia it is critical to look for P waves to make sure first that the tachycardia diagnosis is compatible with circus movement tachycardia using a bypass tract and then to determine, if possible, where the site of atrial activation is beginning. Careful analysis of the ECG suggests a P wave following each QRS with a very short RP interval.[2] A short RP interval is most commonly seen with circus movement tachycardia but does not exclude atrial tachycardia with a long PR or atypical forms of atrioventricular (AV) nodal tachycardia.[3] Carefully analysis of the P wave morphology, however, shows that in lead 1 and AVL it is negative and in lead 3 it is positive. This activation sequence is consistent with activation beginning in the lateral left atrium and is consistent with retrograde conduction over a left-sided bypass tract. It is inconsistent

Cardiovascular Division, Beth Israel Deaconess Medical Center, 185 Pilgrim Road, West Baker 4, Boston, MA 02215, USA
E-mail address: mjoseph2@bidmc.harvard.edu

Card Electrophysiol Clin 2 (2010) 183–185
doi:10.1016/j.ccep.2010.02.003
1877-9182/10/$ – see front matter

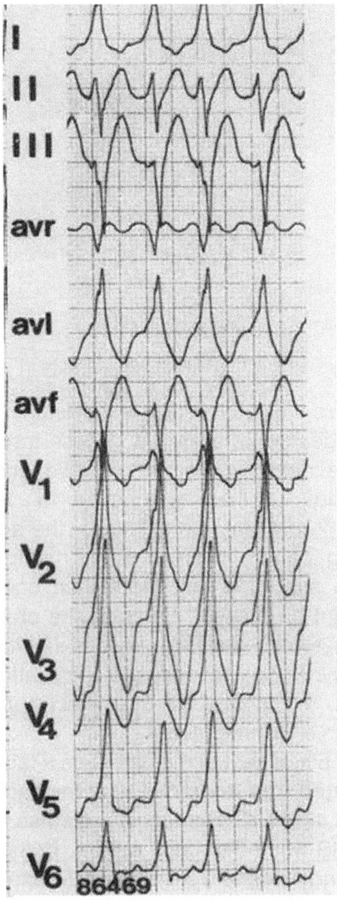

Fig. 1. Patient's electrocardiogram on presentation.

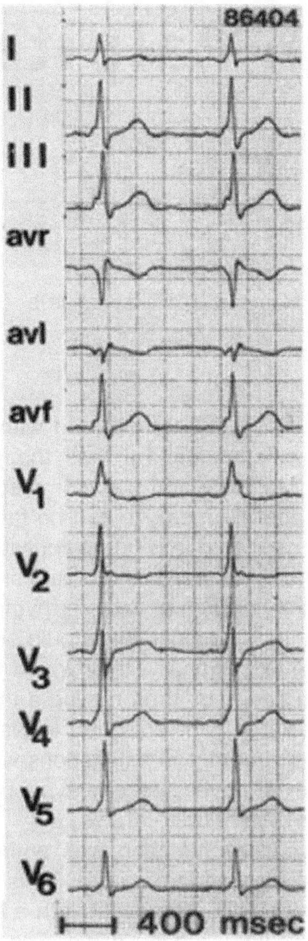

Fig. 2. A 12-lead electrocardiogram of tachycardia.

with AV nodal tachycardia, but does not rule out an atrial tachycardia. One important clue that this is circus movement tachycardia and not atrial tachycardia is the description of the onset of tachycardia by the patient. The description of the initiating premature beat, as a thump in his chest associated with shortness of breath and a pulsation in his neck, is consistent with a ventricular premature beat. The initiation of a tachycardia by a spontaneous ventricular premature beat during sinus rhythm is nearly diagnostic of circus movement tachycardia.[4] Atrial tachycardia would not be initiated by a spontaneous ventricular premature beat.

A wide complex tachycardia was also induced during the electrophysiologic study (**Fig. 3**). This tachycardia has a QRS morphology that is different from the sinus rhythm ECG pattern of pre-excitation and is not a typical right bundle branch block pattern that was seen during the circus movement tachycardia. The QRSs across the precordium are positive and slurred, suggesting that this tachycardia is arising somewhere in the posterior left ventricle. Positive concordance is seen. In the inferior leads the axis is superior, suggesting that this is coming from the inferior part of the left ventricle, from anarea that would be called "left inferior paraseptal." This is clearly different than the QRS during pre-excitation in sinus rhythm and also does not match the P wave morphology during orthodromic circus movement tachycardia. The atrial activation sequence in the orthodromic tachycardia showed a negative P wave in leads 1 and L and positive P in the inferior leads, opposite of the QRS vectors, which were negative in the inferior leads and positive in 1 and L. This mismatch in atrial and ventricular activation confirms the presence of two left-sided bypass tracts.

Multiple bypass tracts are not uncommon.[5] They may be seen in 5% to 15% of patients with Wolff-Parkinson-White syndrome (WPW). To complicate matters, dual AV nodal pathways may be observed in 30% of such patients. This gives rise to the possibility of multiple types of AV and ventriculo atrial conduction and AV nodal

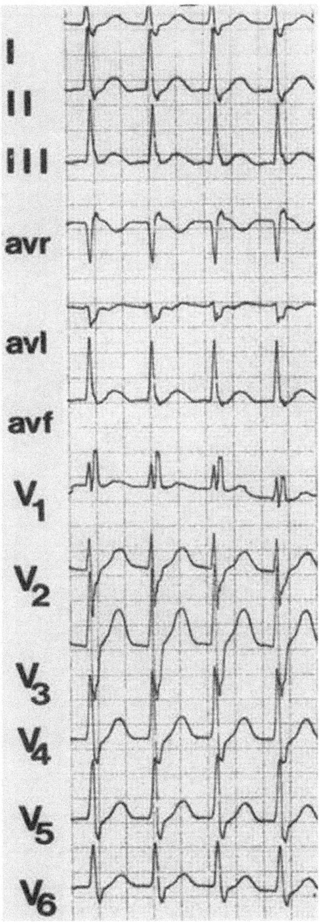

Fig. 3. Wide complex tachycardia.

reentry in patients with WPW. One should always remember the possibility of multiple bypass tracts and coexisting different arrhythmias when evaluating patients with WPW. Thorough analysis of ECG and a detailed electrophysiology study are necessary to cure the patient of the symptoms. This patient did not have AV nodal arrhythmias. Ablation of both the left inferior periseptal and left lateral bypass tracts eliminated his symptoms.

REFERENCES

1. Josephson ME. Preexcitation syndromes. In: Clinical cardiac electrophysiology: techniques and interpretations. 4th edition. Philadelphia: Wolters Kluwer/Lippincott Williams and Wilkins; 2008.
2. Zimetbaum PJ, Josephson ME. Wolff-Parkinson-White syndrome and variants. In: Practical clinical electrophysiology. Philadelphia: Wolters Kluwer/Lippincott Williams and Wilkins; 2009.
3. Cardiovascular Medicine/Cardiac Arrhythmias/Preexcitation-WPW. Up-To-Date On-Line. Available at: www.uptodate.com. Accessed February 12, 2010.
4. Bar-Cohen Y, Khairy P, Morwood J, et al. Inaccuracy of Wolff-Parkinson-White accessory pathway localization algorithms in children and patients with congenital heart defects. J Cardiovasc Electrophysiol 2006; 17:712–6.
5. Wellens HJJ, Conover M. Narrow QRS tachycardia. In: The ECG in emergency decision making. 2nd edition. Philadelphia: Saunders Elsevier; 2006.

Patient with Long RP Tachycardia

Mark E. Josephson, MD

KEYWORDS

- Tachycardia • Palpitations • Congestive heart failure
- Electrocardiogram

A 50-year-old man presented with a history of palpitations over the previous 9 years. These palpitations occurred daily, with increasing frequency of palpitations on exertion. He had no history of Wolff-Parkinson-White syndrome. For the prior 6 months he had increasing shortness of breath and signs of congestive heart failure. An echocardiogram showed biventricular dilatation and a left ventricular ejection fraction of 28%. No focal wall motion abnormalities were present. He used β-blockers, angiotensin-converting enzyme inhibitors, and diuretics with minimal effect on his palpitations or shortness of breath. Catheterization revealed normal coronary arteries and elevated right and left sided pressures.

The patient was then referred to electrophysiology for further work-up. In the office, he had obvious congestive heart failure and a heart rate of approximately 150 beats/min. **Fig. 1** shows the electrocardiogram (ECG), which demonstrates a narrow complex tachycardia and approximately 160 beats per minute. One P wave is seen before each QRS with a longer RP than PR interval. The P wave is inverted in leads II, III, and AVF is slightly upright in R and L. The P wave is also negative in precordial leads. The QRS is notable for alternation of R-wave amplitude. QRS alternans is seen in all 12 ECG leads, most pronounced in the precordial leads. The differential diagnosis of a long RP includes (1) circus movement tachycardia using a slowly conducting bypass tract, (2) atrial tachycardia, (3) the uncommon form of atrioventricular (AV) nodal tachycardia, or (4) a His bundle tachycardia.[1–5] These are schematically shown in **Fig. 2**. Each of these tachycardias can give rise to long RP tachycardias with negative P waves in the inferior leads. P-wave morphology is critical because positive P waves in the inferior leads exclude junctional tachycardia or AV nodal tachycardia. The P wave morphology is important in localizing the origin of atrial activation. In this case, the P wave is not narrow but somewhat broad and has a W-shaped configuration in lead 3. Moreover, it is negative across the precorium. This latter observation suggests it is anteriorly located.

The diagnosis of a long RP tachycardia can be challenging if careful attention is not given to clinical history and close examination of the ECG. The clinical history is important in finding out whether or not the tachycardia is incessant (occurs up to 50% of the day) or is intermittent and paroxysmal. This piece of clinical history is important because incessant tachycardias virtually exclude AV nodal tachycardia, and, in the absence of digitalis or a surgical procedure, in an adult makes junctional tachycardia unlikely. A Holter monitor can be used in deciding how incessant such a tachycardia is. In this case, the patient's clinical history suggested an incessant nature. The increase in rate associated with exercise also suggests that this is catecholamine dependent. Automatic or triggered atrial tachycardias, as well as tachycardias involving the AV node, and slowly conducting bypass tracts are extremely sensitive to catecholamines, and resting heart rates can be only 100 beats a minute and rise to greater than 200 beats a minute during exertion.

There are several maneuvers that can distinguish between the tachycardias (summarized in

Cardiovascular Division, Beth Israel Deaconess Medical Center, 185 Pilgrim Road, West Baker 4, Boston, MA 02215, USA
E-mail address: mjoseph2@bidmc.harvard.edu

Card Electrophysiol Clin 2 (2010) 187–190
doi:10.1016/j.ccep.2010.02.005
1877-9182/10/$ – see front matter

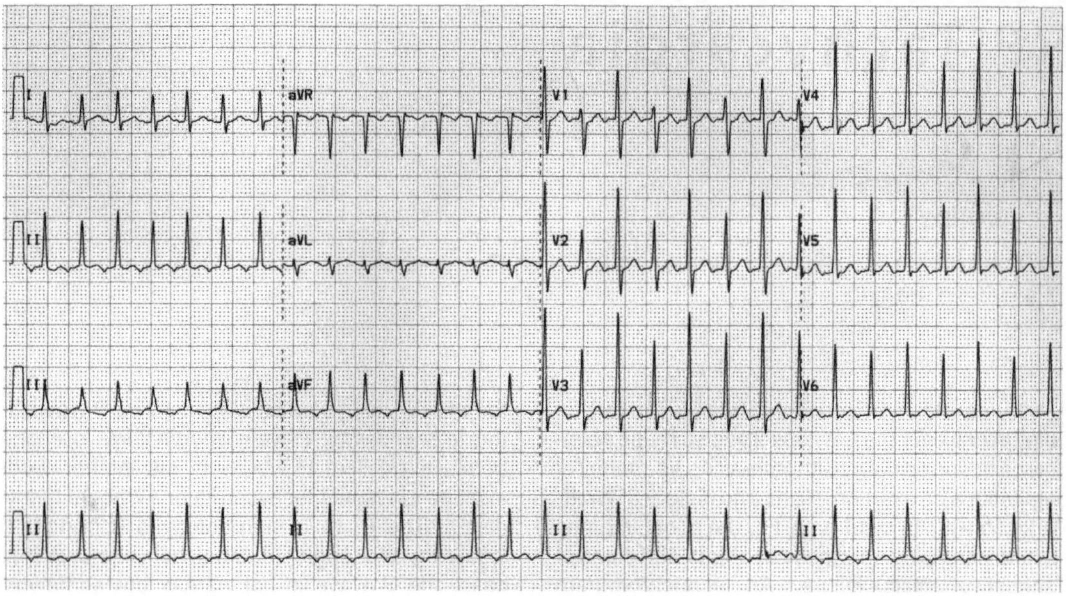

Fig. 1. Initial ECG of the patient is shown.

Table 1). In atrial tachycardia, adenosine or carotid pressure can produce AV nodal block, yet the tachycardia will continue. The presence of continued P waves in the absence of a QRS is diagnostic of atrial tachycardia because His bundle tachycardias have block in the AV node and more QRS than P waves; circus movement tachycardia cannot exist without both atrial and ventricular activation; and AV nodal tachycardia is virtually impossible once complete AV block has occurred. In this patient, the response to carotid sinus pressure is shown in **Fig. 3** (top) carotid sinus pressure produces prolongation of the PR interval followed by AV block and Wenckebach block before resumption of 1:1 conduction.

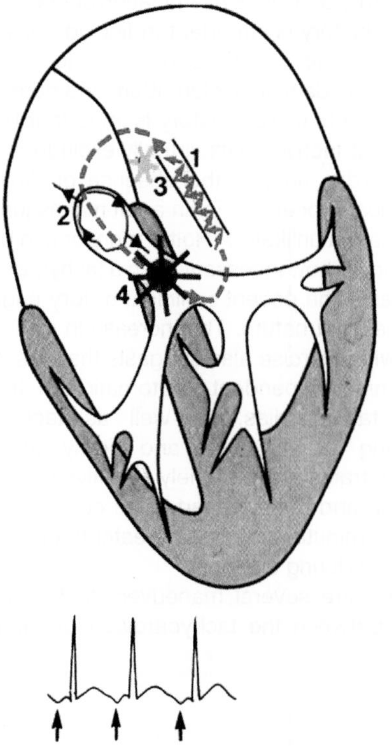

Fig. 2. Schematic diagram shows the differential diagnosis of a long RP. (1) Circus movement tachycardia using slow AP. (2) AV nodal tachycardia (uncommon type). (3) Low atrial tachycardia. (4) His bundle tachycardia.

Table 1
Long RP tachycardia (negative P in leads II, III, AVF)

Effects of carotid sinus massage (CSM) or Adenosine	
Circus movement tachycardia (CMT) using concealed low atrial tachycardia AP with long conduction time	Increase in RP and/or PR interval
	Termination in AV node (AVN) or AP
Uncommon AV nodal reentrant tachycardia (AVNRT)	Increase in RP
	Termination in slow AV nodal path
Low atrial tachycardia	More Ps than QRS
His bundle tachycardia	More QRS than Ps

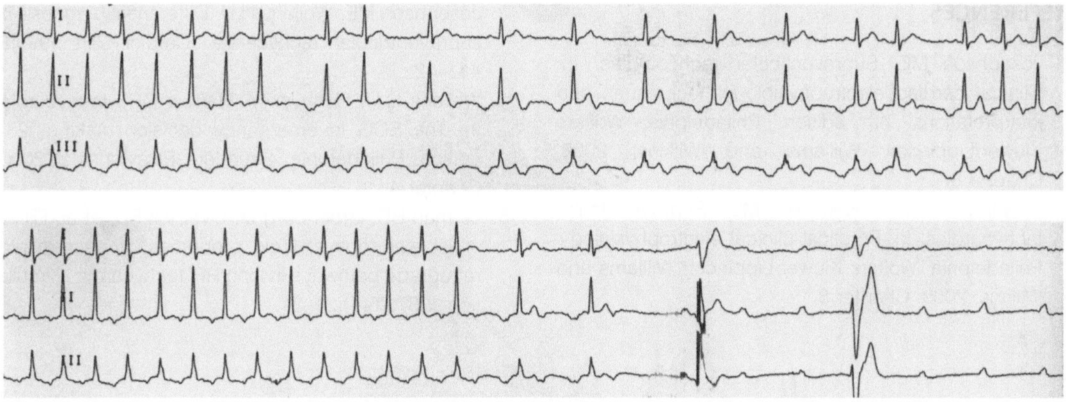

Fig. 3. 2:1 AV block produced by adenosine. Response to carotid sinus pressure (*top*) and response to adenosine (*below*).

The atrial rate minimally slows and P waves continue in the presence of AV block. This never occurs with the other differential diagnoses. In **Fig. 4**, adenosine is given. In this particular instance, adenosine produces 2:1 AV block. The tachycardia transiently terminates and sinus rhythm takes over while complete AV block is present. The tachycardia resumed 2 seconds later with 1:1 conduction. Again, continuation of the tachycardia in the absence of AV conduction is diagnostic of AV block.

Because of his low ejection fraction, his referring doctor suggested an implantable cardioverter defibrillator. The electrophysiology group thought this was inappropriate at this time because incessant tachycardias can cause a dilated cardiomyopathy. As such, he underwent an electrophysiology study. The tachycardia was located to the lateral tricuspid annulus and ablation was performed successfully abolishing the tachycardia (**Fig. 4**). Within 1 month, the patient's ejection fraction had normalized and signs of congestive heart failure dissipated. He has remained free of symptoms of tachycardia or heart failure, off all medications, for the past 3 years. Incessant nature of tachycardia is a known cause of tachymyopathy and, in patients with heart failure and dilated cardiomyopathy, attention to treating the arrhythmia should be given first.

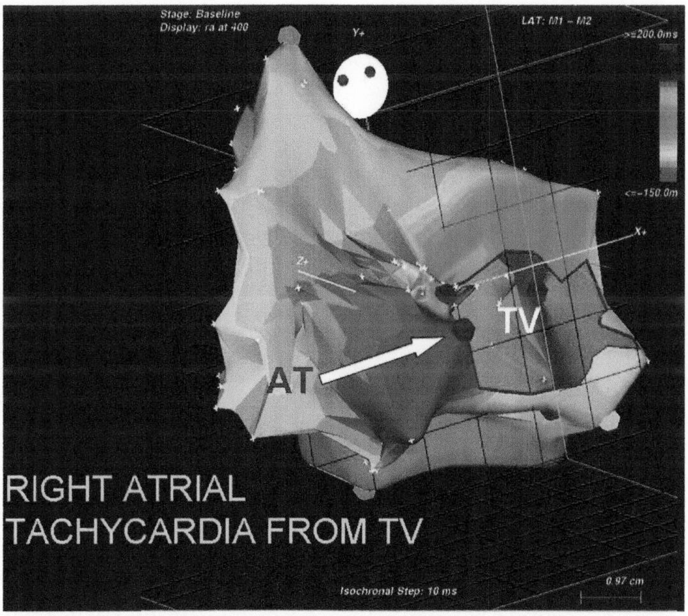

Fig. 4. Patient's response to carotid sinus pressure. AT, SC of atrial tachycardia (shown by *arrow*). TV, tachycardia valve (*arrowhead*).

REFERENCES

1. Josephson ME. Supraventicular tachycardias. In: Clinical cardiac electrophysiology: techniques and interpretations. 4th edition. Philadelphia: Wolters Kluwer/Lippincott Williams and Wilkins; 2008. Chapter 8.
2. Zimetbaum PJ, Josephson ME. Supraventricular tachycardias. In: Practical clinical electrophysiology. Philadelphia: Wolters Kluwer/Lippincott Williams and Wilkins; 2009. Chapter 8.
3. Josephson ME, Wellens HJJ. Differential diagnosis of supraventricular tachycardia. Cardiol Clin 1990;8: 411–42.
4. Wellens HJJ, Conover M. Narrow QRS tachycardia. In: The ECG in emergency decision making. 2nd edition. Philadelphia: Saunders Elsevier, Inc; 2006. Chapter 4.
5. Lerman BB, Greenberg M, Overholt ED, et al. Differential electrophysiologic properties of decremental retrograde pathways in long RP' tachycardia. Circulation 1987;76(1):21–31.

Tachycardia-Mediated Cardiomyopathy

Mark E. Josephson, MD

KEYWORDS

- Tachycardia-mediated cardiomyopathy
- Progressive congestive heart failure
- Group beating pairs • Non-reentrant tachycardia

A 35-year-old woman presented with progressive congestive heart failure 1 month after her pregnancy. A diagnosis of peripartum cardiomyopathy was assumed. While she was in biventricular failure and pulmonary edema, a cardiac arrest occurred. She underwent diuresis and was placed on an ace inhibitor and a beta-blocker. Heart failure improved but remained rather difficult to treat. The patient had no history of cardiac disease before her pregnancy. Although she was somewhat short of breath during her pregnancy, she did not think this was unusual. She gained 54 pounds during her pregnancy and believed that was responsible for the shortness of breath and edema she experienced during the pregnancy. A fast heartbeat was noted during pregnancy and at the time of delivery, but her doctors thought this was sinus tachycardia and not unusual. She did not have any preeclampsia or eclampsia during pregnancy and had no known cardiovascular disease.

An echocardiogram revealed an ejection fraction of 25% with biventricular dilatation and enlarged atria. Because of her low ejection fraction and cardiac arrest, the question was whether an implantable cardioverter-defibrillator (ICD) was indicated for secondary prevention. Clearly, the patient was in acute pulmonary edema at the time of the arrest, and one should always consider the possibility that the arrest was a secondary event. Despite the fact that the metabolic and hemodynamic abnormalities associated with acute severe congestive heart failure could induce ventricular tachycardia/ventricular fibrillation as a transient abnormality, an ICD was recommended.

On physical examination, the patient appeared to be a young woman, somewhat tachypneic, with a blood pressure of 100/60 and an irregular, but rapid rhythm in the 130 range. Occasional cannon A waves were noted with a jugular pulse, which was elevated. The carotid pulse was normal. Her lungs revealed basilar crackles. The cardiac examination revealed an irregular rhythm with murmur of mitral regurgitation. S1 and S2 were variable. She had a right ventricular heave and tricuspid regurgitation as well.

The 12-lead ECG at the time of the irregular rhythm is shown in **Fig. 1**. The most striking thing on first glance is the presence of group beating. Groups of three are seen throughout the tracing followed by a pause. The R-R interval of the first pair was always longer than that of the second pair. More interesting, however, was the appearance of sinus P waves that march through the entire tracing. Of import is that that the second QRS in the triad never had a P wave preceding. The P wave was enlarged with biatrial abnormality (broad in II, positive in L, and with a tall positive and broad terminal negative deflection in V1). Nonspecific T wave flattening and ST changes were also observed. During the day, on ambulation her rate accelerated to nearly 170 beats a minute (**Fig. 2**). During ambulation, there was also an irregular rhythm with group beating pairs that are shorter and pairs that are longer with a pause in the middle. Again, there appears to be sinus P waves marching throughout the rhythm strip with every other beat having no P wave associated with it. In Lead 2, in the middle of the tracing there is a pause, followed by a sinus beat and then a QRS that exhibits aberration. The initial thought

Cardiovascular Division, Beth Israel Deaconess Medical Center, 185 Pilgrim Road, West Baker 4, Boston, MA 02215, USA
E-mail address: mjoseph2@bidmc.harvard.edu

Card Electrophysiol Clin 2 (2010) 191–196
doi:10.1016/j.ccep.2010.02.006

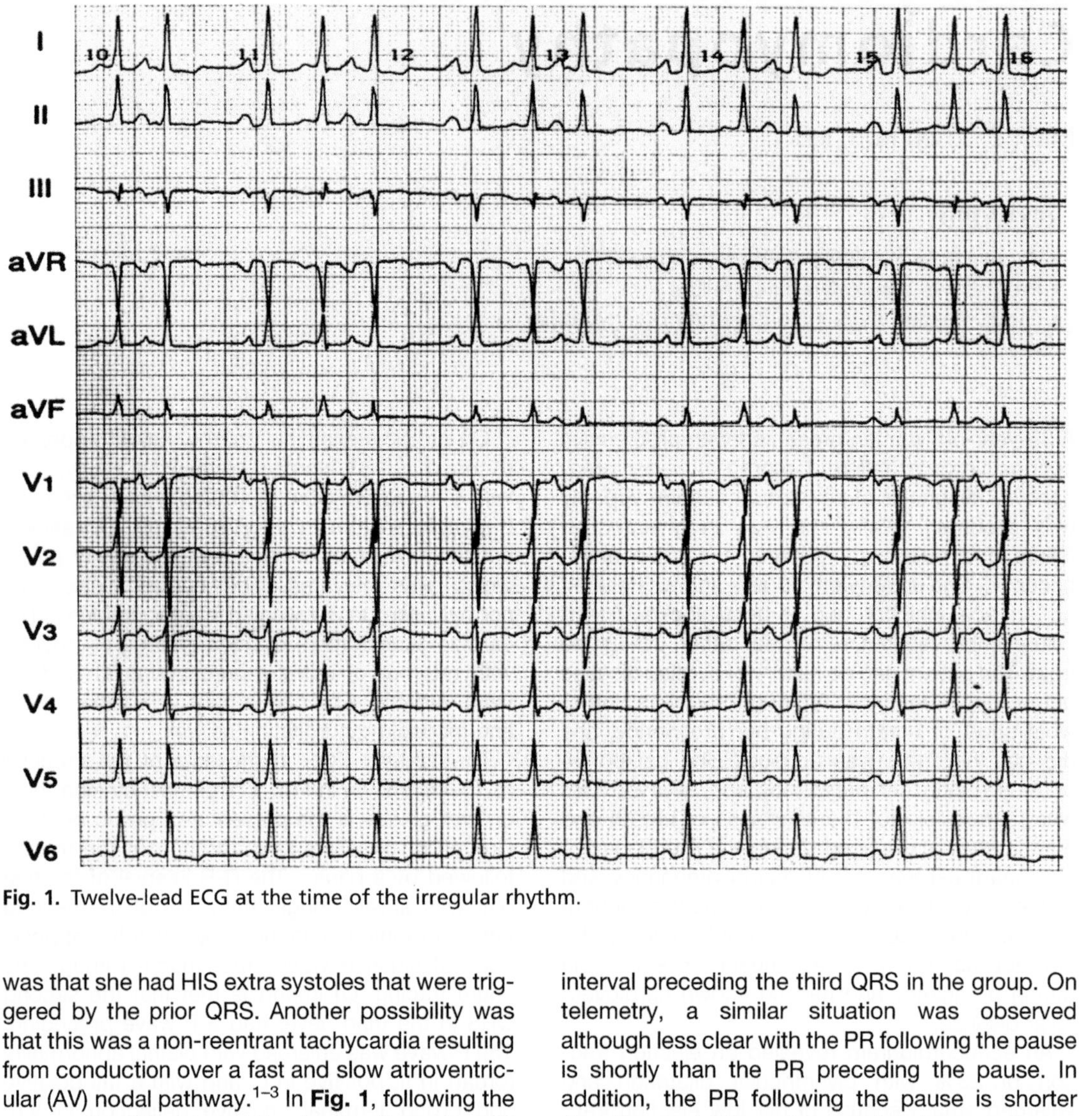

Fig. 1. Twelve-lead ECG at the time of the irregular rhythm.

was that she had HIS extra systoles that were triggered by the prior QRS. Another possibility was that this was a non-reentrant tachycardia resulting from conduction over a fast and slow atrioventricular (AV) nodal pathway.[1–3] In **Fig. 1**, following the pause, the PR interval is shorter than the PR interval preceding the third QRS in the group. On telemetry, a similar situation was observed although less clear with the PR following the pause is shortly than the PR preceding the pause. In addition, the PR following the pause is shorter than the next PR as this rapid rhythm continues.

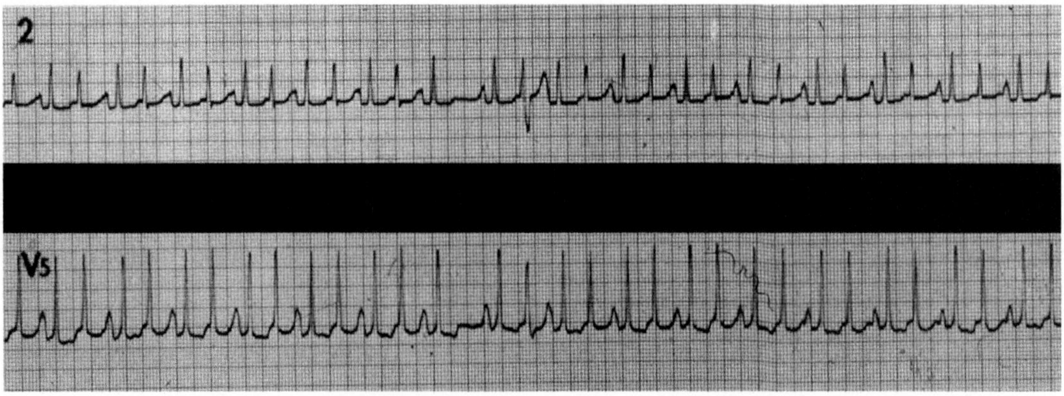

Fig. 2. During ambulation, the patient had an irregular rhythm with group beating pairs that are shorter and pairs that are longer with a pause in the middle.

In view of the rapid rhythm and persistent heart failure, the cardiology team needed to decide on the next step. Should they: (1) add digoxin, (2) increase the diuretic, (3) give intravenous melanoma, (4) evaluate for transplant, or (5) do an electrophysiology consult? In view of the strange pattern of P waves and QRS, an electrophysiology consult was called.

The electrophysiologist believed that this was most likely a non-reentrant 1:2 tachycardia using dual AV nodal pathways. Tracings during the rapid 1:2 tachycardia with intracardiac recordings and a ladder diagram are shown in **Fig. 3**. As in **Figs. 1** and **2**, the sinus rate and rhythm is regular and marches throughout the tracing. Following each P wave are two QRS. The first associated with a short AH and the second with an H in the absence of the preceding P. It was believed that this represented conduction over a fast and a slow pathway shown in the ladder diagram. Conduction over the fast pathway was rapid with PR of about 160 milliseconds and conduction over the slow pathway had a PR of 580 milliseconds. The sinus rate was 632 milliseconds or nearly 100 beats per minute consistent with her heart failure.

A second regular tachycardia was observed that was slower than the non-reentrant tachycardia described in **Fig. 4**. Here a narrow complex tachycardia at a rate of about 125 beats per minute is seen. In this instance, the QRS is totally regular. Atrial activity can be seen at the terminal part of the QRS producing a pseudo S wave in leads 2, 3, and AVF and pseudo R prime in V1. This pattern is typical of AV nodal reentrant tachycardia. At times, the patient ECG would change from the

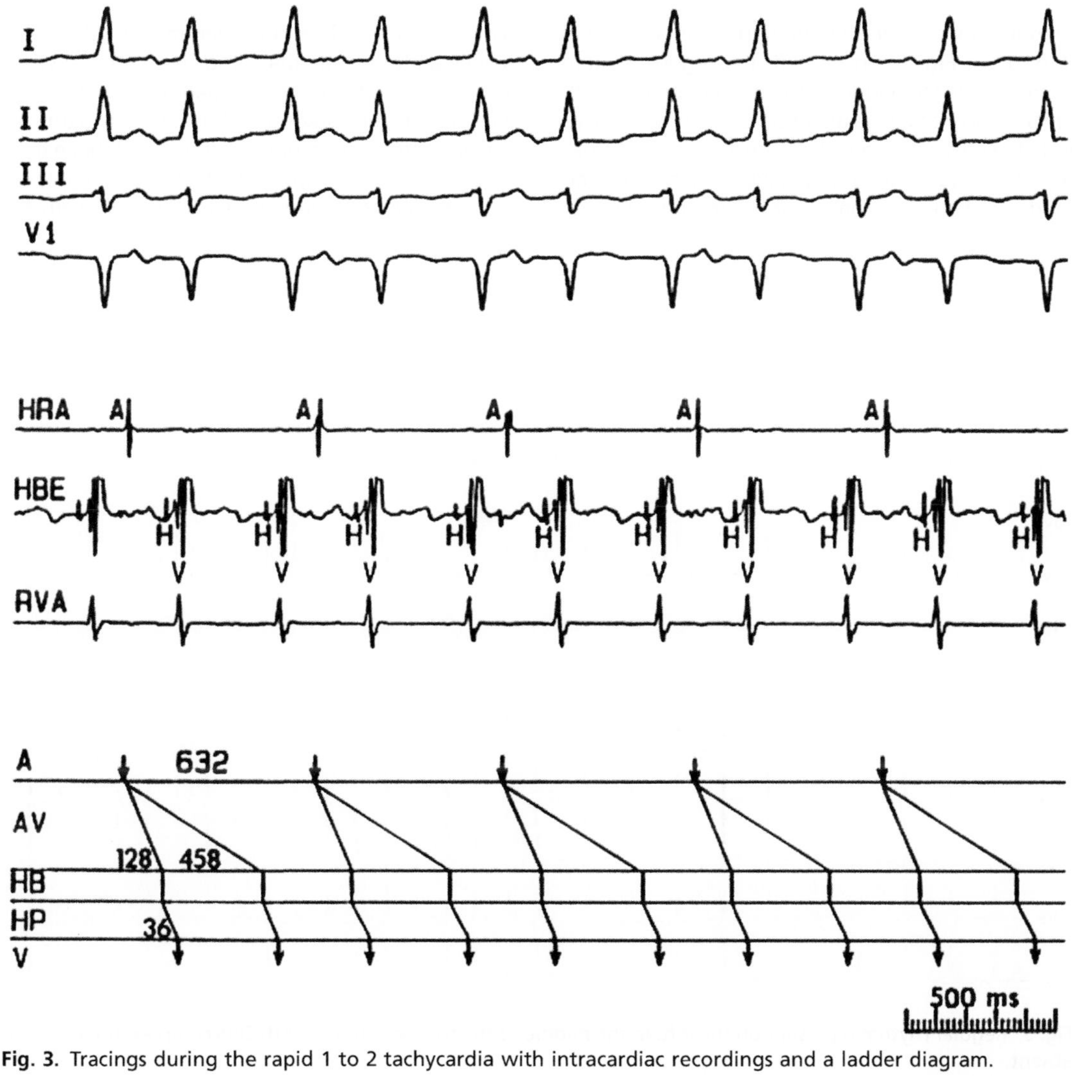

Fig. 3. Tracings during the rapid 1 to 2 tachycardia with intracardiac recordings and a ladder diagram.

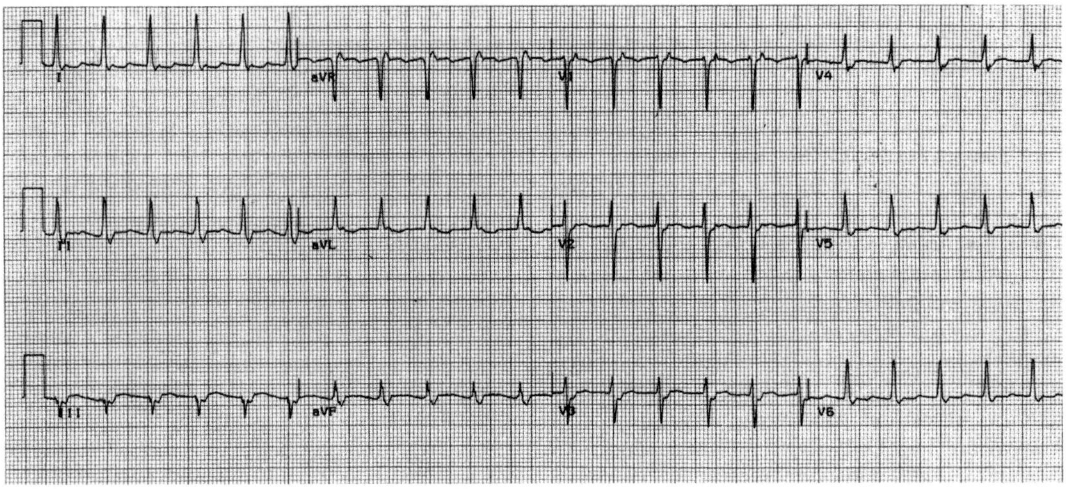

Fig. 4. A second regular tachycardia was observed that was slower than the non-reentrant tachycardia described in **Figs. 1–3**.

irregular to regular rhythm and back and forth (**Fig. 5**). In **Fig. 5**, on the left, the regular rhythm is present. In the middle of the tracing, on the tenth QRS complex there is absence of the P wave. This is followed by the onset of the more rapid non-reentrant tachycardia with sinus rhythm associated with two QRS, one over a fast and one over slow pathway. The non-reentrant rhythm was significantly faster than the reentrant rhythm. Termination of AV nodal reentrant tachycardia was due to retrograde block in the fast pathway. An intracardiac recording during one of these transitions is shown in **Fig. 6**. The first three complexes indicate AV nodal reentrant tachycardia with the

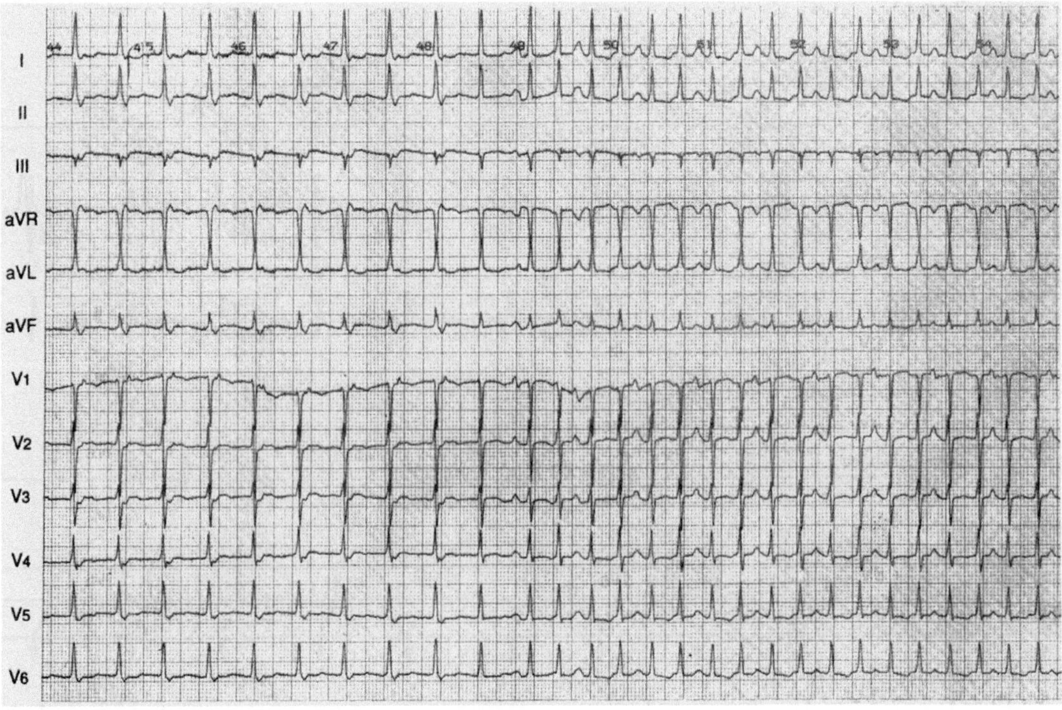

Fig. 5. Regular rhythm is present on the left. In the middle of the tracing, on the tenth QRS complex, the P wave is absent.

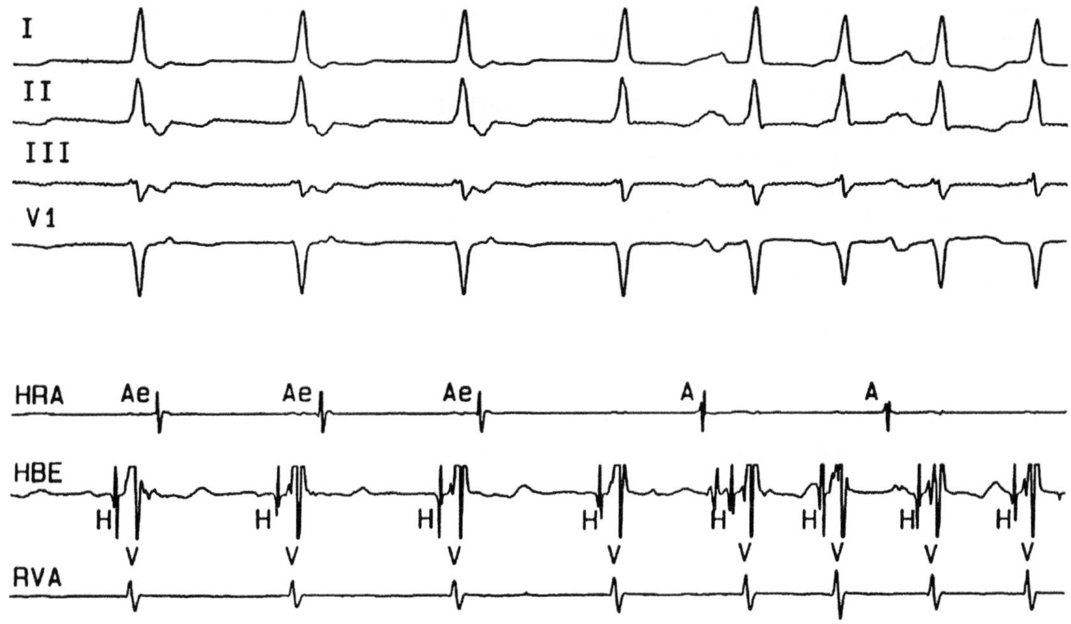

Fig. 6. Intracardiac recording during transition.

atrial activity occurring just at the end of the QRS. After the fourth QRS, atrial activity is not present and the next P wave is a sinus P wave with the ECGs demonstrating a high/low sequence.

The appearance of both AV nodal reentrant tachycardia and non-reentrant 1:2 tachycardia is highly unusual and previously thought not possible. A non-reentrant tachycardia is due to failure of retrograde fast pathway conduction. The 1:2 tachycardia persists instead of AV nodal reentry because each sinus P wave conducts down to fast and down to slow but not back up to fast to complete the reentrant circuit. In fact, there is evidence of linking of the slow and fast pathways. This is demonstrated in **Figs. 1** and **2** by the second PR following a pause being longer than the first PR, suggesting retrograde conduction into the fast pathway. When longer cycles are observed, conduction over the slow pathway is gradually prolonged because of retrograde invasion of the fast pathway into the slow pathway. Less linking is a common element in non-reentrant 1:2 tachycardia. The reason that AV node reentry does not occur is the inability to complete the retrograde activation over the fast and then return over the slow pathway. In this patient, however, that was possible and AV nodal reentry occurred. Note that AV nodal reentry was very slow since it reflects conduction down the slow pathway. Spontaneous termination of AV nodal tachycardia is due to retrograde block in the fast pathway. This is the hallmark of this electrophysiologic situation.

The electrophysiologists believed that the cardiomyopathy might not have been a peripartum cardiomyopathy but rather a tachycardia-mediated cardiomyopathy causing the heart failure. If that were the case, it might be "cured" by eliminating the dual conduction pathway. Nevertheless, an ICD was implanted at the request of the referring cardiologist because of the cardiac arrest. The electrophysiology recommendation was to do an AV nodal modification in an attempt to abolish the slow pathway. This was accomplished and sinus rhythm with one-to-one conduction resumed and no evidence of non-reentrant or AV nodal tachycardia. The patient was then more easily treated for her heart failure and went home 1 week later. Within 6 weeks, her ejection fraction was 55% and her edema had vanished, as had her clinical evidence of heart failure. Over the next 5 years, no ventricular events were observed and she requested that her ICD be removed. It was removed. Her ejection fraction has been normal since the ablation and she went on to have two successful pregnancies. It is now 15 years since the initial cardiac arrest and cardiac myopathy; the patient has a normal heart.

Tachycardia-mediated cardiomyopathy is little appreciated, but highly relevant disorder that is curable, unlike most other cardiomyopathies. Anything that causes incessant rapid rates can do this. The two common causes of cardiomyopathy are the incessant form of SVT using slowly conducting bypass tract or automatic atrial tachycardias. These, in some patients, for reasons that are not well worked out, produce cardiomyopathy after a period of several years. Another rhythm that is often associated with acute and, sometimes, chronic myocardial depression is atrial fibrillation. It is now well established that depressions of ventricular premature beats more than 20% of all impulses can also be associated with a cardiomyopathy. Finally, non-reentrant 1:2 tachycardia are the least common of all of these tachycardia-mediated myopathies. The most important point is to recognize this possibility because all of these myopathies are curable. The author has had the opportunity to cure a patient with an incessant atrial tachycardia who had been accepted for transplantation. The amount of myocardial depression that can be seen with these disorders and the acute cure of them are remarkable.

REFERENCES

1. Josephson ME. Supraventricular tachycardia. In: Clinical cardiac electrophysiology: techniques and interpretations. 4th edition. Philadelphia: Wolters Kluwer/Lippincott Williams and Wilkins; 2008. Chapter 8.
2. Zimetbaum PJ, Josephson ME. Supraventricular tachycardia. In: Practical clinical electrophysiology. Philadelphia: Wolters Kluwer/Lippincott Williams and Wilkins; 2009. Chapter 8.
3. Anselme F, Frederiks J, Boyle NG, et al. An unusual cause of tachycardia-induced myopathy. Pacing Clin Electrophysiol 1996;19(1):115–9.

Paroxysmal Long R-P Tachycardia

David Singh, MD, Nitish Badhwar, MD*

KEYWORDS

• Catheter ablation • Atrial tachycardia • Mitral annulus

A 48-year-old female with a history of hypothyroidism was referred for electrophysiology evaluation for recurrent palpitations. The palpitations were described as paroxysmal and occurred one to two times per week. Her episodes lasted as long as 1.5 hours and terminated spontaneously without specific interventions or maneuvers. They were not correlated with exercise or other identifiable triggers. Propanolol therapy was not effective in suppressing her symptoms and caused excess fatigue. The patient was referred for electrophysiology study and possible ablation.

ELECTROPHYSIOLOGY STUDY

Multipolar electrode catheters were introduced percutaneously from the right femoral and internal jugular veins and positioned into the high right atrium, right ventricular apex, His potential (His) bundle region, and coronary sinus. Bipolar electrograms (30–500 Hz) and unipolar electrograms (0.5–500 Hz) were displayed and stored using a digital recording system (EP MedSystems, West Berlin, NJ, USA). Three-dimensional electroanatomic mapping was performed with Ensite NavX (St Jude Medical, St Paul, MN, USA).

At baseline, the patient was in normal sinus rhythm. Baseline atrial-His and His-ventricular intervals were within normal limits. No ventriculoatrial conduction was observed with or without isoproterenol infusion. Following infusion of isoproterenol at 1 μg/min, the patient was noted to have frequent premature atrial complexes with identical morphologies. Eventually, sustained long R-P tachycardia was reliably induced with both ventricular and atrial overdrive pacing (**Fig. 1**) that had the same atrial activation sequence as the premature atrial complexes.

The diagnosis of atrial tachycardia was confirmed using the following criteria[1]:

- The atrial activation sequence during tachycardia was different from that recorded during sinus rhythm[2]
- Absence of ventriculoatrial conduction at baseline and ventriculoatrial dissociation during tachycardia (**Fig. 2**A)[3]
- Spontaneous changes in the tachycardia cycle length were observed with changes in the A-A interval preceding changes in the H-H interval (see **Fig. 2**B)[4]
- The tachycardia consistently terminated spontaneously with a ventricular complex (see **Fig. 2**B).

QUESTION: WHERE IS THE SITE OF ORIGIN OF THE FOCAL ATRIAL TACHYCARDIA?

During tachycardia, the earliest right atrial activation was noted on the His catheter. However, the coronary sinus had an eccentric activation sequence with the coronary sinus distal preceding the atrial activation at the His position (see **Fig. 1**). This is highly suggestive of a left atrial origin of the atrial tachycardia. Analysis of P wave morphology during tachycardia revealed P waves that were narrower than those during sinus rhythm, suggesting septal origin of the atrial tachycardia. A positive P wave in lead V1 and a negative P wave in AVL also suggested a left atrial focus (**Fig. 3**). The P wave in lead I was difficult to visualize because of its inscription in the preceding T wave. The P waves were noted to be low voltage in the

Division of Cardiology, Department of Cardiac Electrophysiology, University of California, 500 Parnassus Avenue, MU East 4, Box 1354, San Francisco, CA 94143, USA
* Corresponding author.
E-mail address: badhwar@medicine.ucsf.edu

Card Electrophysiol Clin 2 (2010) 197–201
doi:10.1016/j.ccep.2010.01.002
1877-9182/10/$ – see front matter

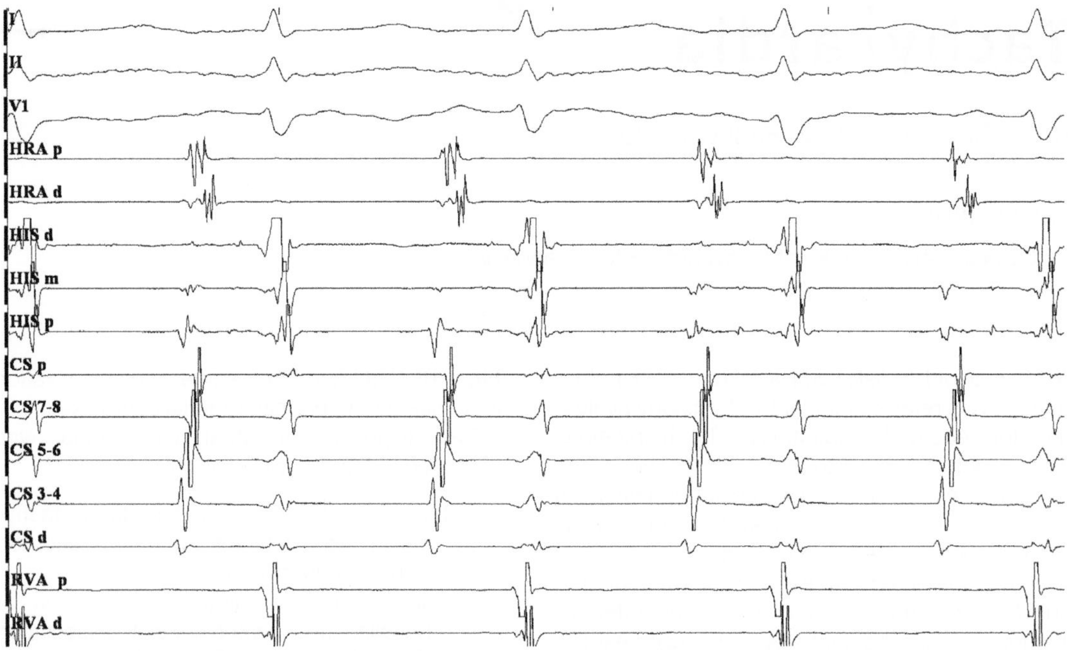

Fig. 1. Intracardiac recording during tachycardia that shows a long R-P tachycardia with eccentric atrial activation in the coronary sinus and earliest atrial activation at coronary sinus distal.

remainder of the limb leads. Hence, a left atrial focus was suspected on the basis of the coronary sinus activation sequence as well as P wave morphology.

Access to the left atrium was obtained through a transseptal approach across an existing patent foramen ovale. A 7F-catheter closed-irrigation ablation catheter with a 4-mm tip (Boston Scientific, Natick, MA, USA) was advanced into the left atrium for mapping and ablation. The earliest bipolar electrogram (relative to P wave onset) associated with a negative unipolar deflection was considered to be the site of atrial tachycardia origin. After detailed mapping of the left atrium, this site was localized to the superior mitral annular region at the 12 o'clock position in a left anterior oblique projection (**Fig. 4**). This region was also characterized by fractionated low-voltage atrial electrogram that preceded the P wave during tachycardia by 30 ms. Transient acceleration followed by termination of the tachycardia was observed after 4 seconds of radiofrequency ablation applied to this region. Tachycardia was not inducible after ablation at this site despite the use of isoproterenol and aggressive atrial pacing. Patient has been symptom-free off medications for 3 months.

DISCUSSION

Atrial tachycardias are uncommon, accounting for approximately 5% to 10% of supraventricular tachycardias in adults referred for electrophysiological evaluation. The origins of focal atrial tachycardias are not random as they tend to cluster in various regions of the right and left atria, including the crista terminalis, the pulmonary veins, the atrial septum, and the tricuspid annulus.[1] Less commonly, atrial tachycardias can originate from the mitral annular region or from the area of mitral annular–aortic continuity.[2] The case presented herein illustrates several features consistent with atrial tachycardia originating from this region.

P Wave Morphology

Analysis of P wave morphology during tachycardia or ectopic atrial impulses (particularly during A-V block) can be useful in localizing the site of focal atrial tachycardias. A number of P wave algorithms have been developed to help determine the atrial tachycardia site of origin.[1,3] Tang and colleagues[3] found that a positive or biphasic P wave in aVL predicted a right atrial focus with a sensitivity of 88%, specificity of 79%, positive predictive value of 83%, and negative predictive value of 85%. They additionally found that a positive P wave in V1 predicted a left atrial focus with a sensitivity of 93%, specificity of 88%, positive predictive value of 87%, and negative predictive value of 94%. An isoelectric or negative P wave in lead I had a specificity of 100% for a left atrial focus, but was only present in 50% of patients with left atrial tachycardias.

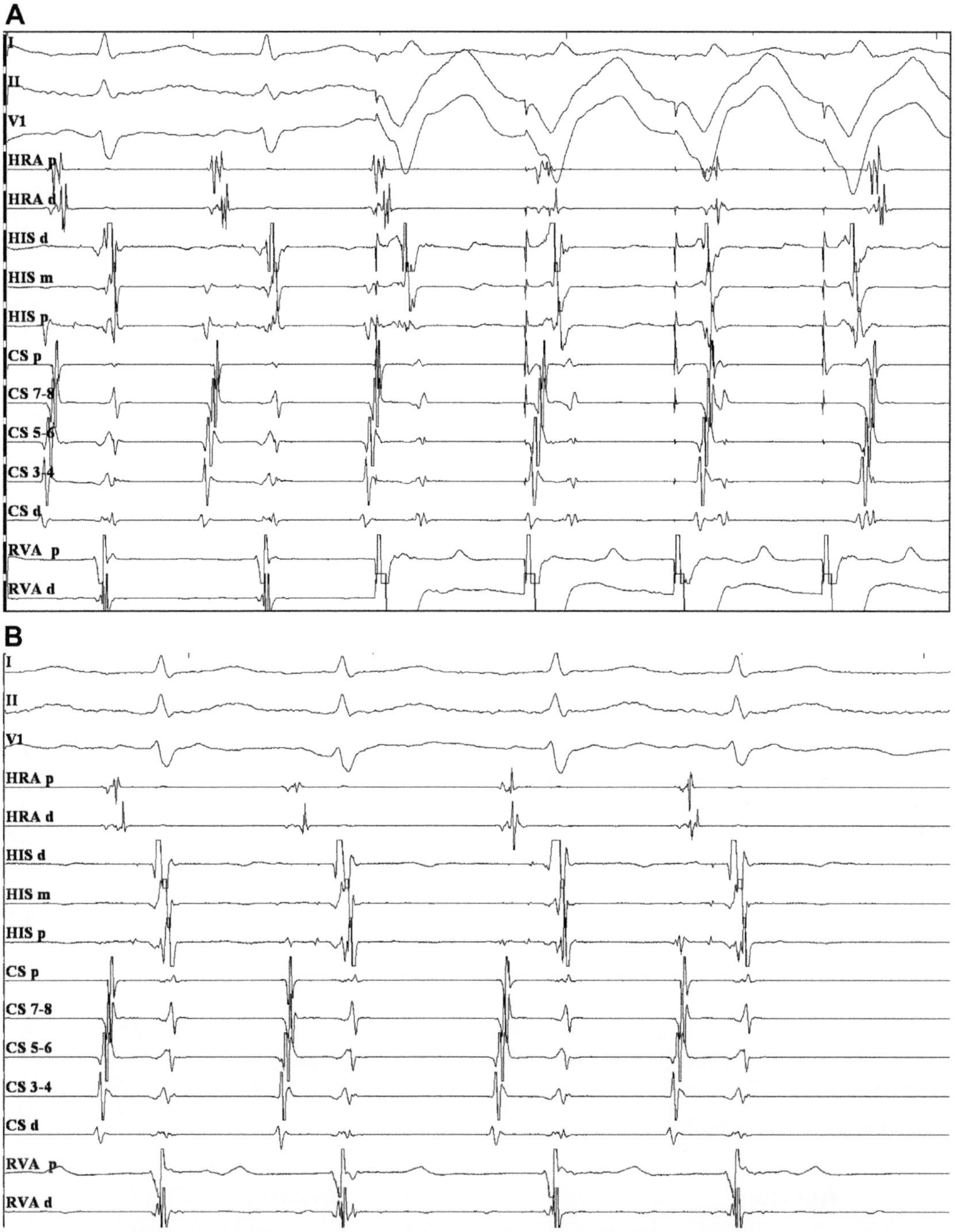

Fig. 2. (*A*) Ventricular overdrive pacing during tachycardia shows ventriculoatrial dissociation. (*B*) Spontaneous termination of tachycardia with a ventricular signal. There is change in the cycle length before termination with change in A-A driving a change in H-H/V-V, suggesting atrial tachycardia as the mechanism of the tachycardia.

In a more recent algorithm, V1 was found to be the most useful lead for distinguishing right from left atrial tachycardias.[1] A V1 lead that was negative or biphasic (positive-negative) predicted a right atrial origin with 69% sensitivity, 100% specificity, 100% positive predictive value, and 66% negative predictive value. A V1 lead that was positive or negative-positive biphasic P wave in V1 had

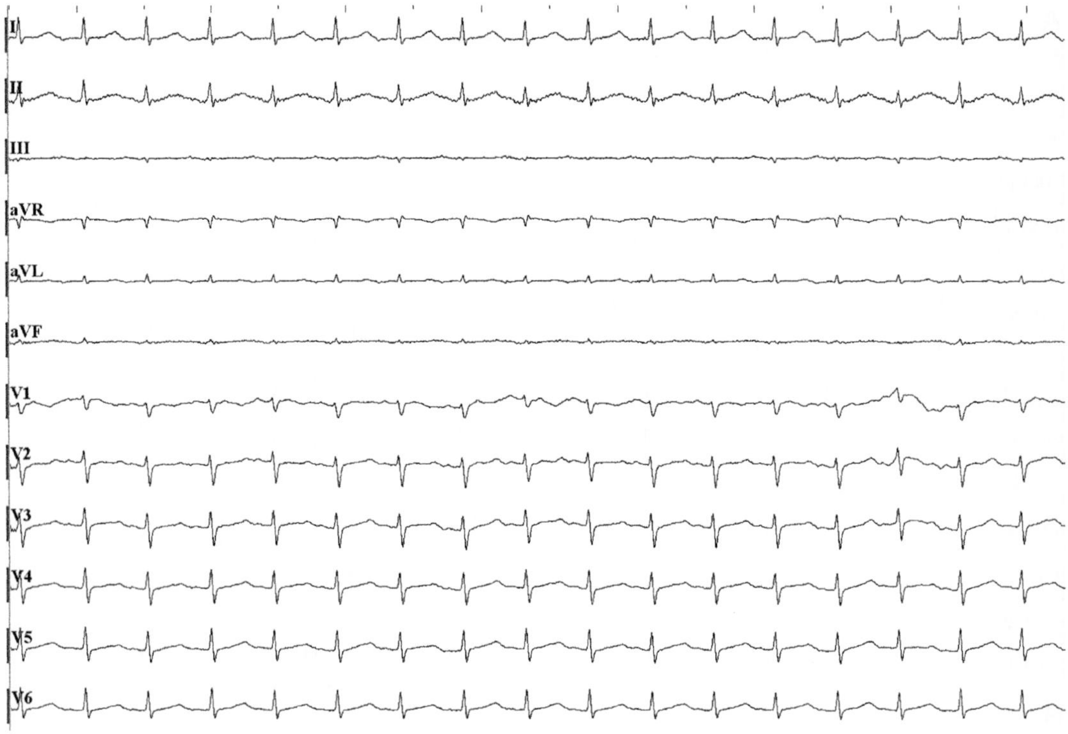

Fig. 3. Twelve-lead electrocardiogram showing P wave morphology during atrial tachycardia. The P waves are positive in V_1, negative in avL, and low voltage in the limb leads.

100% sensitivity, 81% specificity, 76% positive predictive value, and 100% negative predictive value for atrial tachycardias of left atrial origin.

Analysis of P wave morphology for atrial tachycardias originating in the superior mitral annular region has also revealed distinctive features. In a series describing 10 patients with atrial tachycardias with foci in this region, 100% of patients were found to have a positive P wave in V1, and 9 of 10 were found to have a negative P wave in aVL.[2] In another series however, mitral annular atrial tachycardias (MAATs) were universally associated with biphasic (negative-positive) P waves in V1.[4] Another intriguing finding associated with MAATs is the presence of low-voltage P waves in the limb leads during tachycardia.[2,4] Analysis of the P

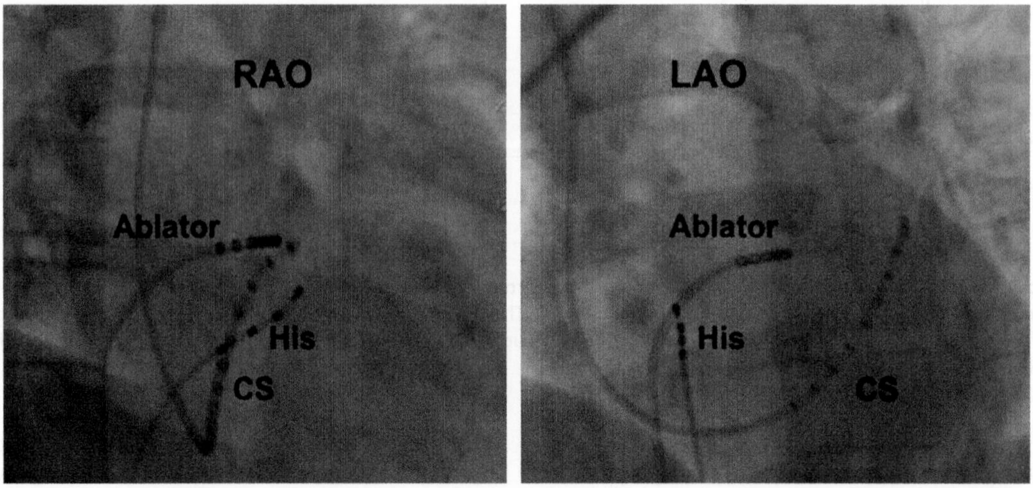

Fig. 4. Fluoroscopic images in right anterior oblique (RAO) and left anterior oblique (LAO) views showing ablator position at the successful site on the mitral annulus. CS, coronary sinus.

wave morphology in our case presented revealed P wave characteristics consistent with some of the features mentioned above: Lead V1 was positive, lead AVL was negative, and low-voltage P waves were observed in the limb leads.

Atrial Activation Sequence

Atrial depolarization during atrial tachycardia depends on a number of factors, including the origin of the atrial tachycardia, the presence of functional or anatomic barriers, the conduction properties of the atria, and the existence of pathways that facilitate interatrial conduction. The latter include Bachmann's bundle, the interatrial septum, and the coronary sinus musculature. MAATs are frequently characterized by proximal-to-distal coronary sinus activation.[2,4,5] MAATs have also been characterized by the finding that the earliest site of atrial activation occurs at the His electrogram position. Recently, Kriatselis and colleagues[5] described a series of 12 patients with atrial tachycardia in whom the earliest atrial activation was recorded at the His site during tachycardia. Of these, 5 patients had atrial tachycardias originating from the mitral annulus and 7 had atrial tachycardias originating from the noncoronary aortic cusp. Therefore, in addition to considering a para-Hisian focus, an operator should also consider mitral annular or noncoronary aortic cusp locations for atrial tachycardias with a concentric coronary sinus activation sequence and earliest His activation.

However, not all MAATs will demonstrate a concentric coronary sinus activation pattern or earliest His activation. In our patient, the coronary sinus distal electrode was the earliest site of activation during tachycardia. While the His electrogram was relatively early, it was consistently activated 10 to 15 seconds after the coronary sinus distal electrode. This finding supports the notion that MAATs may be associated with a variety of atrial activation patterns and cannot be reliably diagnosed on this basis alone.

Radio Frequency Ablation

Typically, atrial tachycardias originating from the mitral annular region are ablated using a transseptal approach. In our patient, we were able to place our catheters in the superior region of the mitral annulus using this technique. However, a retrograde aortic approach has also been described to ablate atrial tachycardias in this region.[5]

SUMMARY

This case highlights characteristic features of atrial tachycardia arising from the mitral annulus. P wave morphologies can provide additional clues regarding the origin of atrial tachycardia on the mitral annulus. The atrial activation sequence is sometimes, but not always, earliest in the His potential electrogram position and may or may not be characterized by proximal-to-distal coronary sinus activation. Careful mapping along the mitral annulus to determine the earliest site of activation with reference to the surface P wave is a reliable method for precisely localizing an atrial tachycardia origin. Catheter ablation can be approached using either a transseptal or retrograde aortic approach.

REFERENCES

1. Kistler PM, Roberts-Thomson KC, Haqqani HM, et al. P-wave morphology in focal atrial tachycardia: development of an algorithm to predict the anatomic site of origin. J Am Coll Cardiol 2006;48(5):1010–7.
2. Gonzalez MD, Contreras LJ, Jongbloed MR, et al. Left atrial tachycardia originating from the mitral annulus-aorta junction. Circulation 2004;110(20):3187–92.
3. Tang CW, Scheinman MM, Van Hare GF, et al. Use of P wave configuration during atrial tachycardia to predict site of origin. J Am Coll Cardiol 1995;26(5): 1315–24.
4. Kistler PM, Sanders P, Hussin A, et al. Focal atrial tachycardia arising from the mitral annulus: electrocardiographic and electrophysiologic characterization. J Am Coll Cardiol 2003;41(12):2212–9.
5. Kriatselis C, Roser M, Min T, et al. Ectopic atrial tachycardias with early activation at His site: radiofrequency ablation through a retrograde approach. Europace 2008;10(6):698–704.

Narrow Complex Tachycardia: What is the Mechanism?

Mohan N. Viswanathan, MD[a,*],
Melvin Scheinman, MD[b], Nitish Badhwar, MD[b]

KEYWORDS

- Supraventricular tachycardia
- Atrioventricular nodal reentrant tachycardia
- Junctional tachycardia • Pacing maneuvers

A 62-year-old woman with recurrent palpitations and a diagnosis of supraventricular tachycardia (SVT) was referred to the authors' attention for further evaluation. She had undergone surgical resection for left atrial myxoma that left her with both right and left atrial surgical scars and a pericardial atrial septal defect patch repair. Shortly after her surgery, she began to experience recurrent palpitations and was thought to have an atrial tachycardia that would last minutes to hours. She had failed treatment with various drugs including beta-blockers, calcium-channel blockers, and, more recently, procainamide. She was ultimately referred for electrophysiology study (EPS) and catheter ablation.

EPS

A four-catheter EPS was performed involving recordings from the high right atrium, His bundle electrogram (HBE), proximal to distal coronary sinus, and right ventricular (RV) apex or base. During normal sinus rhythm, the baseline atrial-His (AH) interval was 61 milliseconds (ms), and His-ventricular interval of 48 ms. There was spontaneous development of a simultaneous atrium (A)-on- ventricle (V) tachycardia with a cycle length of 400 ms after intrinsic premature atrial complexes (PACs). This SVT was noted to repeatedly terminate with an atrial depolarization.

This simultaneous A-on-V tachycardia was also easily initiated with ventricular overdrive (VOD) pacing at 350 ms (**Fig. 1**) and ventricular extrastimulus pacing. Atrial extrastimulus pacing with a drive cycle length of 500 ms with a single extrastimulus at a coupling interval of 350 ms also easily induced the same SVT (**Fig. 2**).

VOD pacing during tachycardia advanced the atrial activation to the pacing cycle length and, upon cessation of pacing, a V-A-V response was demonstrated. Atrial overdrive pacing from the proximal coronary sinus during SVT showed dissociation of the atrial activation from the SVT as the ventricular activation continued at the tachycardia cycle length of 400 ms (**Fig. 3**).

The differential diagnosis included atrioventricular nodal reentrant tachycardia (AVNRT), focal junctional tachycardia (JT), and the rarely seen, concealed nodofascicular tachycardia (NFT). Premature ventricular complexes (PVCs), introduced during tachycardia at the time of His-refractoriness, were unable to advance the following atrial activation or the subsequent His or ventricular activation, eliminating the possibility of a concealed right-sided or septal bypass tract, and argues against the presence of NFT.

Disclosures: None (Viswanathan, Scheinman, and Badhwar).

[a] Division of Cardiology, Section of Cardiac Electrophysiology, University of Washington School of Medicine, 1959 NE Pacific Street, Box 356422, Seattle, WA 98195-6422, USA
[b] Division of Cardiology, Section of Cardiac Electrophysiology, University of California, 500 Parnassus Avenue, Box 1354, San Francisco, CA 94143-1354, USA
* Corresponding author.
E-mail address: viswanam@u.washington.edu

Card Electrophysiol Clin 2 (2010) 203–207
doi:10.1016/j.ccep.2010.01.003

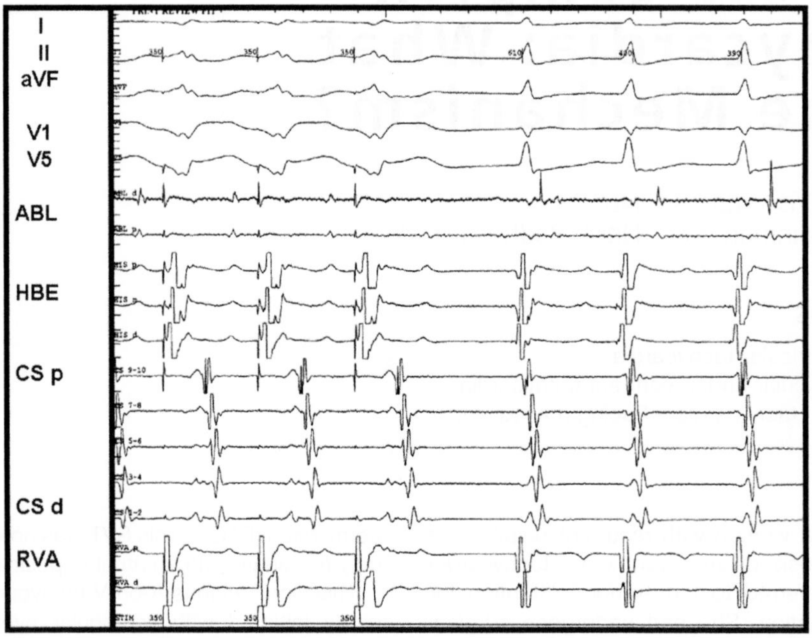

Fig. 1. The supraventricular tachycardia is initiated with ventricular burst pacing at a drive cycle length of 350 ms from the RV basal septum (paced QRS complex is upright in leads II and aVF). ABL, ablator, distal and proximal; CSd, distal coronary sinus; CSp, proximal coronary sinus; RVA, right ventricular catheter, proximal and distal.

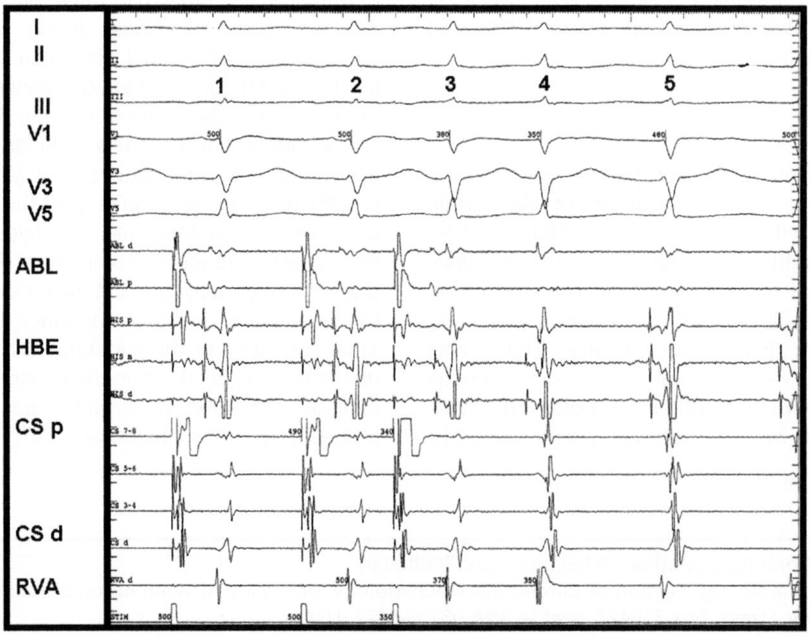

Fig. 2. Supraventricular tachycardia was again initiated easily with atrial extrastimulus pacing at a drive cycle length of 500 ms with the single extrastimulus at a coupling interval of 350 ms. The QRS complexes are labeled 1–5. The generation of QRS complex 4 is discussed in the text. It could be explained based on a 2-for-1 response (ie, "double fire," or due to triggered junctional ectopy after cessation of atrial pacing). ABL, ablator, distal and proximal; CSd, distal coronary sinus; CSp, proximal coronary sinus; RVA, right ventricular catheter, distal.

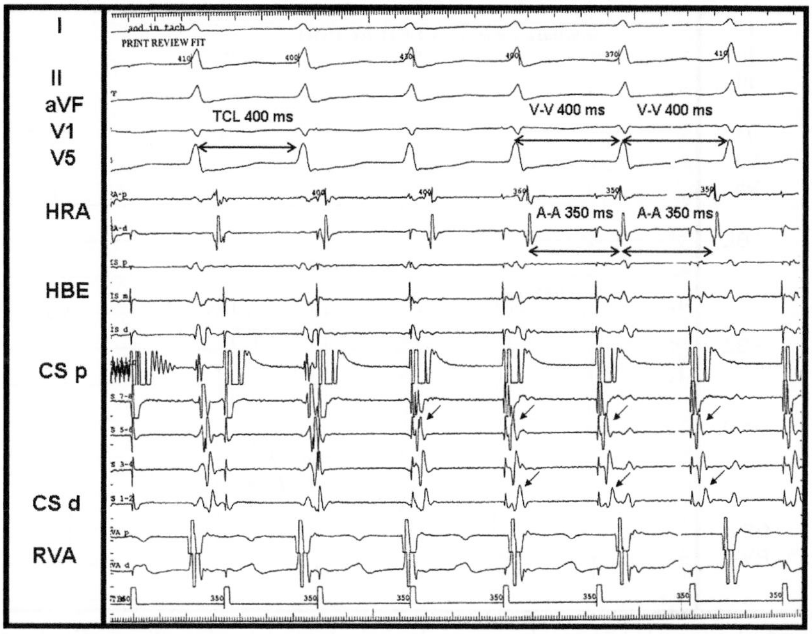

Fig. 3. Atrial overdrive pacing was performed during tachycardia. The tachycardia cycle length is 400 ms and the pacing cycle length is 350 ms. It is evident that there is atrial capture after at least the last four pacing stimuli evidenced by the atrial EGM showing a fixed relationship following the pacing stimuli, as seen on the high right atrium (HRA) recording, or the local CS recording in CS distal, CS 5,6 or CS 3,4 (*oblique arrows*). Despite advancement of the atrial depolarization to the pacing cycle length of 350 ms (labeled as A-A 350 ms), the V-V intervals remain at the tachycardia cycle length of 400 ms (labeled V-V 400 ms), thus demonstrating dissociation of the atrium from the ventricle and the SVT circuit, also eliminating orthodromic AVRT. CSd, distal coronary sinus; CSp, proximal coronary sinus; RVA, right ventricular catheter, proximal and distal.

WHAT DIAGNOSTIC MANEUVER WOULD BE USEFUL IN DIFFERENTIATING AVNRT FROM JT?

We then employed the delivery of a late-coupled PAC when the atrial activation on the HBE recording (His A, or septal A) was committed. This pacing maneuver consistently terminated tachycardia without affecting the subsequent His or ventricular depolarization (**Fig. 4**). This response eliminates JT because with late coupling the junction is already committed and should not be affected by the atrial extrastimulus. Radiofrequency ablation using a 4-mm catheter directed to the slow pathway region resulted in slow junctional ectopy during ablation and the patient was noninducible for SVT after catheter ablation. Clinically, after 2 months of follow up, the patient remains free of palpitations.

DISCUSSION

SVT discrimination in the electrophysiology laboratory remains a challenging but rewarding exercise as it is a key step in determining the appropriate treatment options for many patients.[1,2] Knight and colleagues[3] codified the use of pacing maneuvers, especially the response to cessation of VOD pacing during SVT, and provided evidence for the usefulness of this maneuver in differentiating AVNRT from orthodromic atrioventricular reciprocating tachycardia (AVRT). However, the differentiation of AVNRT from JT continues to perplex clinicians in the electrophysiology laboratory and the development of pacing maneuvers to address this challenge would be welcomed. They pose a diagnostic dilemma given their many similarities such as virtually coincident ventricular and atrial activation (A-on-V tachycardia), the usual evidence of the HBE preceding the atrial and ventricular activation, and a typical concentric retrograde atrial activation sequence (atrial signal on the HBE or the proximal coronary sinus catheter precedes all other atrial electrograms recorded). These features argue for a low atrial septal origin of tachycardia, likely at or near the atrioventricular (AV) node. The differential diagnosis includes AVNRT, JT, parahisian atrial tachycardia, and the rarely seen concealed nodofascicular tachycardia (NFT).[4,5] Because AVNRT

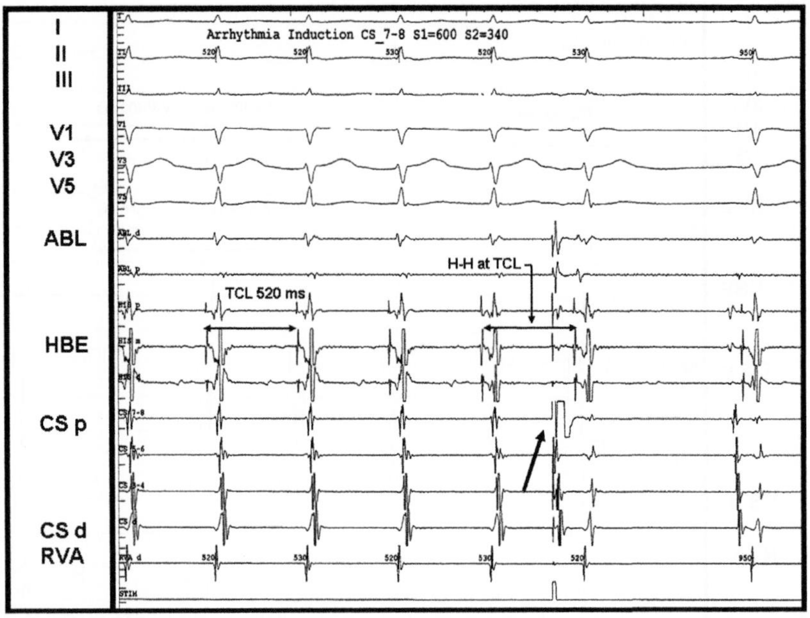

Fig. 4. Delivery of a late-coupled PAC (*oblique arrow*) terminates tachycardia without affecting the immediate His or V (labeled as H-H at TCL). This response was seen repeatedly during tachycardia. ABL, ablator, distal and proximal; CSd, distal coronary sinus; CSp, proximal coronary sinus; RVA, right ventricular catheter, distal.

and JT share many common electrophysiological qualities, they were thought of as the same arrhythmia for many years.[6]

The measurement put forth by Knight and colleagues,[3] the tachycardia cycle length (TCL) subtracted from the post-pacing interval (PPI) after VOD pacing during SVT (PPI-TCL), unfortunately does not differentiate AVNRT from JT. Srivathsan and colleagues[7] looked at the difference between the His-atrial (HA) interval between that seen in tachycardia (HA_{tach})and that seen during ventricular pacing (HA_{pace}) at the basal RV and have found that the magnitude of this difference may be useful to distinguish these arrhythmias. The authors proposed that the insertion of a late PAC during tachycardia from the slow AV nodal pathway region when the septal A was committed would advance the subsequent His in patients with AVNRT and not those with JT.[8] Earlier PACs can potentially affect JT by slowing, accelerating, terminating, or having no effect on the tachycardia focus. However, it is the alternative entry into the junction via the slow AV nodal pathway when the low atrial septum has been rendered refractory by retrograde activation via the fast pathway that allows an appropriately timed late PAC to perturb the next tachycardia beat only in AVNRT. This late PAC can either delay or advance the next His or terminate tachycardia. Termination of tachycardia or delay of the next His are absolutely diagnostic in differentiating AVNRT from JT.[9] Padanilam and colleagues[10] also delivered PACs during tachycardia to differentiate these arrhythmias, with various responses to PACs elicited depending on the timing of the PAC during the tachycardia cycle.

In the case presented above, the A-on-V tachycardia with a very short VA interval (significantly <70 ms) during tachycardia effectively eliminated orthodromic AVRT, as did the key maneuver of atrial overdrive pacing, which dissociated the atrial activation from the tachycardia circuit and ventricular activation (see **Fig. 3**). The V-A-V response during VOD pacing during tachycardia eliminated atrial tachycardia despite the reports of a prior diagnosis of atrial tachycardia. This left AVNRT, JT, or the rare NFT as possibilities to explain the rhythm. Late PVCs (when the His bundle was refractory) failed to affect the subsequent A arguing against NFT. Given that the tachycardia was initiated repeatedly with burst atrial or ventricular pacing and importantly, without a critical AH interval or a classic AH "jump," JT was a distinct possibility (see **Fig. 2**). Upon further analysis of **Fig. 2**, one can postulate whether the fourth ventricular complex (labeled as 4) was created as a result of a "double fire" or 2-for-1 response (ie, an atrial depolarization conducting once down a fast AV nodal pathway and simultaneously down a slow AV nodal pathway resulting in two

QRS complexes for one atrial complex, thus providing evidence of dual AV nodal physiology). The other possibility is that it is explained by triggered junctional ectopy. In the first scenario, a 2-for-1 response would argue in favor of AVNRT as the diagnosis. However, in the second scenario, this would favor JT. This phenomenon was seen occasionally, and the coupling interval of the second ventricular complex was not always the same, also suggesting that it may be more in keeping with JT.

However, the use of appropriately timed PACs proved useful in this case to confirm AVNRT as the diagnosis. Repeated termination of tachycardia with PAC delivery during septal atrial refractoriness (coincident with septal atrial activation) without affecting the immediate tachycardia beat was seen. This suggests the presence of a slow AV nodal pathway that was participating in the tachycardia circuit and when engaged by the late-coupled PAC, perturbed the circuit and terminated the rhythm. Similarly, an atrial extrastimulus inserted when the AV node or His bundle is refractory and terminates the SVT is strong evidence against a nodofascicular pathway.

REFERENCES

1. Morady F. Catheter ablation of supraventricular arrhythmias: state of the art. J Cardiovasc Electrophysiol 2004;15(1):124–39.
2. Nakagawa H, Jackman WM. Catheter ablation of paroxysmal supraventricular tachycardia. Circulation 2007;116(21):2465–78.
3. Knight BP, Ebinger M, Oral H, et al. Diagnostic value of tachycardia features and pacing maneuvers during paroxysmal supraventricular tachycardia. J Am Coll Cardiol 2000;36(2):574–82.
4. Hamdan MH, Kalman JM, Lesh MD, et al. Narrow complex tachycardia with VA block: diagnostic and therapeutic implications. Pacing Clin Electrophysiol 1998;21(6):1196–206.
5. Lau EW. Infraatrial supraventricular tachycardias: mechanisms, diagnosis, and management. Pacing Clin Electrophysiol 2008;31(4):490–8.
6. Josephson ME. Supraventricular tachycardias. In: Josephson ME, editor. Clinical cardiac electrophysiology: techniques and interpretations. 4th edition. Philadelphia: Lippincott Williams & Wilkins; 2008. p. 175–284.
7. Srivathsan K, Gami AS, Barrett R, et al. Differentiating atrioventricular nodal reentrant tachycardia from junctional tachycardia: novel application of the delta H-A interval. J Cardiovasc Electrophysiol 2008;19(1):1–6.
8. Hamdan MH, Badhwar N, Scheinman MM. Role of invasive electrophysiologic testing in the evaluation and management of adult patients with focal junctional tachycardia. Card Electrophysiol Rev 2002; 6(4):431–5.
9. Viswanathan MN, Scheinman MM, Badhwar N. A new diagnostic maneuver to differentiate atrioventricular nodal reentrant tachycardia from junctional tachycardia: a difficult distinction [abstract]. Heart Rhythm 2007;4(5):S288.
10. Padanilam BJ, Manfredi JA, Steinberg LA, et al. Differentiating junctional tachycardia and atrioventricular node re-entry tachycardia based on response to atrial extrastimulus pacing. J Am Coll Cardiol 2008;52(21): 1711–7.

Tachycardia-Induced Cardiomyopathy

Gaetano Barbato, MD[a,*], Valeria Carinci, MD[a], Nitish Badhwar, MD[b]

KEYWORDS

- Cardiomyopathy • Supraventricular tachycardia
- Nonreentrant atrioventricular nodal tachycardia

A 52-year-old female presented with exertional shortness of breath and palpitations over a 3-year period. The echocardiogram revealed a minimal mitral incompetence and moderately reduced global ejection fraction of 42%. ECG at presentation showed an irregular narrow complex tachycardia with more QRS complexes than the P waves (**Fig. 1**). She was referred for electrophysiology study and ablation.

ELECTROPHYSIOLOGY STUDY

At electrophysiology study, multipolar catheters were placed in the right atrium, His-bundle region, right ventricle, and coronary sinus. Careful analysis of the 12-lead ECG shows a stable pattern of a single P wave followed by two QRS complex with PR interval of 240 milliseconds (msec) and 720 msec, respectively. The subsequent P wave was conducted to a single QRS with a PR interval of 360 msec. The EP study confirmed the presence of one atrial (A) signal with dual antegrade conduction to two ventricular (V) complexes followed by an A conducted to a single V. Every V was preceded by a His potential. The A-H interval was 190 msec between the A and the first His, and 660 msec between the same A and a second His potential. The next A was followed by a single V with an A-H interval of 300 msec (**Fig 2**).

WHAT IS THE MECHANISM OF THE VARIABLE VENTRICULAR RESPONSE?

We assumed that the two consecutive V potentials were activated through the fast (FP) and slow (SP) pathways, respectively (double fire) in **Fig. 2**. The following V was also activated through the FP but the A-H interval was longer owing to concealed retrograde conduction of the preceding SPs activation. The "long" FP activation was not followed by SP V activation owing to antegrade block caused by the previous longer FP activation. The antegrade block in the SP after concealed retrograde conduction over the fast in the previous complex was not constant. Sometimes we observed block in the FP (**Fig. 3**) while the A-H interval through the SP remained the same. Concealed retrograde conduction into the FP was followed sometimes by double fire activity after the following A complex (**Fig. 4**). In this case, both FPs and SPs were able to conduct to the His, but when the impulse of the SP reached the His-Purkinje system it was still partially refractory and the QRS has a left bundle branch block pattern.

Based on the diagnosis of incessant nonreentrant atrioventricular nodal tachycardia it was decided to do a SP ablation. A 4-mm ablation catheter was advanced to the tricuspid annulus just anterior to the coronary sinus ostium at the traditional SP region. Ablation at this site led to slow junctional beats without evidence of His-atrial

[a] Cardiology Division, Cardiology Department, Maggiore Hospital, Largo Nigrisoli 2, Bologna 40133, Italy
[b] Division of Cardiology, Department of Cardiac Electrophysiology, University of California, 500 Parnassus Avenue, MU East 431, Box 1354, San Francisco, CA 94143, USA
* Corresponding author.
E-mail address: gaetano.barbato@ausl.bologna.it

Card Electrophysiol Clin 2 (2010) 209–212
doi:10.1016/j.ccep.2010.01.004
1877-9182/10/$ – see front matter

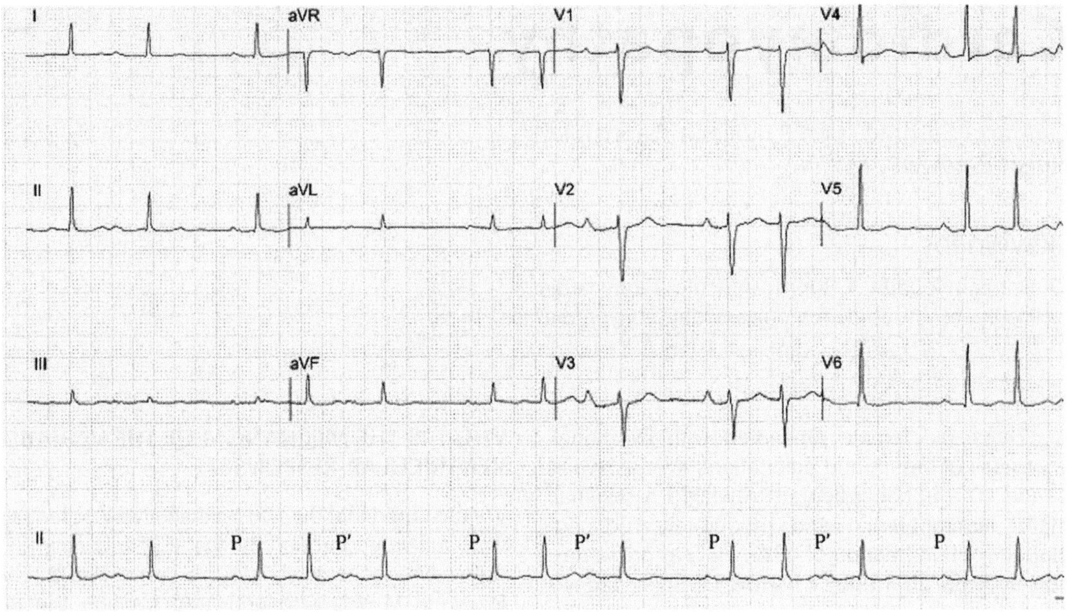

Fig. 1. Twelve-lead ECG at presentation showing a P wave (P) that is followed by two QRS complex and the subsequent P wave (P') that is followed by a single QRS. V, ventricle.

block. The procedure was successful and no double fire was noted after the ablation. The patient underwent an echocardiogram after 2 months of follow up and an improvement of the ejection fraction from 42% to 57% was documented. She also had significant improvement of effort tolerance and quality of life.

DISCUSSION

Atrioventricular nodal reentrant tachycardia is usually associated with dual AV node physiology. Manifestations of longitudinal AV dissociation can be present during sinus rhythm.[1] The least common manifestation is synchronous conduction

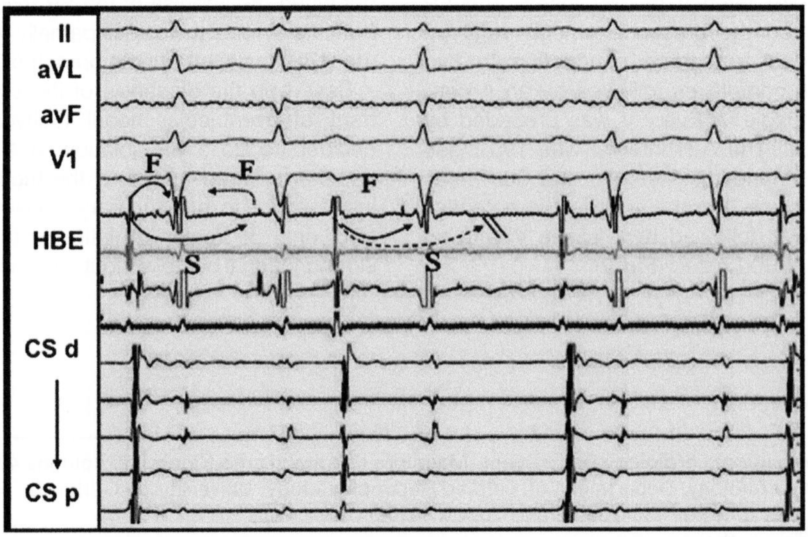

Fig. 2. Intracardiac recording showing fast (F) and slow (S) antegrade conduction at baseline. The dotted lines indicate the retrograde concealed conduction over the FP and the subsequent antegrade block over the SP. CSd, coronary sinus distal; CSp, coronary sinus proximal, HBE, His bundle electrogram.

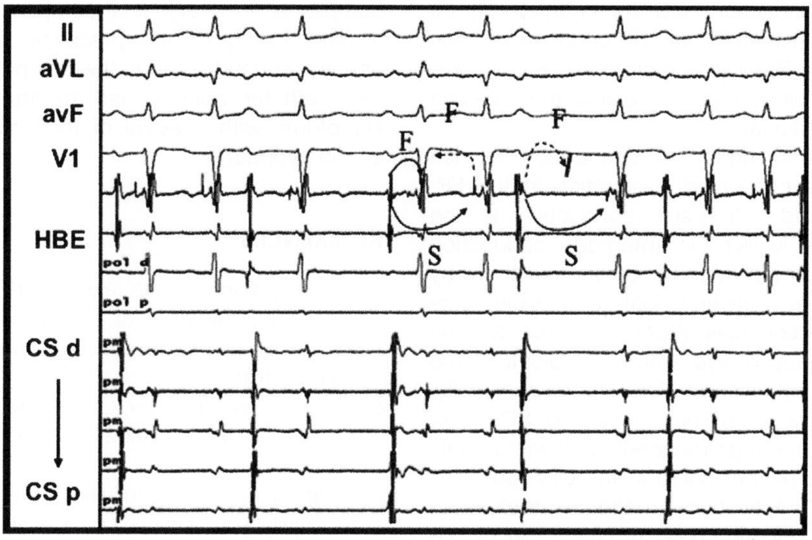

Fig. 3. Fast (F) and slow (S) antegrade conduction. The dotted lines indicated the retrograde concealed conduction over the FP and the subsequent antegrade block over the FP. The antegrade conduction over the SP was constant: 660 msec. CSd, coronary sinus distal; CSp, coronary sinus proximal, HBE, His bundle electrogram.

of a single sinus impulse along the FPs and SPs, inscribing two QRS complexes.[2,3] After the initial description of this phenomenon by Wu and colleagues,[2] Csapo[3] was the first to report a case of paroxysmal nonreentrant nodal tachycardia due to this mechanism.

Later several cases were described.[4–7] The following clinical features were noted: the arrhythmia has an irregular pattern, it is usually refractory to antiarrhythmic therapy, and, if incessant, can lead to cardiomyopathy. A recent report[6] tried to identify the underlying electrophysiological determinants of double firing, describing the following criteria: (1) sufficient antegrade dissociation of AV node, (2) absence of retrograde conduction over each AV nodal pathway following

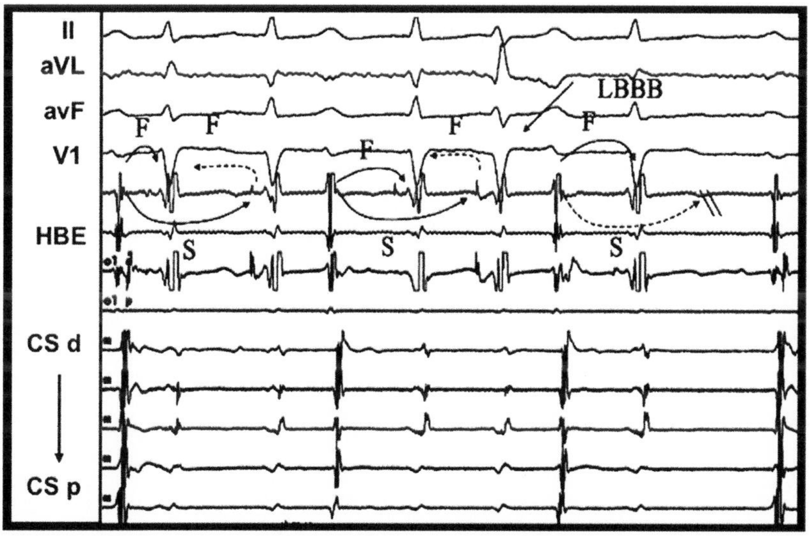

Fig. 4. Two consecutive sinus beats are conducted with longitudinal dissociation. Fast (F) and slow (S) pathway conduction annotated. Note that FP conduction of the second beat is longer than FP conduction of the first beat because of the retrograde concealed conduction (*dotted lines*). The SP conduction of the second beat meets refractoriness in the distal His-Purkinje system leading to a QRS with a left bundle branch pattern (LBBB). CSd, coronary sinus distal; CSp, coronary sinus proximal, HBE, His bundle electrogram.

antegrade conduction over its counterpart, (3) differences between FP and SP conduction times exceeding His-Purkinje refractoriness, and (4) critical timing of sinus impulses relative to preceding AV nodal conduction.

The unique finding in this case is the presence of retrograde concealed conduction in the FP. The concealed retrograde conduction is the cause of the longer FP antegrade conduction (300msec vs the previous 190msec). In this way the difference between fast and slow time conduction decreases (from 470msec to 360 msec), with successive antegrade block in the His-Purkinje system via the SP. Occasionally, there is activation of both FPs and SPs after the concealed retrograde conduction with bundle branch block pattern noted in the QRS complex noted with SP activation. An alternative explanation posits conduction delay or block over the FP due to delay or block in the AV nodal final common pathway. This is unlikely because block in the final common pathway after expected FP conduction leads to marked delay in SP conduction to the ventricle (see **Fig 3**). The next V would have to show an even longer delay during FP conduction but in fact the opposite occurred, thus confirming electrotonic interaction between the FP and the SP.

SUMMARY

This is a typical example of a tachycardia-induced cardiomyopathy due to incessant tachycardia with moderately increased ventricular rate. This was due to nonreentrant atrioventricular nodal tachycardia that gave rise to two ventricular complexes for every atrial complex. It describes a rare finding of the presence of retrograde concealed conduction in the fast pathway. Curative catheter ablation led to improvement of symptoms with reversal of tachycardia-induced cardiomyopathy.

REFERENCES

1. Fisch C, Mandrola JM, Rardon DP. Electrocardiographic manifestations of dual atrioventricular node conduction during sinus rhythm. J Am Coll Cardiol 1997;29:1015–22.
2. Wu D, Denes P, Dhingra R, et al. New manifestations of dual A-V nodal pathways. Eur J cardiol 1975;2: 459–66.
3. Csapo G. Paroxysmal nonreentrant tachycardias due to simultaneous conduction in dual atrioventricular nodal pathways. Am J Cardiol. 1979;43(5):1033–45.
4. Sutton FJ, Lee YC. Supraventricular nonreentrant tachycardia due to simultaneous conduction through dual atrioventricular nodal pathways. Am J Cardiol 1983;51:897–900.
5. Anselme F, Frederiks J, Boyle N, et al. An unusual cause of tachycardia-induced myopathy. Pacing Clin Electrophysiol 1996;19:115–9.
6. Gaba D, Pavri BB, Greenspon AJ, et al. Dual antegrade response tachycardia induced cardiomyopathy. Pacing Clin Electrophysiol. 2004;27(4):533–6.
7. Mansour M, Marrouche N, Ruskin J, et al. Incessant nonreentrant tachycardia due to simultaneous conduction over dual atrioventricular nodal pathways mimicking atrial fibrillation in patients referred for pulmonary vein isolation. J Cardiovasc Electrophysiol. 2003;14(7):752–5.

Recurrent Accessory Pathway Conduction in a Patient with Wolff-Parkinson-White Syndrome: How to Ablate?

Daniel Y. Wang, MD, Shepard D. Weiner, MD, Hasan Garan, MD, William Whang, MD*

KEYWORDS

- Catheter ablation • Wolff-Parkinson-White syndrome
- Supraventricular tachycardia

A 24-year-old man presented to the emergency department with sudden-onset, sustained palpitations. His medical history was notable for intermittent palpitations beginning several months before presentation, lasting a few seconds to minutes at a time. Electrocardiogram (ECG) demonstrated preexcited atrial fibrillation (AF) with an average ventricular rate of 208 beats per minute (**Fig. 1**), ultimately causing hemodynamic instability and requiring defibrillation to sinus rhythm. The ventricular preexcitation pattern was suggestive of a right-sided accessory pathway (AP) (**Fig. 2**). On admission, physical examination, chest radiograph, and laboratory evaluation were unremarkable. Transthoracic echocardiography revealed no significant structural abnormalities and preserved left and right ventricular systolic function. He was referred for electrophysiology study (EPS).

During EPS, the pattern of activation during sinus rhythm and ventricular pacing was consistent with a right anterolateral AP, and orthodromic atrio-ventricular re-entry tachycardia was induced. During induced atrial fibrillation, the shortest RR interval was 210 milliseconds. Radiofrequency (RF) ablation at multiple sites of early ventricular activation at the 10 o'clock position on the tricuspid annulus failed to eliminate pre-excitation. A site with short local ventriculo-atrial (VA) time during ventricular pacing was found at the base of the right atrial appendage (RAA), and an 8 mm tip catheter was used to ablate at this site, with loss of pre-excitation (**Fig. 3**).

The patient returned 4 weeks later with palpitations and was found to have recurrence of pre-excitation by ECG. EPS was performed, and a 3.5 mm open-tip irrigated catheter (Navistar ThermoCool, Biosense Webster, Diamond Bar, CA, USA) was used to perform repeat ablation of the atrial insertion of the AP at the base of the RAA. Approximately 24 hours after the ablation, however, pre-excitation recurred.

QUESTION: WHAT SHOULD BE THE NEXT ABLATION STRATEGY?

The patient returned for a repeat EPS using an epicardial approach. Epicardial access was obtained via a subxyphoid approach under fluoroscopic guidance with injection of contrast to visualize entry into the pericardial space.[1] A deflectable 4 mm ablation catheter (Navistar,

Department of Medicine, Columbia University Medical Center, Harkness 366, 180 Fort Washington Avenue, New York, NY 10032, USA
* Corresponding author.
E-mail address: ww42@columbia.edu

Card Electrophysiol Clin 2 (2010) 213–216
doi:10.1016/j.ccep.2010.01.005
1877-9182/10/$ – see front matter

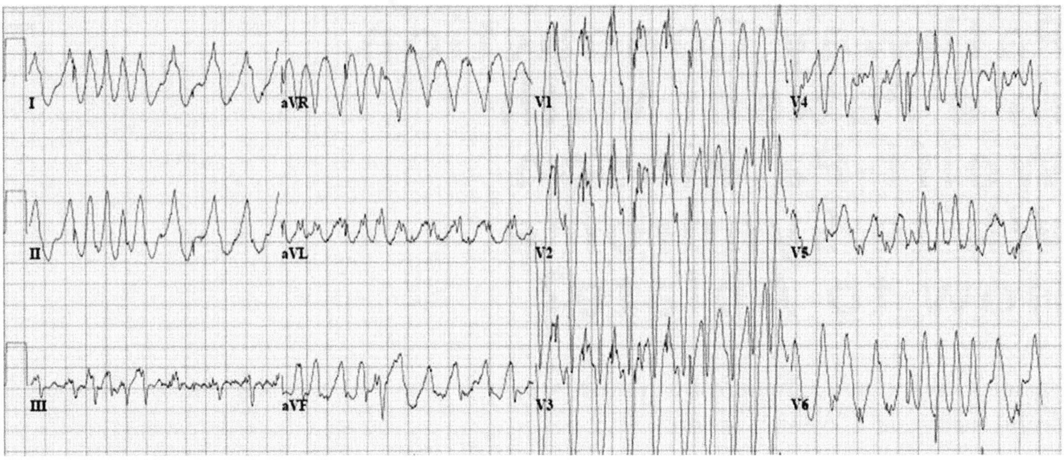

Fig. 1. Pre-excited atrial fibrillation.

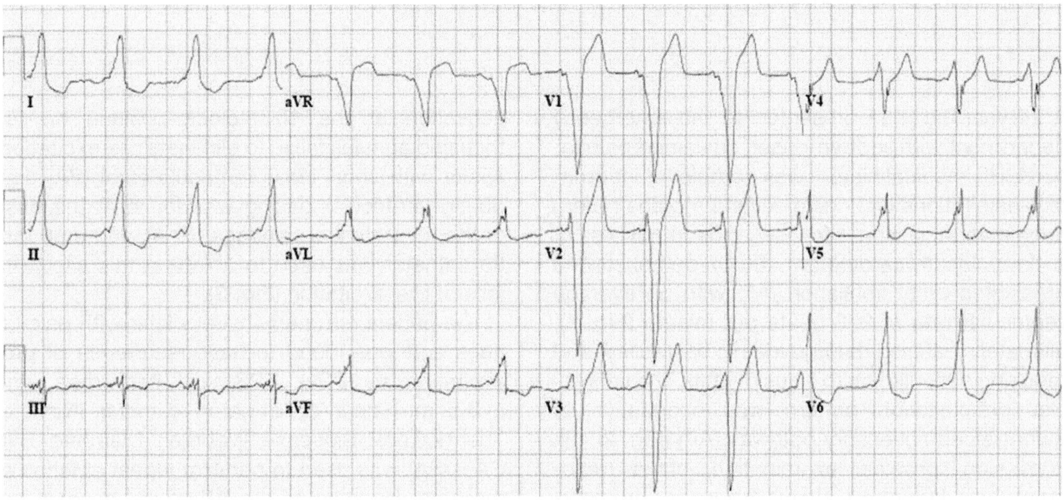

Fig. 2. Sinus rhythm with ventricular pre-excitation pattern suggestive of right-sided accessory pathway.

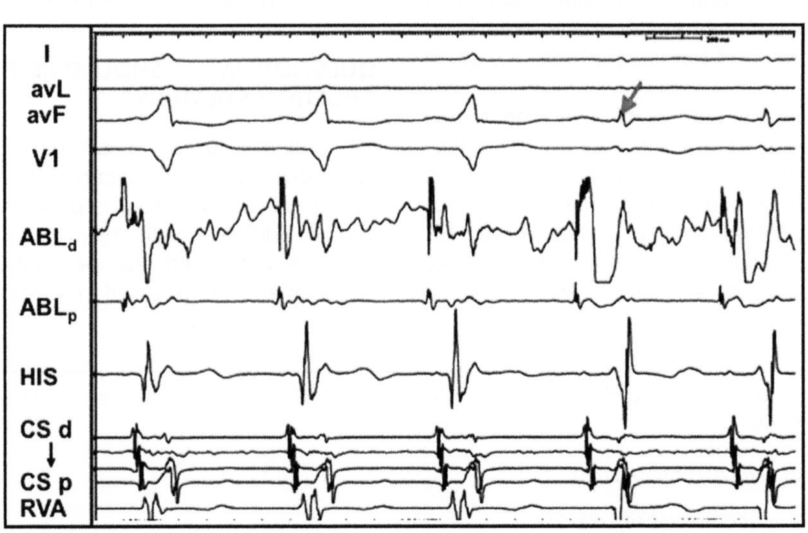

Fig. 3. Intracardiac electrogram in sinus rhythm during successful ablation *(arrow)* showing surface ECG, ablator (ABL), bundle of His (HIS), coronary sinus (CS), and right ventricular (RV) recordings.

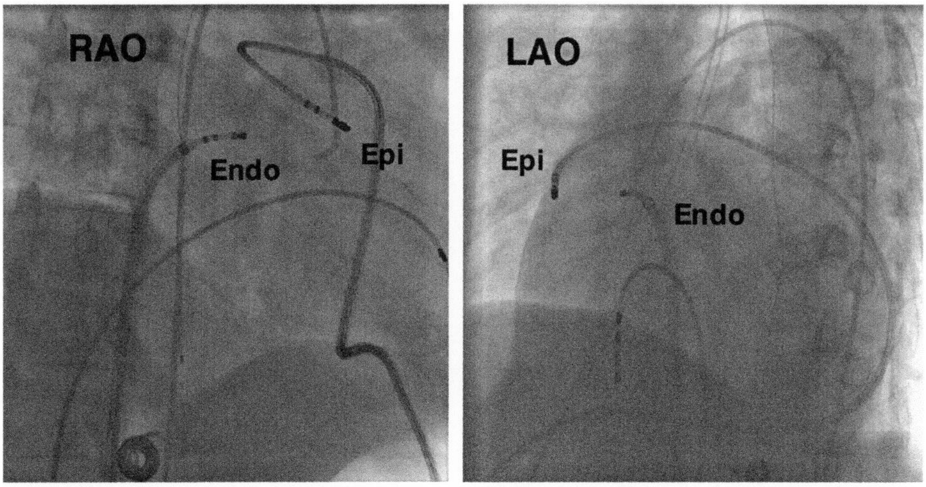

Fig. 4. Fluoroscopic catheter positioning in right anterior oblique and left anterior oblique projections. Ablator is epicardial (Epi), and a second mapping catheter sits at the prior successful endocardial ablation site (Endo). A diagnostic coronary catheter is positioned in the right coronary artery.

Biosense Webster, Diamond Bar, CA, USA) was advanced through an 8 French sheath into the pericardial space. Coronary angiography was performed to localize the right coronary artery. During ventricular pacing, a site with short local VA time was identified adjacent to the prior endocardial ablation site at the base of the RAA. Ablation at this site in sinus rhythm (30 W) resulted in sustained loss of pre-excitation. Fluoroscopic catheter positions are shown in **Fig. 4**. After ablation, the patient remained asymptomatic with no evidence of pre-excitation on ECG after 24 months of follow-up.

DISCUSSION

RF ablation is a first-line therapy for AP mediated tachycardias. Variant APs arising from the RAA, treated with endocardial or surgical ablation, have been reported previously.[2–4] Ablation of APs from the tricuspid or mitral annulus or in a branch of the coronary sinus has been associated with success rates greater than 90%.[5,6] In cases of prolonged or failed AP ablation, an epicardial approach was used in 8% to 18% of cases, including the right atrial free wall.[7,8] Epicardial ablation of RAA to right ventricle APs has been reported previously.[9,10] For APs that originate from the RAA, this case illustrates that successful ablation may be performed far from the annulus at the atrial insertion site. A lack of AP potential in the annulus may indicate the need to explore elsewhere in the right atrium.[9] In this case, the short VA time during ventricular pacing allowed identification of a successful site for epicardial ablation.

REFERENCES

1. Sosa E, Scanavacca M. Epicardial mapping and ablation techniques to control ventricular tachycardia. J Cardiovasc Electrophysiol 2005;16(4): 449–52.
2. Milstein S, Dunnigan A, Tang C, et al. Right atrial appendage to right ventricle accessory atrioventricular connection: a case report. Pacing Clin Electrophysiol 1997;20(7):1877–80.
3. Soejima K, Mitamura H, Miyazaki T, et al. Catheter ablation of accessory atrioventricular connection between right atrial appendage to right ventricle: a case report. J Cardiovasc Electrophysiol 1998; 9(5):523–8.
4. Goya M, Takahashi A, Nakagawa H, et al. A case of catheter ablation of accessory atrioventricular connection between the right atrial appendage and right ventricle guided by a three-dimensional electroanatomic mapping system. J Cardiovasc Electrophysiol 1999;10(8):1112–8.
5. Jackman WM, Wang XZ, Friday KJ, et al. Catheter ablation of accessory atrioventricular pathways (Wolff-Parkinson-White syndrome) by radiofrequency current. N Engl J Med 1991;324(23):1605–11.
6. Calkins H, Sousa J, el-Atassi R, et al. Diagnosis and cure of the Wolff-Parkinson-White syndrome or paroxysmal supraventricular tachycardias during a single electrophysiologic test. N Engl J Med 1991;324(23):1612–8.

7. Morady F, Strickberger A, Man KC, et al. Reasons for prolonged or failed attempts at radiofrequency catheter ablation of accessory pathways. J Am Coll Cardiol 1996;27(3):683–9.
8. Valderrábano M, Cesario DA, Ji S, et al. Percutaneous epicardial mapping during ablation of difficult accessory pathways as an alternative to cardiac surgery. Heart Rhythm 2004;1(3):311–6.
9. Lam C, Schweikert R, Kanagaratnam L, et al. Radiofrequency ablation of a right atrial appendage–ventricular accessory pathway by transcutaneous epicardial instrumentation. J Cardiovasc Electrophysiol 2000;11(10):1170–3.
10. Schweikert RA, Saliba WI, Tomassoni G, et al. Percutaneous pericardial instrumentation for endo-epicardial mapping of previously failed ablations. Circulation 2003;108(11):1329–35.

Supraventricular Tachycardia: Where to Ablate?

Colleen Johnson, MD, MS*, Melvin Scheinman, MD

KEYWORDS

- Atrioventricular nodal reentrant tachycardia
- Catheter ablation • Coronary sinus

A 60-year-old woman with diabetes, hypertension, and hypothyroidism experienced palpitations for 7 years. Her palpitations were acute in onset and associated with rapid rates. She was seen initially in an emergency room where she was found to have a narrow complex tachycardia with a heart rate of approximately 200 beats per minute. Intravenous adenosine and β-blockers had no effect. Direct current cardioversion was performed to terminate tachycardia.

She was subsequently able to terminate her palpitations with vagal maneuvers. She underwent an electrophysiology study during which no arrhythmias could be provoked, although there was evidence of dual atrioventricular (AV) nodal function. She was referred for repeat electrophysiology study with possible ablation.

ELECTROPHYSIOLOGY STUDY AND CATHETER ABLATION

The electrophysiology study began with placement of multipolar catheters in the high right atrium (HRA), His, coronary sinus (CS), and right ventricular apex. At baseline, the patient was in normal sinus rhythm at a cycle length of 800 milliseconds with normal atrial-His and His-ventricular intervals, 128 and 50 milliseconds, respectively. Overdrive pacing of the right ventricular apex at a cycle length of 450 milliseconds elicited an echo complex suggestive of dual AV nodal physiology. Decremental double extrastimuli delivered to the HRA revealed a jump in the atrial-His interval consistent with dual AV node physiology. Narrow complex tachycardia was first induced with double extrastimuli delivered to the HRA at 500 and 320 milliseconds. Retrograde atrial activation during tachycardia was earliest on the His channel; however, there was eccentric retrograde activation of the CS, with CS 5,6 being the earliest (**Fig. 1**). The timing from the surface V to septal A during tachycardia was approximately 30 milliseconds. Tachycardia terminated spontaneously with an atrial depolarization. Sustained tachycardia at a cycle length of 300 milliseconds was induced with a single extrastimulus delivered to the HRA at 250 milliseconds at a drive train of 450 milliseconds in the setting of isoproterenol infusion at 1.5 μg/min. Overdrive pacing from the right ventricular apex at a cycle length of 270 milliseconds led to entrainment of the tachycardia with acceleration of the atrial electrogram to the pacing cycle length and resumption of the original tachycardia cycle length with a V-A-V response on cessation of pacing (**Fig. 2**). The difference between V-A timing in tachycardia (30 milliseconds) and Stim-A timing in ventricular overdrive pacing (138 milliseconds) was 108 milliseconds. The difference between the postpacing interval (480 milliseconds) and the tachycardia cycle length (300 milliseconds) was 180 milliseconds. These findings argue against either an atrial tachycardia or an accessory pathway–mediated tachycardia. As such, the diagnosis of AV nodal reentrant tachycardia (AVNRT) was made.

An ablation of the slow AV nodal pathway was attempted using a combined anatomic and electrophysiologic approach. During sinus rhythm,

Division of Cardiology, Department of Cardiac Electrophysiology, University of California San Francisco, 500 Parnassus Avenue, MU 434, Box 1354, San Francisco, CA 94143, USA
* Corresponding author.
E-mail address: Colleen.J.Johnson@ucsfmedctr.org

Card Electrophysiol Clin 2 (2010) 217–220
doi:10.1016/j.ccep.2010.01.006

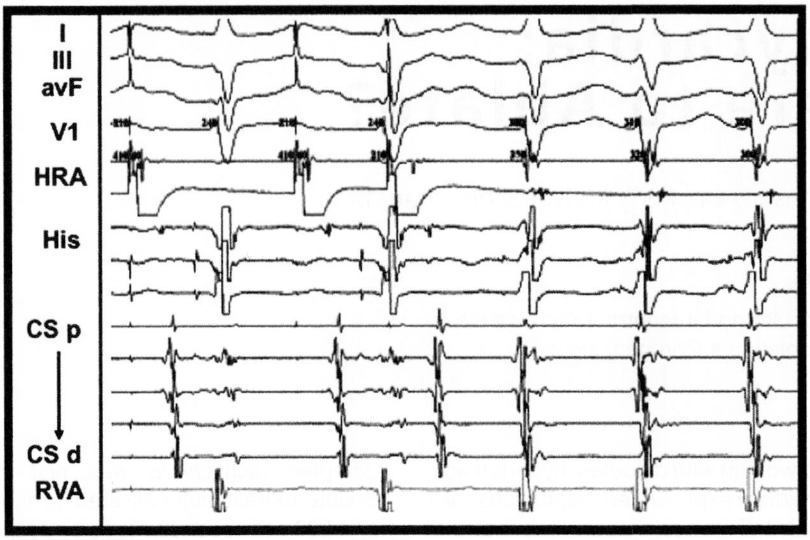

Fig. 1. Intracardiac recording showing initiation of tachycardia with atrial extrastimuli. The initiation is dependent on a critical interval. The tachycardia exhibits an eccentric atrial activation pattern in the coronary sinus.

a 4-mm ablation catheter was placed at a site anterior to the CS ostium and inferior to the His location (**Fig. 3**, blue points). The signal at this place had a small A and large V signal. Radiofrequency ablations were made in this location at a temperature of 50°C and power of 40 W. No junctional complexes occurred during radiofrequency ablation. The ablation catheter was then brought incrementally anterior and superior toward the His catheter (see **Fig. 3**, red points). Radiofrequency ablations were then made in this location at a temperature of 50°C and power of 40 W. Again, no junctional complexes occurred during ablation. After ablation at both sites, decremental double extrastimuli were delivered to the HRA. Tachycardia was reinitiated with double extrastimuli to the HRA at 500 and 200 milliseconds with the same characteristics discussed previously.

QUESTION: WHERE SHOULD ONE ATTEMPT TO ABLATE NOW?

It was hypothesized that this was AVNRT using left-sided AV nodal extensions. As such, the

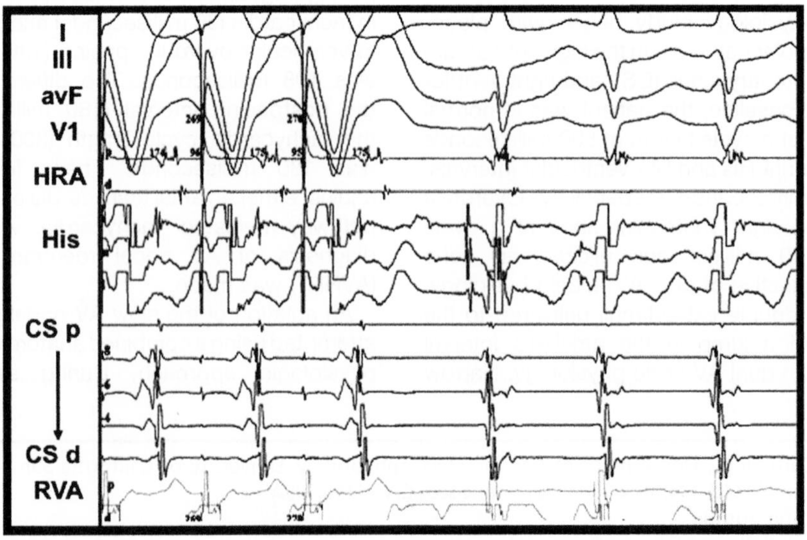

Fig. 2. Ventricular overdrive pacing during tachycardia displaying V-A-V response that rules out atrial tachycardia.

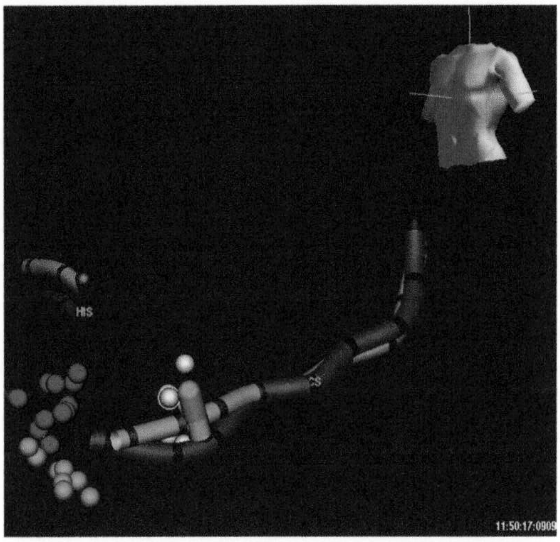

Fig. 3. Left anterior oblique view showing the location of His catheter (*yellow*) and CS catheter (*aqua*) using the Ensite NavX navigation system (St Jude Medical, Inc, St Paul, MN, USA). Ablation sites are shown as initial slow pathway modification (*blue points*), further anterior ablation (*red points*), and site of successful ablation within the CS (*white points*).

4-mm ablation catheter was moved into the proximal CS, 1 cm past the CS ostium (see **Fig. 3**, white points). During the first radiofrequency ablation applied with an average power of 20 W, there was a flurry of accelerated junctional beats. Postablation, however, tachycardia was again initiated. As such, two more radiofrequency ablations were made approximately 2 cm within the CS. Accelerated junctional beats were elicited with both ablations. After this, one could not initiate tachycardia with aggressive pacing nor elicit evidence of dual AV nodal physiology.

DISCUSSION

Typical AVNRT arises in the setting of functional dual AV nodes, most commonly using an antegrade slow and retrograde fast pathway. The slow pathway is believed to be located anatomically as a right posterior extension from the compact AV node within the triangle of Koch.[1] The fast pathway is usually found more anterior, closer to the His bundle. Catheter ablation of typical (antegrade slow, retrograde fast) AVNRT targets slow pathway ablation. Ablation of the slow pathway is based on the anatomic placement of a radiofrequency catheter in the right inferior septum between the tricuspid annulus and the ostium of the CS. Ablation begins posteriorly and proceeds anteriorly until either tachycardia cannot be initiated or concern relative to proximity of the ablation to the compact AV node. Ablation at this site has been found to successfully eradicate AVNRT in more than 90% of patients with typical AVNRT.[2]

The AV node in AVNRT, however, is a much more complex structure than represented by the anatomic dual AV node model and the region of the compact node. Inoue and Becker[3] performed autopsy studies on human hearts that showed the existence of left-sided posterior AV nodal extensions. Nam and colleagues[4] found eccentric activation with earliest activation 1 cm distal to the CS ostium in 6% of typical AVNRT cases. Katritsis and colleagues[5] performed detailed mapping of retrograde atrial activation in typical AVNRT showing that the earliest retrograde activation was on the left side of the septum in 53% of patients. Hwang and colleagues[6] showed that although 6% of patients with atypical AVNRT have eccentric retrograde atrial activation starting from various points in the CS, all were successfully treated with standard slow pathway modification. Similarly, Chen and colleagues[7] found 8% of patients with both typical and atypical AVNRT to have earliest retrograde activation in the CS; however, these were cured with traditional right-sided slow pathway modification ablation. Contrary to this, cases of typical AVNRT requiring catheter ablation on the left side of the septum after failure with traditional slow pathway modification have been reported.[8,9]

In the case detailed herein, the patient had earliest retrograde activation at the His channel recording consistent with most patients with typical AVNRT but also displayed evidence of left-sided AV nodal extensions with the eccentric retrograde activation seen in the CS. Regardless, traditional slow pathway modification did not result in eradication of tachycardia or evidence of dual nodal conduction. Rather, ablation 1 to 2 cm within the CS was required. This suggests the antegrade slow pathway had a critical component within the proximal CS, in close continuity with left-sided posterior nodal extensions, rather than at the apex of the triangle of Koch. Although there are reports of ablation within the CS necessary to terminate AVNRT[4] these are of atypical forms of AVNRT (slow-slow and fast-slow AVNRT).

REFERENCES

1. Lee PC, Chen SA, Hwang B. Atrioventricular node anatomy and physiology: implications for ablation of atrioventricular nodal reentrant tachycardia. Curr Opin Cardiol 2009;24(2):105–12.
2. Kwaku KF, Josephson ME. Typical AVNRT: an update on mechanisms and therapy. Card Electrophysiol Rev 2002;6(4):414–21.

3. Inoue S, Becker AE. Posterior extensions of the human compact atrioventricular node: a neglected anatomic feature of potential clinical significance. Circulation 1998;97(2):188–93.
4. Nam GB, Rhee KS, Kim J, et al. Left atrionodal connections in typical and atypical atrioventricular nodal reentrant tachycardias: activation sequence in the coronary sinus and results of radiofrequency catheter ablation. J Cardiovasc Electrophysiol 2006; 17(2):171–7.
5. Katritsis DG, Ellenbogen KA, Becker AE. Atrial activation during atrioventricular nodal reentrant tachycardia: studies on retrograde fast pathway conduction. Heart Rhythm 2006;3(9):993–1000.
6. Hwang C, Martin DJ, Goodman JS, et al. Atypical atrioventricular node reciprocating tachycardia masquerading as tachycardia using a left-sided accessory pathway. J Am Coll Cardiol 1997;30(1): 218–25.
7. Chen J, Anselme F, Smith TW, et al. Standard right atrial ablation is effective for atrioventricular nodal reentry with earliest activation in the coronary sinus. J Cardiovasc Electrophysiol 2004;15(1):2–7.
8. Altemose GT, Scott LR, Miller JM. Atrioventricular nodal reentrant tachycardia requiring ablation on the mitral annulus. J Cardiovasc Electrophysiol 2000; 11(11):1281–4.
9. Jais P, Haissaguerre M, Shah DC, et al. Successful radiofrequency ablation of a slow atrioventricular nodal pathway on the left posterior atrial septum. Pacing Clin Electrophysiol 1999;22(3): 525–7.

Rare Diagnosis of a Common Supraventricular Tachycardia

David S. Kwon, MD, PhD, Nitish Badhwar, MD*

KEYWORDS

• Nodoventricular • Nodofascicular • Mahaim
• Supraventricular tachycardia

The patient is a 54-year-old woman who has had intermittent palpitations over the preceding 15 years. These episodes have lasted for minutes to hours and have been accompanied by chest discomfort and shortness of breath, but without any history of syncope or presyncope. She presented for consultation because of a recent increase in the frequency of her episodes, occurring now at rest. One episode of supraventricular tachycardia (SVT) terminated when she placed a cold towel on her face. An electrocardiogram (ECG) was obtained revealing a narrow complex tachycardia at a rate of 170 beats per minute with a pseudo R' noted in V1. She had normal left ventricular function by two-dimensional ECG. A Holter monitor obtained in 2006 revealed only occasional premature atrial and ventricular contractions.

ELECTROPHYSIOLOGY STUDY

The patient was brought to the electrophysiology laboratory in sinus rhythm without evidence of pre-excitation on the surface electrocardiogram. Multipolar catheters were placed in standard positions: right ventricular apex (RVA), His bundle (His), high right atrium (HRA), and the coronary sinus (CS). Baseline atrio-His (AH) and His-ventricular (HV) intervals were 70 milliseconds and 35 milliseconds, respectively. Dual AV node physiology was observed with decremental atrial extrastimuli, and a concentric CS activation pattern was noted with pacing from the RVA catheter. An A on V tachycardia was induced easily with atrial overdrive pacing or with atrial extrastimuli that were dependent on a critical AH.

The septal V–A timing of the tachycardia was less than 70 milliseconds. Ventricular overdrive pacing (VOD) from the RVA entrained the tachycardia with a V-A-V response after cessation of pacing. Tachycardia was sustained and allowed for further diagnostic pacing maneuvers. Single ventricular beats were given during SVT at the time of His bundle refractoriness (V on His), and the timing of the subsequent atrial activation was advanced with reset of tachycardia (**Fig. 1**). Early premature ventricular complex (initiated from the CS branch vein) terminated tachycardia without activating the atrium. Single atrial beats (from the CS ostium) given late during SVT when the septal A was committed terminated the SVT. Differential RV pacing comparing the RV base with the RV apex revealed similar ventriculoatrial (VA) timing, suggesting the presence of a septal accessory pathway rather than retrograde AV nodal conduction. Parahisian pacing at high output that captured the His during SVT was able to capture the atrium within two beats (**Fig. 2**). Finally, HRA pacing during SVT dissociated the A from the tachycardia.

QUESTION: WHAT IS THE DIAGNOSIS?

An A on V supraventricular tachycardia with septal VA timing less than 70 milliseconds rules out

Section of Cardiac Electrophysiology, Division of Cardiology, University of California, 500 Parnassus Avenue, MU 434, San Francisco, CA 94143, USA
* Corresponding author.
E-mail address: badhwar@medicine.ucsf.edu

Card Electrophysiol Clin 2 (2010) 221–224
doi:10.1016/j.ccep.2010.01.007
1877-9182/10/$ – see front matter

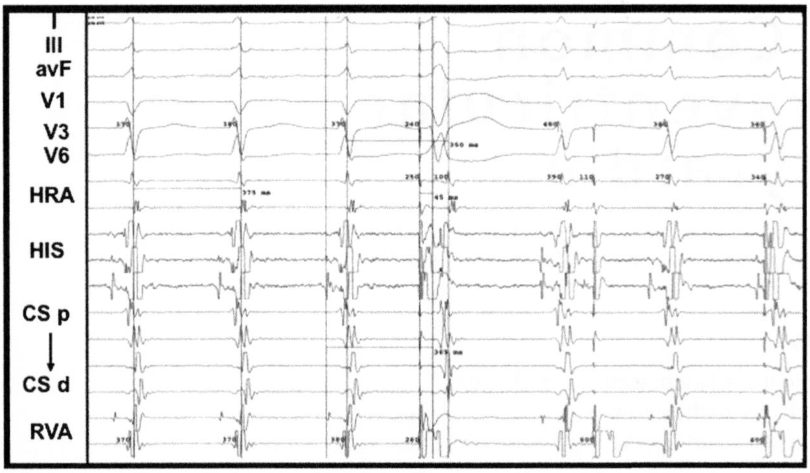

Fig. 1. Intracardiac electrograms during supraventricular tachycardia. Depicted are the surface leads (I, III, avF, V1, V3, V6), high right atrium intracardiac electrograms (HRA), His bundle electrograms (HIS), coronary sinus (CS) (d—distal poles; 7, 8—proximal poles), right ventricular apex catheter (RVA). A His-synchronous ventricular extrastimulus that advances the subsequent atrial electrogram is shown. The tachycardia cycle length is 375 milliseconds, and the HRA electrogram following the V on His is advanced by 25 milliseconds and resets tachycardia. The ventricular extrastimulus is given within 45 milliseconds of the expected His depolarization.

extranodal accessory pathway-mediated SVT. The differential diagnosis of an A on V SVT is focal junctional tachycardia (JT), atrial tachycardia, atrioventricular nodal re-entrant tachycardia (AVNRT), concealed nodofascicular (NF)/nodoventricular (NV) tachycardia, and intrahisian reentrant tachycardia. VOD during tachycardia showing a V-A-V response and PVC terminating tachycardia with VA block rules out atrial tachycardia. A late PAC that terminates tachycardia when the His A is committed argues against JT as the mechanism. Finally, a His synchronous PVC that pulls in the A and resets tachycardia argues against both AVNRT and JT as the mechanism of the SVT. This pacing maneuver during A on V tachycardia proves the participation of a concealed NF/NV accessory pathway as the retrograde limb.

Radiofrequency catheter ablation was conducted in the region of the slow AV nodal pathway to target the proximal insertion of the NF/NV pathway using a deflectable tip 4 mm EPT (Boston Scientific, Natick, Massachusetts) catheter along the medial tricuspid annulus approximately one third of the way between the CS ostium and the His bundle position (**Fig. 3**). Electroanatomical

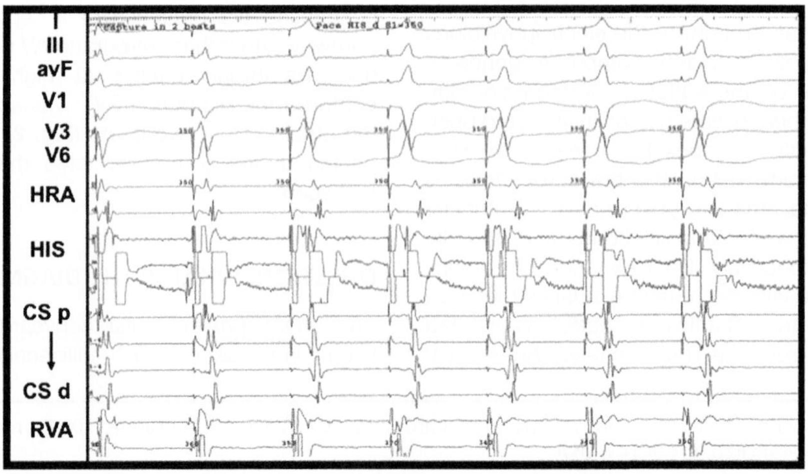

Fig. 2. Intracardiac electrograms are as described previously. His bundle overdrive pacing during tachycardia. Concealed entrainment of the tachycardia is achieved within two paced beats demonstrating that the His bundle is integral to the tachycardia circuit.

mapping with the Ensite NavX (St Jude Medical, St Paul, MN, USA) system was used to record catheter position. Three ablation lesions were delivered during sinus rhythm, with each resulting in junctional beats during ablation. Neither AV block, nor PR prolongation, was observed during radiofrequency ablation. Following a 30-minute waiting period, only rare beats consistent with activation of the slow pathway were observed at baseline and with isoproterenol at 0.5 μg/min. SVT was no longer inducible. The patient has been symptom-free off medications for 10 months.

DISCUSSION

The first description of alternate pathways existing between the AV node and ventricular myocardium, nodoventricular accessory pathways, is attributed to Mahaim and colleagues in the 1930s.[1,2] These and other variants such as nodofascicular pathways are quite rare, and diagnosis of these accessory pathways can be elusive. Furthermore, evaluation of the 12-lead ECG may be equally unrevealing, as minimal pre-excitation may be evident, or there may be retrograde-only conduction in most of these pathways. In this case presentation, a seemingly typical A on V tachycardia was observed, which may have been easily and mistakenly determined to be AVNRT. Closer examination was required to arrive at the correct diagnosis.

A key maneuver performed in this case was a His-synchronous ventricular extrastimulus that was able to advance the ensuing atrial depolarization. This result indicated the presence of an NF or NV pathway and excluded AVNRT, JT, and intrahisian re-entrant tachycardia from the differential diagnosis. As entrainment of supraventricular tachycardias is a standard diagnostic tool for the differentiation of SVT,[3,4] it is possible that with the added maneuver of providing a V on His during tachycardia, the diagnostic accuracy of such A on V tachycardias may increase.

Entrainment mapping of a concealed NV accessory pathway has been described elegantly by Quinn and colleagues[5] with detailed mapping of the circuit. In this case study, His bundle overdrive pacing was used to further define the critical elements of the circuit, as early entry into the circuit with pacing (<two paced beats) demonstrates that the His and the fascicle or ventricle are part of the tachycardia circuit. In the authors' experience, it takes more than two His captured beats to capture the atrium during AVNRT, because the His and ventricle are not integral parts of the circuit.[6] This manner of overdrive pacing may be especially useful if differential RV pacing or parahisian pacing maneuvers are unable to provide clear diagnostic results.

Ablation of these NV fibers previously was described by Grogin and colleagues.[7] These investigators determined the proximal insertion of Mahaim fibers is either from the slow atrioventricular nodal pathway or from the distal final common pathway. Similarly, the patient described here exhibited dual AV nodal physiology, and, indeed, ablation in the slow pathway region was able to successfully eliminate tachycardia and render the patient noninducible.

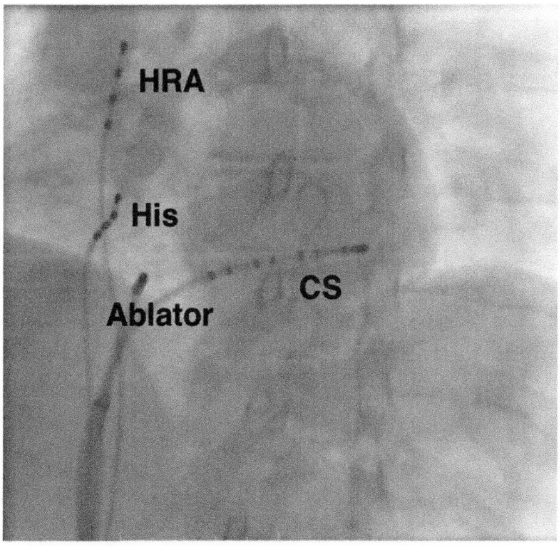

Fig. 3. Catheter positions are described by fluoroscopy. The high right atrium (HRA), His bundle, coronary sinus (CS), and ablation catheter are depicted in the left anterior oblique orientation.

SUMMARY

This case describes diagnostic maneuvers that will lead to an accurate diagnosis of a given A on V supraventricular tachycardia. The list of maneuvers described is not exhaustive but includes techniques to help diagnose a concealed NV/NF pathway mediation tachycardia that is in the differential diagnosis of a failed AVNRT ablation. The practicing electrophysiologist must be prepared to perform these maneuvers in order to ensure the safest and most focused ablation procedures.

REFERENCES

1. Mahaim I, Benatt A. Nouvelles recherches sur les connexions superieures de la branche gauche du faisceau de His-Tawara avec cloison interventriculaire. Cardiologia 1938;1:61–76.

2. Mahaim I, Winston MR. Recherches d'lanatomic comparee et du pathologic experimentale sur les connexions hautes du faisceau de His-Tawara. Cardiologia 1941;5:189–260.
3. Michaud GF, Tada H, Chough S, et al. Differentiation of atypical atrioventricular node re-entrant tachycardia from orthodromic reciprocating tachycardia using a septal accessory pathway by the response to ventricular pacing. J Am Coll Cardiol 2001;38:1163–7.
4. Knight BP, Ebinger M, Oral H, et al. Diagnostic value of tachycardia features and pacing maneuvers during paroxysmal supraventricular tachycardia. J Am Coll Cardiol 2000;36:574–82.
5. Quinn FR, Mitchell LB, Mardell AP, et al. Entrainment mapping of a concealed nodoventricular accessory pathway in a man with complete heart block and tachycardia-induced cardiomyopathy. J Cardiovasc Electrophysiol 2008;19:90–4.
6. Viswanathan MN, Badhwar N, Lee BK, et al. His bundle pacing and entrainment: a single pacing maneuver to differentiate mechanisms of supraventricular tachycardias [abstract]. Heart Rhythm 2007;4(5):S77.
7. Grogin HR, Lee RJ, Kwasman M, et al. Radiofrequency catheter ablation of atriofascicular and nodoventricular Mahaim tracts. Circulation 1994;90:272–81.

Persistent Long R–P Tachycardia

Zian H. Tseng, MD, MAS*, Melvin Scheinman, MD

KEYWORDS

- Permanent junctional reciprocating tachycardia
- Catheter ablation • Coronary sinus

The patient is a 28-year-old man who had an 11-year history of palpitations associated with dyspnea and dizziness. The episodes lasted from minutes to several hours and occurred up to several times a day. Numerous medications, including beta-blockers, calcium channel blockers, and digoxin were ineffective at arrhythmia control. Holter monitoring demonstrated incessant episodes of supraventricular tachycardia (SVT). He then underwent the first of three unsuccessful catheter ablation procedures in June 2000. A long R–P tachycardia with decremental retrograde conduction consistent with permanent junctional reciprocating tachycardia (PJRT) was diagnosed. The shortest ventriculoatrial (VA) interval during tachycardia was mapped to inside the coronary sinus (CS) where ablation was performed. The patient was symptom-free for 10 months and then had a recurrence of palpitations. Two subsequent ablative procedures were performed in 2002 and 2003. They targeted the shortest VA interval during tachycardia with applications of radiofrequency (RF) energy in the right and left posteroseptal regions (via retrograde aortic approach) and again within the CS. These initially were successful, but the arrhythmia recurred the following day. Multiple combination antiarrhythmic drug therapy was ineffective, and the patient then was referred to the authors' institution for a repeat attempt at catheter ablation.

ELECTROPHYSIOLOGY STUDY

Antiarrhythmic agents were discontinued for at least five half-lives, and written informed consent was obtained. The patient underwent electrophysiology study with catheters inserted into the right atrium, His bundle region, CS, and right ventricle. SVT occurred spontaneously and was also easily inducible with multiple maneuvers, including atrial or ventricular overdrive pacing, or with atrial or ventricular extrastimuli. SVT could be initiated without a critical increase in the atrial-His interval. Surface ECG showed a long R–P tachycardia with negative P waves in leads II, III, aVF, and V2 through V6.

Intracardiac recordings during SVT showed earliest retrograde atrial activation in the proximal CS. In addition, during tachycardia a sharp, high-frequency potential (accessory pathway [AP]) was recorded from the proximal CS bipole (CS os) (**Fig. 1**B), which was not present during sinus rhythm (**Fig. 1**A). The AP was recorded 221 milliseconds after the QRS and preceded the succeeding P wave by 61 milliseconds. Mapping of the potential during tachycardia showed that it had maximal amplitude at the os of the CS with progressive decrease in amplitude as the mapping catheter was moved to within the CS. A premature ventricular stimulus during SVT delivered while the His bundle was refractory captured the atrium while maintaining the same sequence of atrial activation. An earlier premature ventricular stimulus terminated tachycardia without conduction to the atrium. The response to ventricular extrastimuli confirmed that the decremental conducting properties of the AP occurred at the ventricle–AP interface (**Fig. 2**A). These observations suggest that the SVT mechanism was indeed atrioventricular re-entry with the retrograde limb consisting of

Section of Cardiac Electrophysiology, Division of Cardiology, Department of Medicine, University of California, San Francisco School of Medicine, 500 Parnassus Avenue, Room MU E-434, Box 1354, San Francisco, CA 94143-1354, USA

* Corresponding author.

E-mail address: zhtseng@medicine.ucsf.edu

Card Electrophysiol Clin 2 (2010) 225–229
doi:10.1016/j.ccep.2010.01.008
1877-9182/10/$ – see front matter

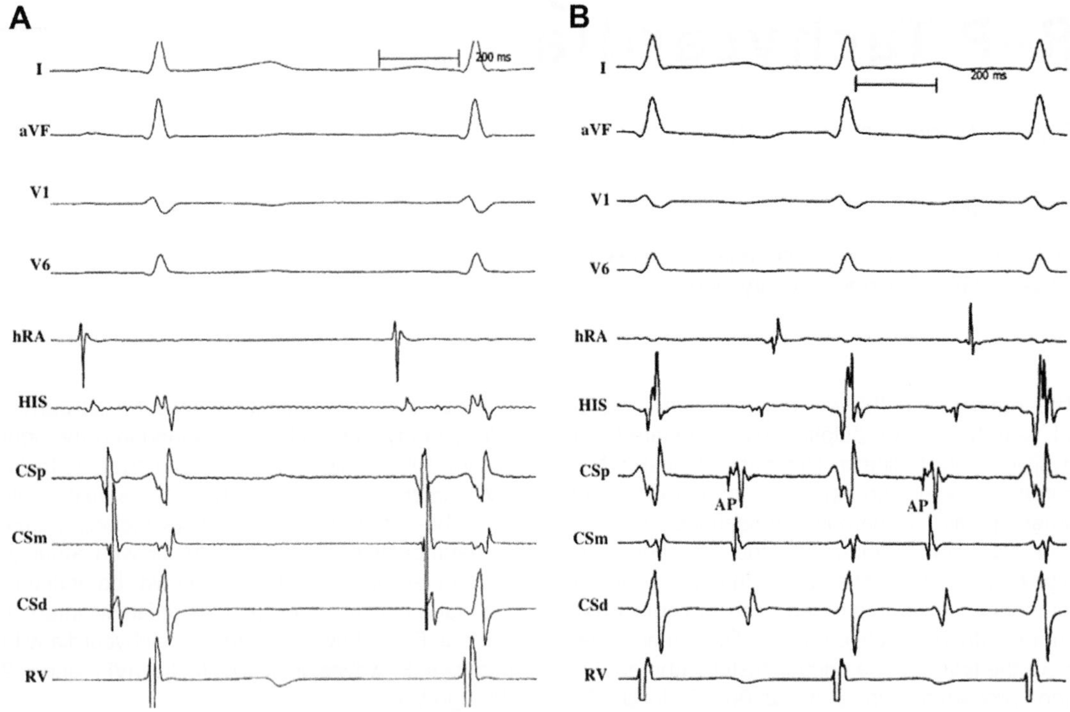

Fig. 1. (*A*) Simultaneous surface and intracardiac recordings from the high right atrium, His bundle region, proximal, middle, and distal CS are shown during sinus rhythm. (*B*) Intracardiac recordings during tachycardia. Note the recording of a distinct accessory pathway potential (AP) in the proximal CS channel that was not present during sinus rhythm. AP was recorded 221 milliseconds after the QRS and preceded the succeeding P wave by 61 milliseconds. *Abbreviations:* CSd, distal coronary sinus channel; CSm, midcoronary sinus channel; CSp, proximal coronary sinus channel; HRA, high right atrial channel; HIS, His bundle channel; I, aVF, V1, and V6 = corresponding surface electrocardiogram leads; RV, right ventricular apex channel.

a decremental conducting AP located in the proximal CS.

QUESTION: WHAT SHOULD BE THE ABLATION STRATEGY GIVEN THE PREVIOUS HISTORY OF RECURRENT SVT AFTER SUCCESSFUL ABLATION?

Catheter Ablation

Mapping of the posterior septum and right atrium during SVT confirmed that the shortest VA interval was located in the proximal CS approximately 1 cm within the os, while the AP potential was recorded maximally at the os. Delivery of radiofrequency energy at the site of earliest atrial activation (1 cm into the CS) initially resulted in an increase in AP–atrial interval and then termination of tachycardia at the AP–atrium interface (**Fig. 2**B). The AP potential persisted, even during sinus rhythm (see **Fig. 2**B), consistent with activation of the AP with block to the atrium. Tachycardia was not possible, because the AP–atrial connection was ablated. Ventricular overdrive pacing after SVT termination demonstrated VA dissociation but persistent ventricle–AP conduction (**Fig. 3**A). The AP potential itself was then targeted for ablation. and the ablation catheter placed just inside the CS os where the maximum AP potential was recorded. During the first several seconds of application of radiofrequency energy, the potential gradually decreased in amplitude and then disappeared (see **Fig. 3**B). After ablation, ventricular pacing again demonstrated VA dissociation without AP potential, and there were no acute or late complications. The patient remains free from tachycardia over a 3-year follow-up.

Discussion

Prior studies have demonstrated that the mechanism of PJRT incorporates a retrograde decremental conducting accessory pathway,[1–7] which is also capable of decremental antegrade conduction following AV junction ablation.[8,9]

The most definitive anatomic study was reported by Critelli and colleagues,[8] who showed the presence of a Kent-bundle type accessory AV connection and proposed that its decremental conduction properties were caused by the tortuous, serpiginous route of fibers connecting

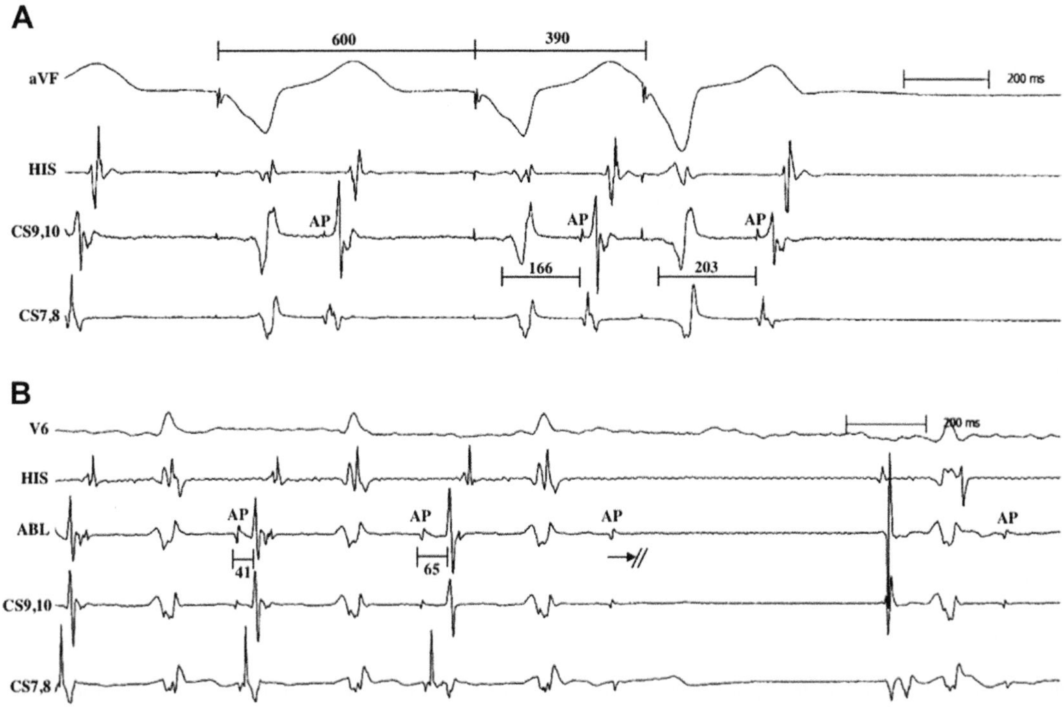

Fig. 2. (*A*) Programmed ventricular pacing demonstrates decrementally conducting properties of the AP occurring at the ventricle–AP interface. A ventricular extrastimulus inserted 390 milliseconds after the last drive train at 600 milliseconds shows prolongation of the V–AP interval from 166 milliseconds to 203 milliseconds. (*B*) Delivery of radiofrequency energy at the site of earliest atrial activation (1 cm into the CS) initially results in an increase in AP–atrial interval and then termination of tachycardia at the AP–atrial interface. During sinus rhythm following tachycardia termination, the AP potential persisted, consistent with activation of the AP with block to the atrium. Intervals in milliseconds. *Abbreviations:* ABL, recording from ablation catheter placed 1 cm inside coronary sinus; aVF, surface electrocardiogram lead; CS7,8, coronary sinus recording from 1 cm inside coronary sinus; CS9,10, coronary sinus recording from near os; HIS, His bundle channel.

the atrium and ventricle across the CS os. They cited the experimental studies by Spach,[10] showing the influence of the geometric features of fibers on the propagation of depolarization to explain the decremental properties of the AP.

In previous studies,[6,7] possible accessory pathway potentials were recorded in over 50% of cases. The recording of an independent AP potential suggests that conduction occurs through a discrete fiber crossing the AV annulus. A recent report by Scaglione and colleagues[11] describes an accessory pathway potential recording in a case of PJRT with decremental conduction demonstrated at the AP–atrial interface. In that and prior studies, however, no definitive validation was made to prove that the AP potential recording was independent of either the atrium or ventricle.

In the present case, a distinct AP potential was recorded within the CS during tachycardia just before atrial activation. The authors further demonstrated that the decremental conduction properties occurred over the V–AP segment. During ablation, the AP–atrium interface first was severed, terminating tachycardia and resulting in VA dissociation. During VA dissociation, the AP potential was linked to the ventricle, confirming that the AP potential was independent of the atrium. The AP–atrial ablation site was 1 cm lateral to the site of maximal AP potential recording. A subsequent RF application resulted in successful ablation of the AP potential; hence this potential was dependent on but not part of ventricular activation.

The authors' observations suggest that the AP potential represents recordings from the AP as it crosses the CS. A more complex relationship between the AP and CS also can be envisioned in which the ventricular segment of the AP attaches to CS musculature at the os while the AP–atrial connection results from CS muscle insertion more distal in the CS, a configuration consistent with that described by Sun and colleagues.[12] A CS muscle to atrial connection, however, is unlikely, however, because after

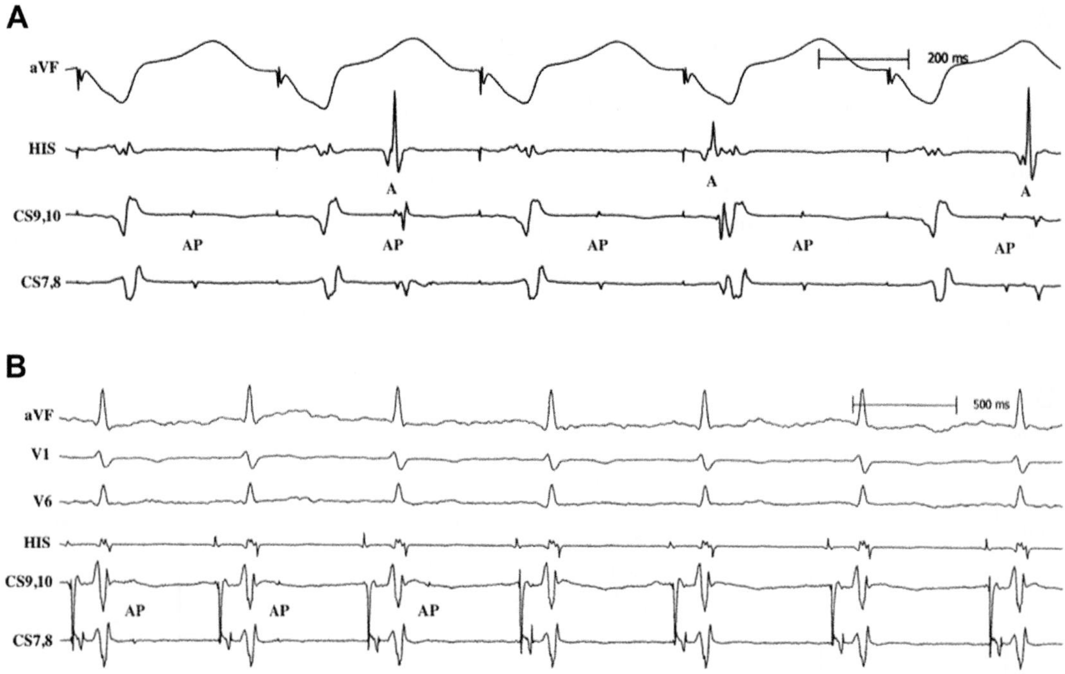

Fig. 3. (*A*) Ventricular overdrive pacing following successful ablation and tachycardia termination demonstrates VA dissociation but persistent ventricle–AP connection. (*B*) Delivery of radiofrequency energy during sinus rhythm targeting the site of maximal AP potential near the CS os demonstrates the gradual decrease in amplitude and then disappearance of AP. *Abbreviations:* aVF, V1, and V6, corresponding surface electrocardiogram leads; CS7,8, coronary sinus recording from 1 cm inside coronary sinus; CS9,10, coronary sinus recording from near os; HIS, His bundle channel.

ablation, the authors found complete VA dissociation that would have required complete disruption of the extensive network of CS muscle to atrial connections.[13,14]

More likely is the possibility that the AP potential recording represents true AP activation with an oblique course from medial to lateral over the CS. Because repeated prior attempts at ablation were directed at the site of earliest atrial activation during tachycardia, successful durable ablation in this case of recalcitrant PJRT may have been dependent upon targeting the AP potential for ablation.

REFERENCES

1. Gallavardin L, Veil P. Tachycardies auriculaires en slaves [Auricular tachycardias]. Arch Mal Coeur 1927;20:1 [in French].
2. Coumel P, Cabrol C, Fabiato A, et al. Tachycardie permamente par rythme reciproque. I—Prevues du diagnosstic parstimulation auriculaire et ventriculaire [Reciprocal permanent tachycardia: diagnosis by auricular and ventricular programmed stimulation]. Arch Mal Coeur 1967;60:1830–64 [in French].
3. Gallagher JJ, Sealy WC. The permanent form of junctional reciprocating tachycardia: further elucidation of the underlying mechanism. Eur J Cardiol 1978;8:413–30.
4. Critelli G, Gallagher JJ, Thiene G, et al. The permanent form of junctional reciprocating tachycardia. In: Benditt D, Benson D, editors. Cardiac pre-excitation syndromes. Boston: Martinus Nijhoff; 1986. p. 233–53.
5. Chien WW, Cohen TJ, Lee MA, et al. Electrophysiological findings and long-term follow-up of patients with the permanent form of junctional reciprocating tachycardia treated by catheter ablation. Circulation 1992; 85(4):1329–36.
6. Ticho BS, Saul JP, Hulse JE, et al. Variable location of accessory pathways associated with the permanent form of junctional reciprocating tachycardia and confirmation with radiofrequency ablation. Am J Cardiol 1992;70(20):1559–64.
7. Gaita F, Haissaguerre M, Giustetto C, et al. Catheter ablation of permanent junctional reciprocating tachycardia with radiofrequency current. J Am Coll Cardiol 1995;25(3):648–54.
8. Critelli G, Gallagher JJ, Monda V, et al. Anatomic and electrophysiologic substrate of the permanent form of junctional reciprocating tachycardia. J Am Coll Cardiol 1984;4(3):601–10.

9. Critelli G, Gallagher JJ, Thiene G, et al. Electrophysiologic and histopathologic correlations in a case of permanent form of reciprocating tachycardia. Eur Heart J 1985;6(2):130–7.
10. Spach M. The electrical representation of cardiac muscle based on discontinuities of atrial resistivity at a microscopic and macroscopic level. A basis for saltatory propagation in cardiac muscle. In: de Carvalho A, Hoffmann B, Liebermann M, editors. Normal and abnormal conduction in the heart. Biophysics, physiology, pharmacology, and ultrastructure. Mount Kisko (NY): Futura; 1982. p. 145–53.
11. Scaglione M, Caponi D, Riccardi R, et al. Accessory pathway potential recording in a case of permanent junctional reciprocating tachycardia with decremental conduction localized on the atrial site. Ital Heart J 2001;2(2):147–51.
12. Sun Y, Arruda M, Otomo K, et al. Coronary sinus–ventricular accessory connections producing posteroseptal and left posterior accessory pathways: incidence and electrophysiological identification. Circulation 2002;106(11):1362–7.
13. von Ludinghausen M, Ohmachi N, Boot C. Myocardial coverage of the coronary sinus and related veins. Clin Anat 1992;5:1–15.
14. Chauvin M, Shah DC, Haissaguerre M, et al. The anatomic basis of connections between the coronary sinus musculature and the left atrium in humans. Circulation 2000;101(6):647–52.

Supraventricular Tachycardia in a Patient with Repaired Congenital Heart Disease

Ronn E. Tanel, MD[a,b,*]

KEYWORDS

• Atrial tachycardia • Congenital heart disease
• Mustard procedure

The patient is a 16-year-old boy who had a Mustard operation for transposition of the great arteries with an intact ventricular septum. In transposition of the great arteries, the intracardiac anatomy is usually normal. The aorta, however, arises from the right ventricle, and the pulmonary artery arises from the left ventricle. The patient was cyanotic as a newborn because of the parallel pulmonary and systemic circulations, with minimal mixing though a patent ductus arteriosus and at an atrial level communication. The Mustard operation is an atrial switch operation in which systemic venous return is redirected to the mitral valve so that the left ventricle can eject deoxygenated blood to the pulmonary artery. The pulmonary venous return is redirected to the tricuspid valve so that the right ventricle can eject oxygenated blood to the aorta.

The patient was doing well in his usual state of health and presented for evaluation when he noticed palpitations and fatigue for several days. He was unsure of exactly when the palpitations began, and reported that the sensation of a racing heart beat was intermittent. He denied chest pain, shortness of breath, dizziness, or syncope. He previously had been well and denied intercurrent illness. He had a pacemaker implanted previously for a history of sinus node dysfunction. He was not taking any medications and denied alcohol or illicit drug use. **Fig. 1** shows the electrocardiogram (ECG) on presentation.

QUESTION: WHAT IS THE DIAGNOSIS OF THE SUPRAVENTRICULAR ARRHYTHMIA?

Fig. 1 shows a narrow QRS complex rhythm without consistent P waves. There are some beats that appear to possibly have a P wave preceding the QRS complex, but these are inconsistent. The ventricular rate is approximately 85 beats per minute, which is faster than the patient's stated usual rate of around 50 beats per minute. The recording otherwise shows right axis deviation and right ventricular hypertrophy, which are typical findings in patients who have had a Mustard operation and, as a result, have a systemic right ventricle. It is possible that this recording represents a junctional rhythm with occasional sinus capture beats, but it would be more typical for

[a] Division of Pediatric Cardiology, Department of Pediatrics, University of California San Francisco School of Medicine, 521 Parnassus Avenue, Box 0632, San Francisco, CA 94143, USA
[b] Pediatric Arrhythmia Center, Division of Pediatric Cardiology, UCSF Children's Hospital, 505 Parnassus Avenue, San Francisco, CA 94143, USA
* Division of Pediatric Cardiology, Department of Pediatrics, University of California San Francisco School of Medicine, 521 Parnassus Avenue, Box 0632, San Francisco, CA 94143.
E-mail address: ronn.tanel@ucsf.edu

Card Electrophysiol Clin 2 (2010) 231–234
doi:10.1016/j.ccep.2010.01.009
1877-9182/10/$ – see front matter

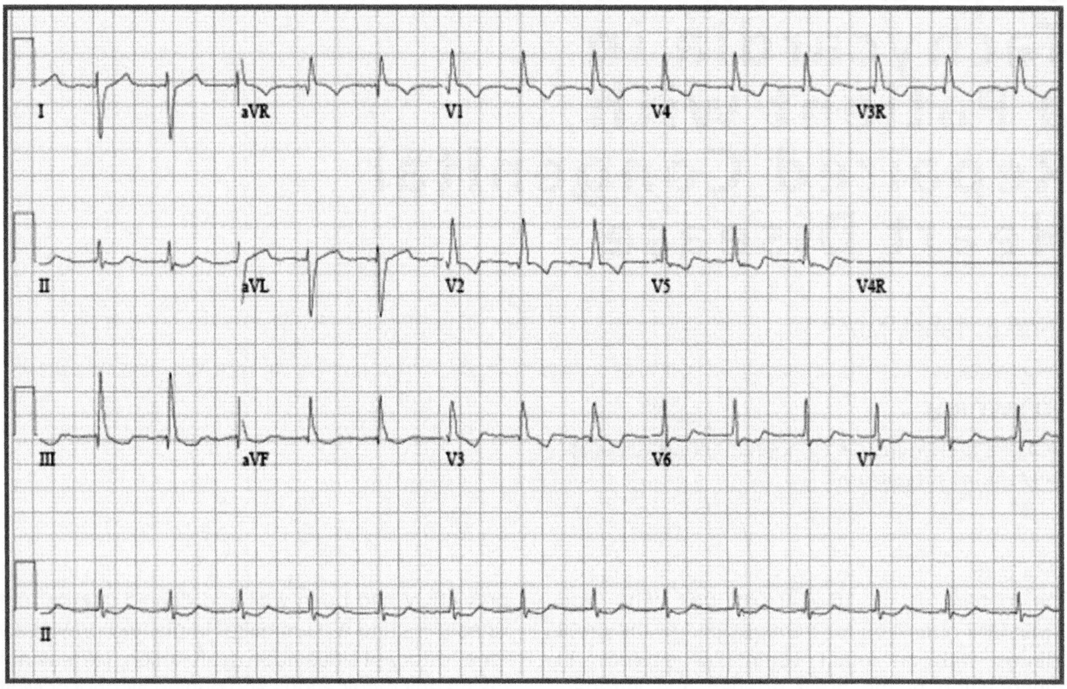

Fig. 1. 12-lead electrocardiogram on presentation showing a ventricular rate of 85 beats per minute. It is difficult to identify distinct P waves. There is right ventricular hypertrophy with right axis deviation that is characteristic of patients after Mustard procedure.

junctional rhythm in a postoperative patient to be slow as a result of sinus node dysfunction.

Despite the fact that there is no clear, consistent atrial activity, it is important to consider an atrial tachycardia in any patient with repaired congenital heart disease who has a heart rate faster than his or her usual baseline rate. Atrial arrhythmias may be very difficult to detect in patients with repaired congenital heart disease for various reasons. For example, in those with a large, dilated atrium, the atrial cycle length may be very slow so that P waves may not be observed easily between QRS complexes. In addition, the P waves during an atrial tachycardia may have very different morphologies than those seen in patients with a structurally normal heart. For example, it is uncommon for patients with repaired congenital heart disease to have typical flutter waves during intra-atrial re-entrant tachycardia. Finally, young patients with repaired congenital heart disease frequently have intact atrioventricular node conduction, so that a rapid ventricular response may preclude the ability to see P waves, especially when the conducted QRS complex is wide.

In order to recognize P waves during a suspected atrial tachycardia in a patient with repaired congenital heart disease, it may be beneficial to analyze the rhythm during spontaneous or induced atrioventricular block. Sometimes spontaneous atrioventricular block occurs during initial examination of the patient. If this does not occur, admitting the patient for continuous telemetry or outpatient evaluation with a Holter monitor could be helpful. Methods by which atrioventricular block can be induced include vagal maneuvers performed by the patient and the administration of adenosine during the atrial tachycardia.

Fig. 2 shows recordings from a 24-hour Holter monitor in this patient. The beginning of the top strip shows an atrial rhythm with a ventricular rate of 83 beats per minute and a slightly prolonged PR interval, which is not unusual for a patient with a history of extensive atrial surgery. The recordings occur while the patient is asleep. Midway through the top recording strip, the patient has atrioventricular block, resulting in a slower ventricular response. As a result, his pacemaker is activated, and he begins to pace the ventricle. This change to a slower ventricular response with ventricular pacing allows for the underlying atrial rhythm to be analyzed more easily. In this case, there is an atrial tachycardia at a cycle length of approximately 240 milliseconds that was not apparent during the faster ventricular response.

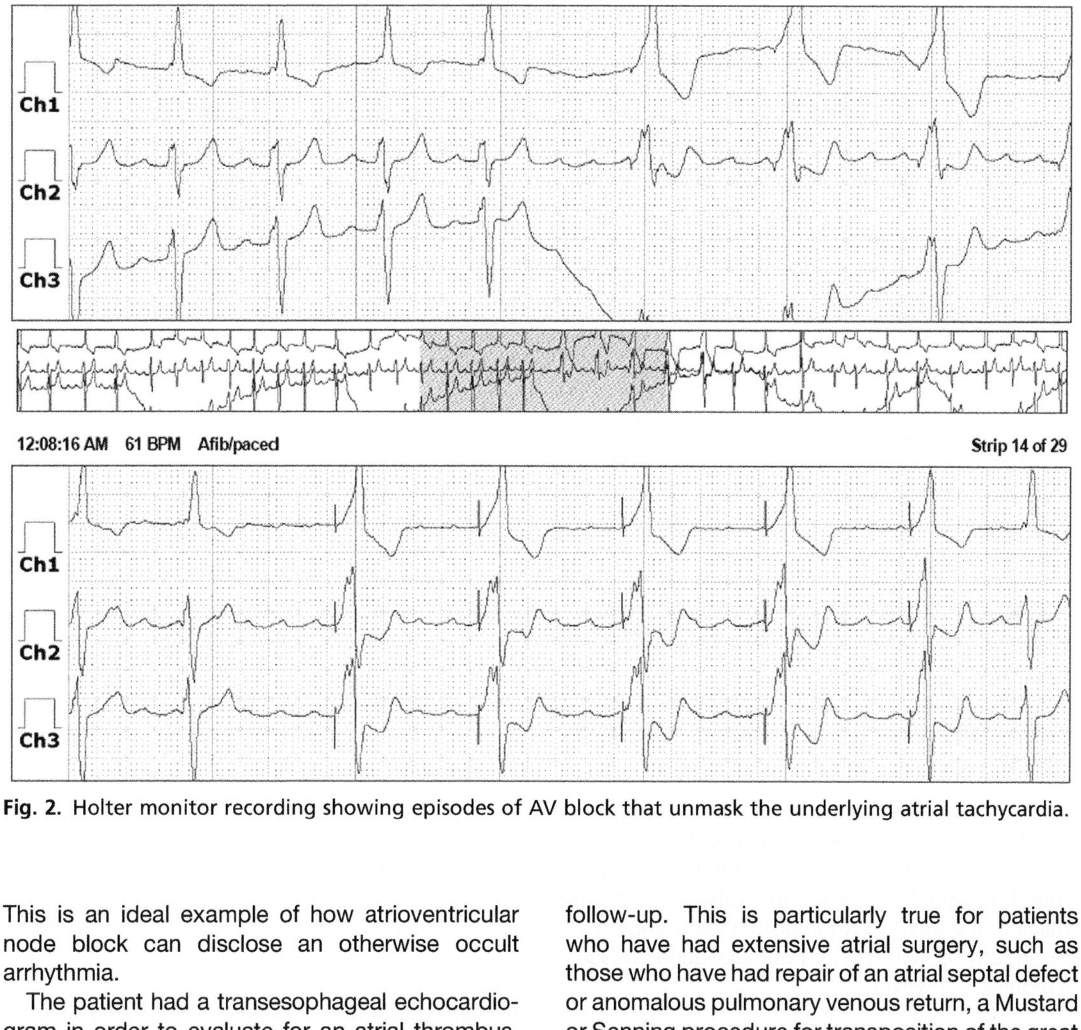

Fig. 2. Holter monitor recording showing episodes of AV block that unmask the underlying atrial tachycardia.

This is an ideal example of how atrioventricular node block can disclose an otherwise occult arrhythmia.

The patient had a transesophageal echocardiogram in order to evaluate for an atrial thrombus, because his symptoms were present for several days. When the echocardiogram showed no sign of thrombus, cardioversion was performed with overdrive atrial pacing through the atrial pacing lead. This resulted in sinus bradycardia at a rate of 57 beats per minute. Although the ventricular rate of the tachycardia was not very fast, it is important to note that it was significantly faster than the rate of his baseline sinus bradycardia. **Fig. 3** shows the resultant rhythm with first-degree atrioventricular block, right axis deviation, left atrial enlargement, right ventricular hypertrophy, and poor R wave progression across the precordial leads. These are all common electrocardiographic findings in a patient who has had a prior Mustard procedure.

DISCUSSION

Patients who have had surgery for congenital heart disease are at increased risk for the development of supraventricular arrhythmias during long-term follow-up. This is particularly true for patients who have had extensive atrial surgery, such as those who have had repair of an atrial septal defect or anomalous pulmonary venous return, a Mustard or Senning procedure for transposition of the great arteries,[1,2] or a Fontan procedure for single ventricle physiology.[3,4] Patients may develop bradyarrhythmias, tachyarrhythmias, or both.

Based on the clinical history, electrocardiogram appearance, and response to atrial overdrive pacing, the diagnosis made was an intra-atrial re-entrant tachycardia, or incisional flutter. Intra-atrial re-entrant tachycardia is a common long-term follow-up problem in patients who have had a Mustard operation. The arrhythmia can result in minor symptoms as in this patient or in more worrisome symptoms, such as syncope, if the atrial tachycardia is rapid and is associated with a rapid ventricular response (1:1 atrioventricular conduction). Patients who have had a Mustard procedure may be at particular risk if their systemic right ventricle has depressed systolic function.[5,6] The flutter waves in these patients are sometimes atypical, representing alternative flutter circuits than the usual isthmus-dependent counterclockwise circuit observed in patients without congenital

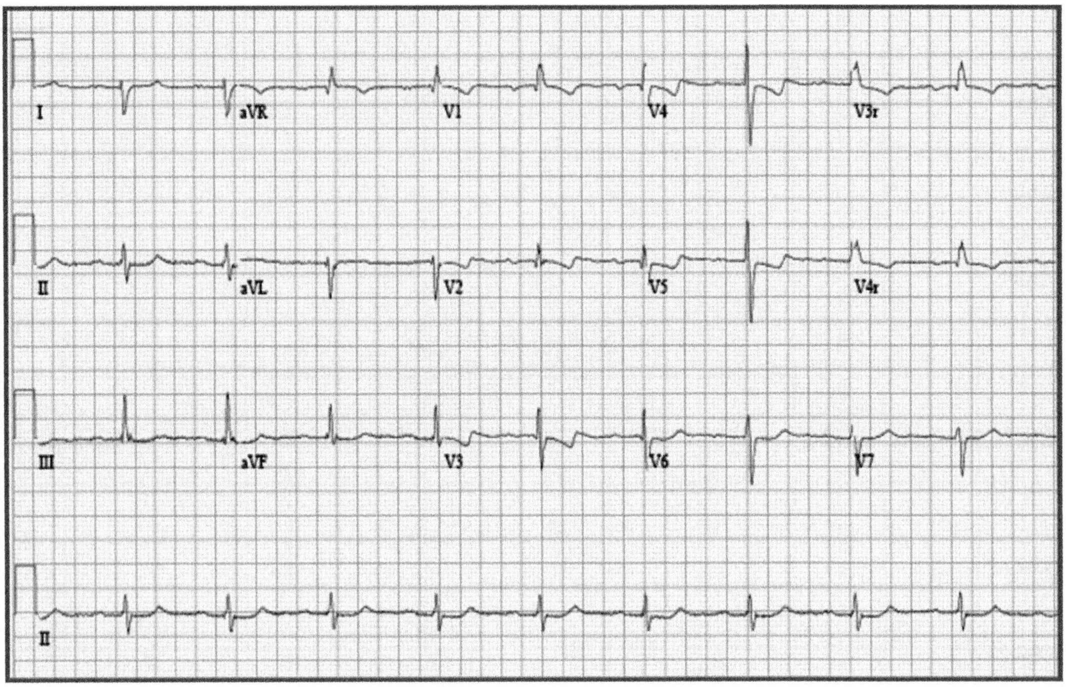

Fig. 3. 12-lead ECG after conversion to sinus rhythm showing a slower sinus rate with prolonged PR interval and similar QRS morphology as in tachycardia (see **Fig. 1**).

heart disease. Intra-atrial reentrant tachycardia may be treated with medications, but it is usually a rather refractory arrhythmia. Patients with postoperative atrial flutter are candidates for catheter ablation therapy.[7] A thorough understanding of the underlying anatomy and vascular access issues is required, however.

REFERENCES

1. Puley G, Connelly M, Harrison D, et al. Arrhythmia and survival in patients >18 years of age after the Mustard procedure for complete transposition of the great arteries. Am J Cardiol 1999;83(7):1080–4.
2. Gelatt M, Hamilton RM, McCrindle BW, et al. Arrhythmia and mortality after the Mustard procedure: a 30-year single-center experience. J Am Coll Cardiol 1997;29(1):194–201.
3. Fishberger SB, Wernovsky G, Gentles TL, et al. Factors that influence the development of atrial flutter after the Fontan operation. J Thorac Cardiovasc Surg 1997;113:80–6.
4. Driscoll DJ, Offord KP, Feldt RH, et al. Five- to fifteen-year follow-up after Fontan operation. Circulation 1992;85:469–96.
5. Kammeraad JA, van Deurzen CH, Sreeram N, et al. Predictors of sudden cardiac death after Mustard or Senning repair for transposition of the great arteries. J Am Coll Cardiol 2004;44:1095–102.
6. Kanter RJ, Garson A Jr. Atrial arrhythmias during chronic follow-up of surgery for complex congenital heart disease. Pacing Clin Electrophysiol 1997;20:502–11.
7. Triedman JK, Saul JP, Weindling SN, et al. Radiofrequency ablation of intra-atrial re-entrant tachycardia after surgical palliation of congenital heart disease. Circulation 1995;91:707–14.

Supraventricular Tachycardia and Atrioventricular Block

Duy Thai Nguyen, MD, Nitish Badhwar, MD*

KEYWORDS

- Catheter ablation
- Supraventricular tachycardia
- Atrioventricular block

An 85-year-old woman with hypertension presented with palpitations and presyncope for several years. A Holter by her referring cardiologist showed frequent atrial premature beats and bursts of nonsustained supraventricular tachycardia (SVT). Attempts with medical therapy to control her palpitations had resulted in bradycardia. She was, therefore, referred to the authors' center for electrophysiology study and possible ablation.

ELECTROPHYSIOLOGY STUDY

At electrophysiology study, multipolar catheters were placed in the right atrium, His-bundle region, right ventricle, and coronary sinus (CS). At baseline, the patient was in normal sinus rhythm with normal atrial-His and His-ventricular intervals. Multiple episodes of a mid- to long-RP SVT occurred spontaneously (**Fig. 1**). The differential diagnosis included atrial tachycardia (AT), atypical atrioventricular nodal reentrant tachycardia (AVNRT), and atrioventricular reentrant tachycardia (AVRT) utilizing a slowly conducting concealed accessory pathway and concealed nodoventricular tachycardia (NVT). On further review of **Fig. 1**, the tachycardia initiated with an atrial premature beat, followed by two beats of atrioventricular (AV) block, which would rule out AVRT and NVT. This was further substantiated when the SVT spontaneously converted to 2:1 AV block (**Fig. 2**).

Hence, the differential diagnosis was narrowed to AT versus atypical AVNRT. There was concentric atrial activation during tachycardia with earliest atrial signal at the CS ostium. Initial attempts to ventricular overdrive pace during SVT resulted in AV dissociation, another feature that would rule out AVRT.

WHAT MANEUVERS SHOULD UTILIZED TO DISTINGUISH AT FROM AVNRT?

To demonstrate ventriculoatrial (VA) linking, atrial overdrive pacing from various locations during tachycardia was performed at a cycle length that was 20 ms faster than the tachycardia cycle length (TCL). The VA interval of the return beat, after pacing was completed, was similar to the VA interval during tachycardia and was similar regardless of where atrial overdrive pacing was performed, thus linking the ventricle and atrium (**Fig. 3**). Establishing VA linking was therefore most consistent with AVNRT (or AVRT if it were still in the differential but it had already been ruled out).[1,2] VA linking would not be expected with atrial tachycardia, as atrial activation is not dependent on ventricular activation.

Several other pacing maneuvers were also performed. Ventricular burst pacing was performed during tachycardia at a faster cycle length than TCL to terminate the tachycardia. Termination of the tachycardia during ventricular pacing, without depolarization of the atrium, excluded atrial tachycardia.[3] Finally, ventricular overdrive pacing (VOD) during tachycardia was eventually able to capture the atrium, and the atrial activation sequence was similar to the atrial activation sequence during tachycardia. After VOD was completed, the

Division of Cardiology, Section of Cardiac Electrophysiology, University of California-San Francisco, 500 Parnassus Avenue, MU East 4, Box 1354, San Francisco, CA 94143, USA
* Corresponding author.
E-mail address: badhwar@medicine.ucsf.edu

Card Electrophysiol Clin 2 (2010) 235–238
doi:10.1016/j.ccep.2010.01.010
1877-9182/10/$ – see front matter

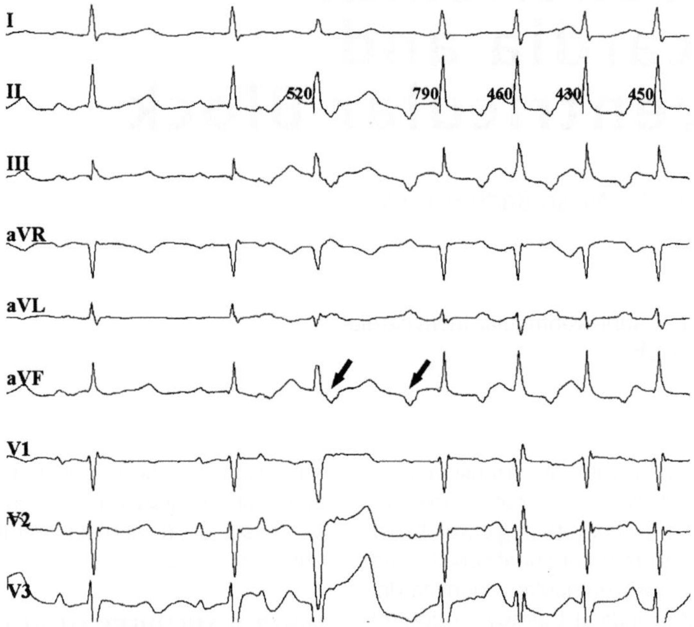

Fig. 1. ECG of SVT initiation. After a premature atrial beat that initiated tachycardia, there were two beats of AV block (*arrows*).

sequence following the last ventricularly paced beat was an atrial-ventricular response. This response was consistent with AVNRT (or AVRT, although this was no longer in the differential diagnosis for the patient's tachycardia).[4] Hence, AT was definitively excluded.

Once the diagnosis of atypical, slow-slow AVNRT was confirmed, an asymmetric 4 mm ablation catheter was advanced to the tricuspid annulus just anterior to the CS ostium (**Fig. 4**). Ablation was directed at the site of earliest retrograde atrial activation near the CS ostium and immediately elicited junctional beats without evidence of His-atrial block. After ablation was completed, no further spontaneous tachycardia was present. In addition, SVT could not be induced despite addition of Isuprel and atrial or ventricular extrastimuli. The patient has been symptom-free without evidence of recurrence.

DISCUSSION

A mid- to long-RP SVT, which is diagnosed as atypical AVNRT, can be described as a fast-slow or slow-slow AVNRT. In slow-slow AVNRT, a slow AV nodal pathway is utilized as the

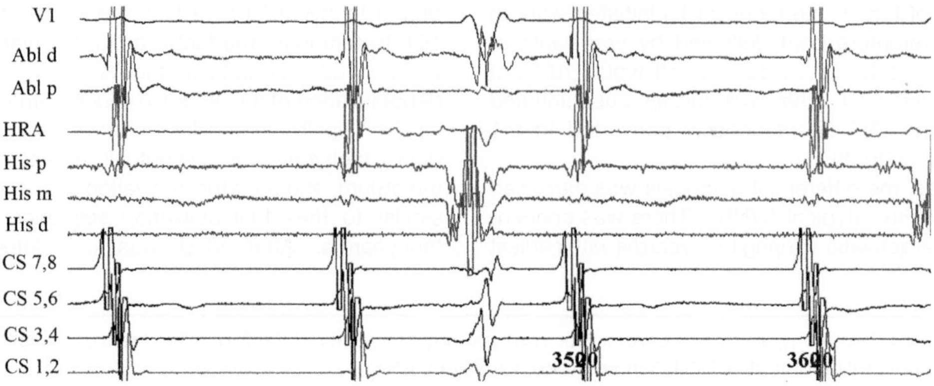

Fig. 2. Baseline intracardiac electrograms during SVT with 2:1 AV block. Ablator (Abl) was placed along the tricuspid annulus and anterior to the CS ostium; CS with 1–2 most distal and 7–8 most proximal. CS, coronary sinus; d, distal; His, His bundle; HRA, high right atrium; m, mid; p, proximal; V1, electrocardiogram lead V1.

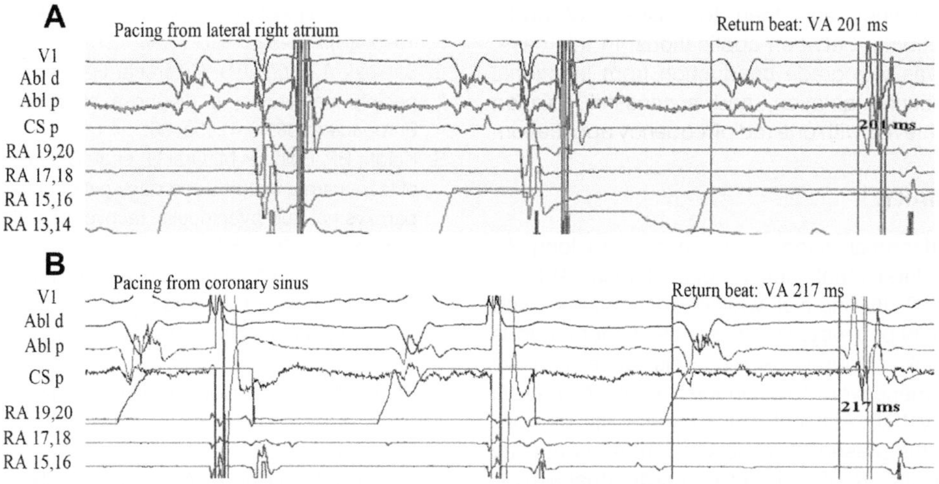

Fig. 3. Atrial overdrive pacing during tachycardia at a cycle length that was 20 ms faster than TCL from two sites: pacing from lateral right atrium (*A*) and pacing from the CS (*B*). The VA interval of the return beat, after pacing was completed, was similar to the VA interval of tachycardia (200 ms) and remained fixed regardless of site of pacing. Ablator (Abl) or was placed along the tricuspid annulus and anterior to the CS ostium; multipolar catheter in right atrium (RA) along lateral wall. p, proximal; d, distal.

anterograde pathway and another slow AV nodal pathway is the retrograde limb. It is relatively rare, accounting for 10% to 15% of all patients with AVNRT.[5] Characteristics of slow-slow AVNRT include the presence of a lower common pathway and the fact that the site of earliest retrograde atrial activation is near the CS ostium.[6] Both features were present in this case, because the patient had spontaneous 2:1 AV block during AVNRT, which strongly supported the existence of a lower common pathway.[7] Furthermore, the site of successful ablation was near the CS ostium, which was also the site of earliest retrograde atrial activation. It is important to recognize that patients with slow-slow AVNRT often lack retrograde conduction over the fast AV nodal pathway. Hence, junctional beats may not have retrograde conduction over the fast pathway and AV node conduction cannot be evaluated during ablation.[6] It is therefore prudent to deliver only short applications of

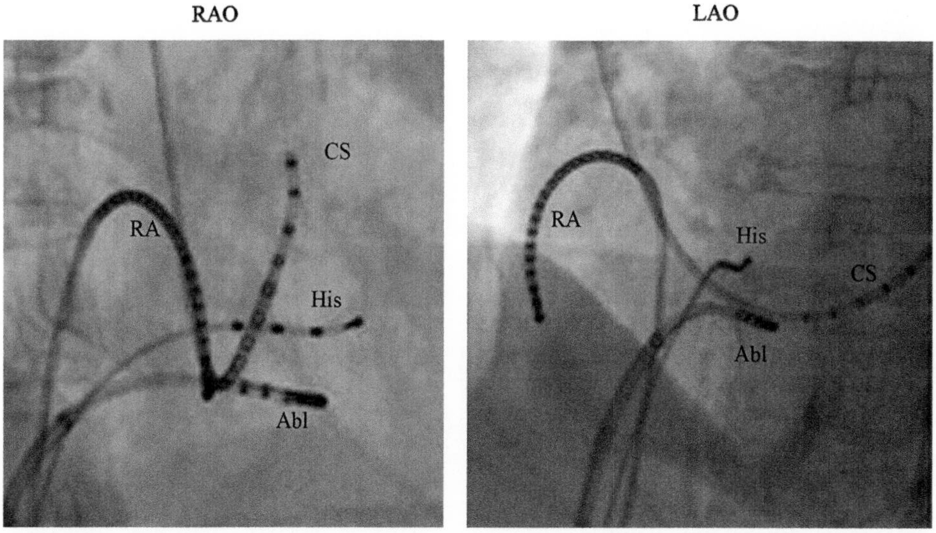

Fig. 4. Fluoroscopic views (LAO, left anterior oblique; RAO, right anterior oblique) of successful site of ablation. The ablator (Abl) was located along the medial tricuspid annulus, just anterior to the CS. His, His bundle catheter; RA, multipolar catheter placed around the lateral RA.

radiofrequency and then to assess AV nodal conduction in between applications. In this case, there was retrograde conduction from junctional beats during ablation, and successful ablation was achieved with one radiofrequency application.

SUMMARY

The differential diagnosis for a mid- to long-RP SVT include atrial tachycardia, atypical AVNRT, and AVRT utilizing a slowly conducting concealed accessory pathway. The presence of spontaneous AV block excludes AVRT. This case reviews pacing maneuvers to distinguish atrial tachycardia from AVNRT. Atypical AVNRT generally demonstrates the presence of a lower common pathway and has its site of earliest retrograde atrial activation near the coronary sinus ostium, which would be the target for ablation.

REFERENCES

1. Kadish AH, Morady F. The response of paroxysmal supraventricular tachycardia to overdrive atrial and ventricular pacing: can it help determine the tachycardia mechanism? J Cardiovasc Electrophysiol 1993;4(3):239–52.
2. Sarkozy A, Richter S, Chierchia G-B, et al. A novel pacing manoeuvre to diagnose atrial tachycardia. Europace 2008;10(4):459–66.
3. Knight BP, Ebinger M, Oral H, et al. Diagnostic value of tachycardia features and pacing maneuvers during paroxysmal supraventricular tachycardia. J Am Coll Cardiol 2000;36(2):574–82.
4. Knight BP, Zivin A, Souza J, et al. A technique for the rapid diagnosis of atrial tachycardia in the electrophysiology laboratory. J Am Coll Cardiol 1999;33(3):775–81.
5. Heidbuchel H, Jackman WM. Characterization of subforms of AV nodal reentrant tachycardia. Europace 2004;6(4):316–29.
6. Gonzalez M, Jaime R. Ablation of AVNRT and variants guided by intracardiac recordings. In: Huang SKS, Wood M, editors. Catheter ablation of cardiac arrhythmias. Philadelphia: Saunders; 2006. p. 347–67.
7. Wellens HJ, Wesdorp JC, Duren DR, Lie KI. Second degree block during reciprocal atrioventricular nodal tachycardia. Circulation 1976;53(4):595–9.

Changing QRS Morphology in a Patient with Wolff-Parkinson-White Syndrome

Vasanth Vedantham, MD, PhD, Zian H. Tseng, MD, MAS*

KEYWORDS

- Supraventricular tachycardia • Atrioventricular reentry
- Accessory pathway • Atriofascicular pathway

CLINICAL PRESENTATION

A 28-year-old otherwise healthy man with a history of palpitations was referred to the electrophysiology clinic after a 12-lead electrocardiogram (ECG) revealed ventricular preexcitation. Given the history of recurrent palpitations and the importance of risk stratification for sudden cardiac death in patients with ventricular preexcitation, electrophysiologic study with possible ablation was recommended.

ELECTROPHYSIOLOGIC STUDY

Evaluation of the initial ECG with Wolff-Parkinson-White syndrome (**Fig. 1**) shows left bundle branch block QRS morphology, early precordial R-wave transition, and left inferior axis suggesting an anteroseptal accessory pathway.[1,2] The rhythm strip in V_1 shows a changing QRS morphology with a positive delta wave, which might suggest a left-sided pathway. Initial findings on intracardiac electrograms (**Fig. 2**A) demonstrated ventricular preexcitation with a negative His-ventricular (HV) interval (−10 milliseconds). The surface ECG showed a right bundle branch block QRS morphology (note the difference in lead V_1 from the ECG in **Fig. 1**), with the earliest intracardiac ventricular activation seen in the distal coronary sinus electrode, suggesting the presence of a left lateral accessory pathway rather than a septal pathway. Consistent with this finding, ventricular overdrive pacing (see **Fig. 2**B) showed eccentric atrial activation, with the site of earliest activation in the distal coronary sinus while atrial overdrive pacing at progressively shorter cycle lengths resulted in a wide right bundle branch block QRS morphology with precordial concordance and inferior axis (see **Fig. 2**C). With continued decremental atrial overdrive pacing, the QRS complex abruptly changed from right bundle branch block to left bundle branch block morphology with a left superior axis (see **Fig. 2**D).

WHAT IS THE REASON FOR THE CHANGE IN THE QRS PATTERN?

At first, aberrant conduction in the left bundle was considered as an explanation for this finding, but no His bundle electrogram could be identified on the His channel preceding the onset of the QRS complex. With still shorter atrial pacing cycle lengths, the *atrioventricular* (AV) relationship exhibited decremental timing, but again no electrogram consistent with normal conduction system depolarization was identified preceding the QRS. Furthermore, a late precordial transition (after V_4) and superior axis are inconsistent with typical left bundle branch block. This constellation of findings (left bundle morphology, late transition,

Cardiac Electrophysiology Section, Cardiology Division, University of California, 500 Parnassus Avenue, MU-433, Box 1354, San Francisco, CA, USA
* Corresponding author.
E-mail address: zhtseng@medicine.ucsf.edu

Card Electrophysiol Clin 2 (2010) 239–243
doi:10.1016/j.ccep.2010.01.011
1877-9182/10/$ – see front matter

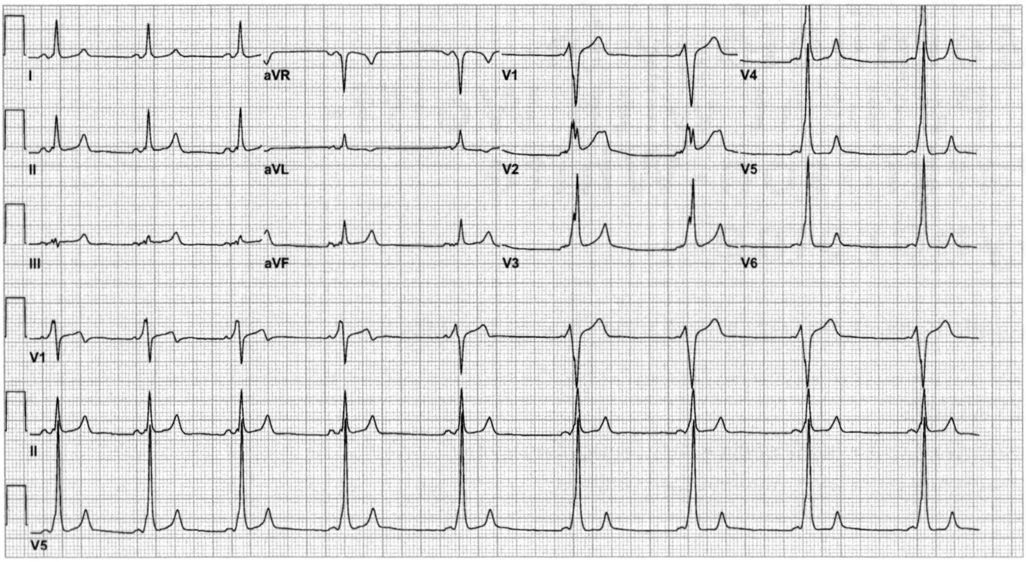

Fig. 1. 12-lead ECG. Ventricular preexcitation is present. Note the extremely short PR interval with fusion between P wave and QRS in the precordium.

superior axis, negative HV interval, decremental conduction) raised the possibility of a second, right-sided accessory pathway inserting into the right ventricular conduction system (atriofascicular).[3] The existence of a second pathway also accounts for the discordance between the original 12-lead ECG (suggesting a left-sided or septal pathway) and the ECG recorded on the day of the procedure (suggesting a left lateral pathway). With these possibilities in mind, we proceeded to tachycardia induction.

Two regular tachycardias were induced during the procedure. Tachycardia No. 1 was induced with ventricular overdrive pacing and exhibited

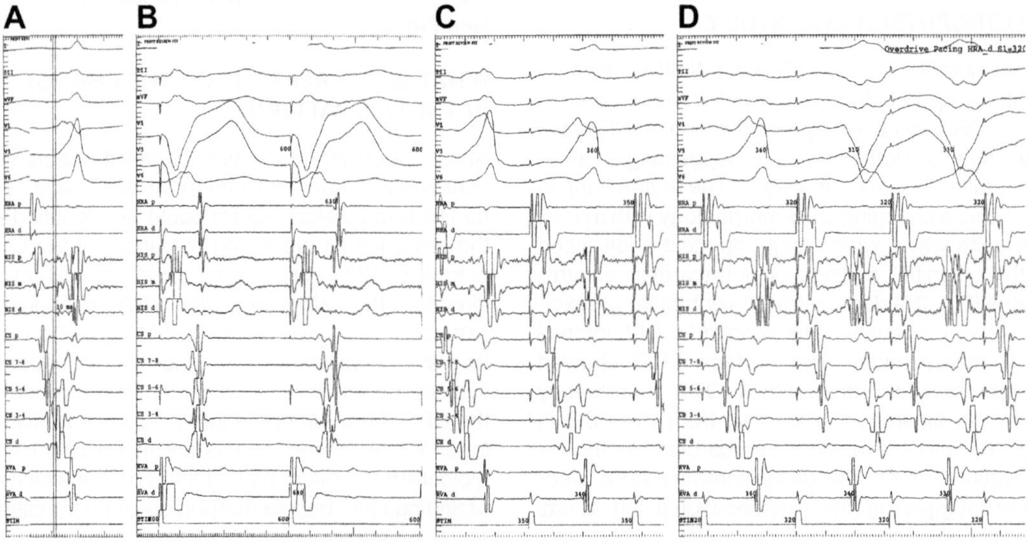

Fig. 2. (*A*) Sinus rhythm shows ventricular preexcitation with a different QRS morphology than in the ECG of **Fig 1**. The HV interval of −10 milliseconds is shown. (*B*) Ventricular overdrive pacing results in eccentric retrograde conduction with the atrial electrogram in CS 1–2 earliest. (*C*) Atrial overdrive pacing shows a pattern of preexcitation that is most consistent with a left lateral accessory pathway. (*D*) Pacing at shorter coupling intervals caused block with an abrupt change in the QRS complex and a small change in the AV interval. The absence of a His deflection and decremental conduction suggested the presence of an atriofascicular accessory pathway. (Scale: large divisions correspond to 100 milliseconds.)

a narrow QRS complex and eccentric atrial activation (**Fig. 3**A). The narrow QRS complex indicates that the AV node is the antegrade limb of this tachycardia, while the eccentric activation suggested the left lateral accessory pathway as the retrograde limb (orthodromic atrioventricular reciprocating tachycardia [AVRT]). In addition, ventricular overdrive pacing was used to entrain this tachycardia, and on cessation of pacing and resumption of tachycardia, a ventricular-atrial-ventricular (V-A-V) response was observed, ruling out atrial tachycardia. The postpacing interval–tachycardia cycle length (PPI-TCL) of 70 milliseconds, along with the eccentric atrial activation pattern, excluded AV node reentry as the mechanism of the tachycardia. Subsequently, this tachycardia was observed to occur with right bundle branch block at a longer cycle length (see **Fig. 3**B). Inspection of intracardiac electrograms, however, revealed that the ventricular-atrial (VA) interval (measured from the surface QRS to the earliest identifiable atrial electrogram) was similar with and without right bundle branch block. This observation argues against a right-sided accessory pathway as the retrograde limb and is consistent with a left-sided accessory pathway. The change in tachycardia cycle length was therefore attributed to delay in the antegrade limb (AV node), illustrating the importance of measuring VA interval as opposed to cycle length when assessing the effect of bundle branch block on AV reentrant circuits.[4]

Fig. 4A shows induction of tachycardia No. 2 with a ventricular extrastimulus delivered at a coupling interval of 300 milliseconds. The extrastimulus captures the ventricle and results in conduction retrograde via the left lateral pathway to the atrium (eccentric atrial activation), which is followed by a single bundle branch reentry complex, as evidenced by the His bundle electrogram and the right bundle branch potential on the right ventricular channel (arrows 1 and 2) preceding the ventricular depolarization. Once again, the ventricular depolarization is followed by eccentric atrial activation via the left lateral accessory pathway, which is followed by another QRS complex (the first beat of tachycardia). Neither a His bundle electrogram nor a right bundle potential precedes this ventricular depolarization, and the QRS axis is distinct from the previous 2 ventricular depolarizations, making bundle branch reentry or catheter-induced premature ventricular depolarization very unlikely.

This initiation, together with basic features of the tachycardia, strongly suggests AV reentry tachycardia as the mechanism. First, eccentric atrial activation matching that observed during ventricular overdrive pacing (identical to tachycardia No. 1) excludes typical AV node reentry. Second, initiation of tachycardia with a V-A-V sequence effectively rules out atrial tachycardia. Ventricular tachycardia with 1:1 retrograde conduction should also be considered, but the fact that the tachycardia QRS morphology is identical to that observed with rapid

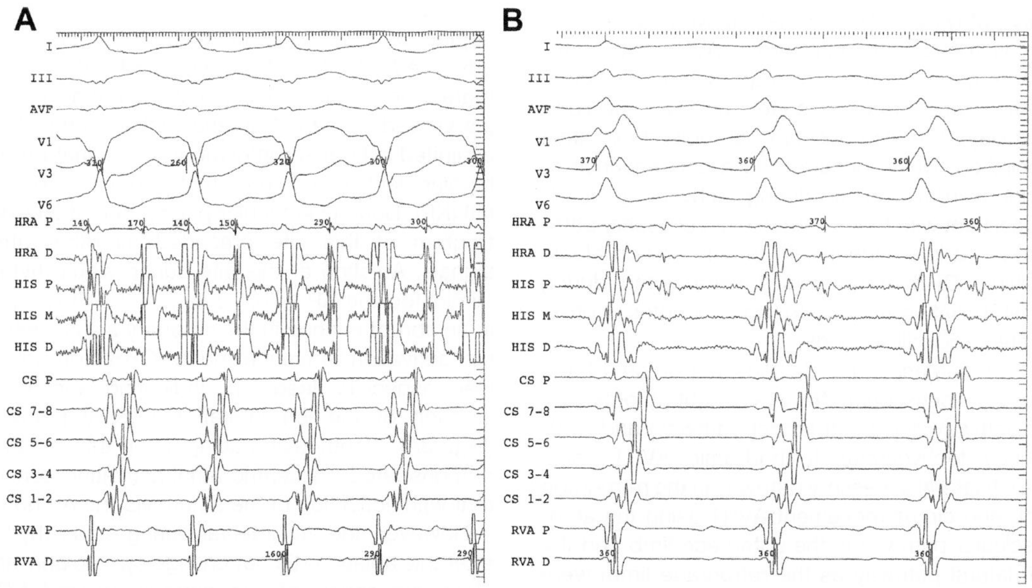

Fig. 3. Tachycardia No. 1. (*A*) Narrow complex with eccentric atrial activation. (*B*) Right bundle branch block with eccentric retrograde activation. There is no change in the ventricular-atrial interval. Antegrade limb was the AV node, and the retrograde limb was the left lateral pathway.

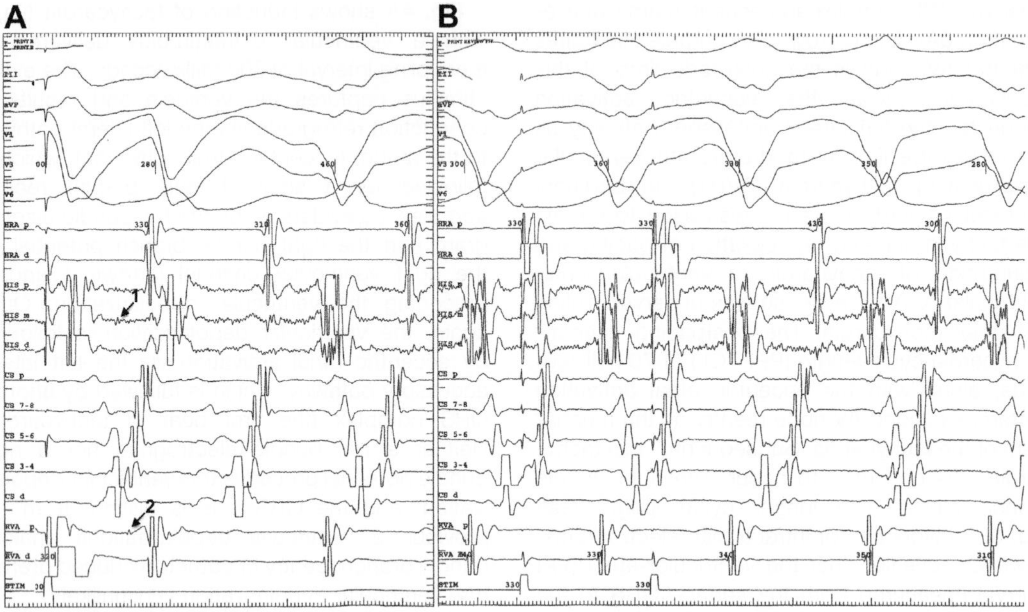

Fig. 4. Tachycardia No. 2. (*A*) Initiation with a ventricular extrastimulus followed by bundle branch reentry. Arrow 1 is the His deflection, and arrow 2 is the right bundle branch potential. (*B*) Initiation with atrial overdrive pacing. No His signal could be identified during tachycardia. Antegrade limb was the atriofascicular pathway, and the retrograde limb was the left lateral pathway.

atrial pacing makes this possibility highly unlikely. In addition, initiation of tachycardia with atrial overdrive pacing showed an atrial-ventricular-atrial response, providing more evidence against ventricular tachycardia (see **Fig. 4**B). The absence of an identifiable His depolarization preceding the QRS, together with the finding of a second accessory pathway, indicated that tachycardia No. 2 is circus movement tachycardia (AVRT with antegrade conduction via a right-sided accessory pathway and retrograde conduction via a left-sided pathway). We also observed an episode of atrial fibrillation, which occurred as a consequence of atrial overdrive pacing during tachycardia No. 1. Consistent with the presence of 2 accessory pathways and intermittent right bundle branch block, multiple QRS morphologies were noted during atrial fibrillation with shortest cycle lengths approximately 250 milliseconds.

To summarize the diagnostic portion of the study, 2 accessory pathways (a right atriofascicular pathway and a left lateral pathway) and 2 AV reentry tachycardias (orthodromic AVRT using the left lateral accessory pathway in the retrograde limb and circus movement AVRT using the atriofascicular pathway in the antegrade limb and the left lateral pathway as the retrograde limb) were observed. Rapid atrial fibrillation in which most ventricular complexes were preexcited was also observed.

CATHETER ABLATION

Because both accessory pathways participated in tachycardia circuits and both were capable of antegrade conduction at short cycle lengths, both pathways were targeted for mapping and ablation, beginning with the left lateral pathway. Transseptal puncture was performed using standard techniques and a mapping/ablation catheter was advanced into the left atrium. A site at approximately the 3 o'clock position on the mitral annulus (as viewed in the left anterior oblique projection) exhibited a tight AV interval with a signal on the bipolar electrogram consistent with a Kent potential (KP). During ventricular pacing, the atrial electrogram at this site preceded all other atrial signals. Ablation at this site during sinus rhythm eliminated the KP within 2 seconds and resulted in an abrupt change in the coronary sinus ventricular activation sequence and the QRS morphology (see especially lead V_1), indicating successful ablation of the left lateral accessory pathway (**Fig. 5**A). Ventricular pacing after this ablation demonstrated concentric atrial activation consistent with activation of the atrium via the AV node.

However, the HV interval during sinus rhythm after this ablation did not change appreciably and close inspection of the surface 12-lead ECG revealed persistent ventricular preexcitation, confirming the presence of a second accessory

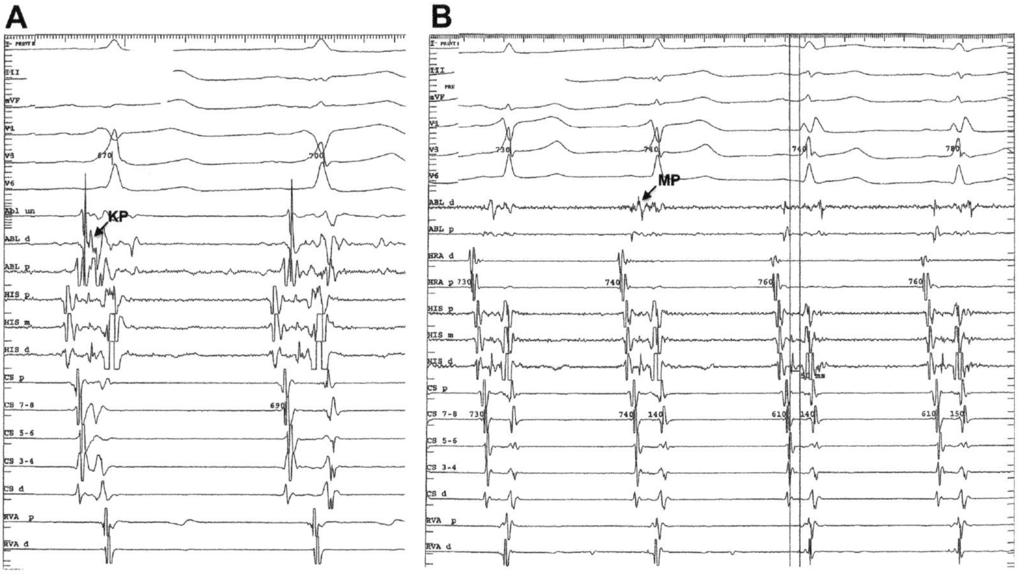

Fig. 5. Successful ablation sites. (*A*) A site at the 3 o'clock position on the mitral annulus exhibited a KP. *Radiofrequency* (RF) ablation abruptly changed the QRS complex and ventricular activation pattern, but the HV interval remained short with ventricular preexcitation. (*B*) Identification of an M potential (atriofascicular pathway potential) at the 7 o'clock position on the tricuspid annulus. RF ablation eliminated preexcitation and normalized the HV interval.

pathway. Atrial overdrive pacing confirmed a decremental right-sided accessory pathway. Retrograde conduction via this pathway was never observed with ventricular pacing. The ablation catheter was then withdrawn to the right atrium, and mapping was undertaken at the tricuspid annulus. Mapping was guided by searching for potentials between the atrial and ventricular electrograms that could be consistent with activation of the atriofascicular accessory pathway (M potential or MP).[5] After extensive mapping, a site at approximately the 7 o'clock position on the tricuspid annulus was identified, which exhibited a low-amplitude, low-frequency complex signal between the atrial and ventricular depolarization consistent with an MP. Ablation at this site resulted in disappearance of the MP and nearly immediate loss of ventricular preexcitation (see **Fig. 5**B). The HV interval increased from 30 to 50 milliseconds (normal). The surface ECG after this ablation showed no ventricular preexcitation, and accessory pathway conduction could not be demonstrated with either atrial or ventricular pacing. No tachycardia was inducible at the end of the procedure, and the patient has experienced complete resolution of his palpitations at 1 year after the procedure.

REFERENCES

1. Fitzpatrick AP, Gonzales RP, Lesh MD, et al. New algorithm for the localization of accessory atrioventricular connections using a baseline electrocardiogram. J Am Coll Cardiol 1994;23(1):107–16.
2. Arruda MS, McClelland JH, Wang X, et al. Development and validation of an ECG algorithm for identifying accessory pathway ablation site in Wolff-Parkinson-White syndrome. J Cardiovasc Electrophysiol 1998;9(1):2–12.
3. Tchou P, Lehmann MH, Jazayeri M, et al. Atriofascicular connection or a nodoventricular Mahaim fiber? Electrophysiologic elucidation of the pathway and associated reentrant circuit. Circulation 1988;77(4):837–48.
4. Kerr CR, Gallagher JJ, German LD. Changes in ventriculoatrial intervals with bundle branch block aberration during reciprocating tachycardia in patients with accessory atrioventricular pathways. Circulation 1982;66(1):196–201.
5. McClelland JH, Wang X, Beckman KJ, et al. Radiofrequency catheter ablation of right atriofascicular (Mahaim) accessory pathways guided by accessory pathway activation potentials. Circulation 1994;89(6):2655–66.

Ventricular Tachycardia

Masood Akhtar, MD

KEYWORDS

- Ventricular tachycardia spectrum
- Bundle branch re-entry • Coronary artery disease

The understanding of ventricular tachycardia (VT) has evolved from a simple entity of an arrhythmia of subjunctional origin to one with an ever increasing variety of locations and mechanisms.[1–10] The once frequently published monomorphic (MM) VT of coronary artery disease origin now is replaced in part by polymorphic VT, and MMVT of noncoronary origin.[1–10]

For a clinician to arrive at a reasonable diagnosis from the myriad of possibilities, some systematic approach is desirable. One possibility is to classify according to clinical presentation. Aside from cardiac arrest, however, the symptoms of VT often are shared by less ominous arrhythmias such as most forms of supraventricular tachycardia (SVT). Even the so-called cardiac arrest may not be caused by VT, unless documented by electrocardiogram (ECG). The most practical classification incorporates a combination of ECG patterns and the underlying substrate.

Table 1 is an attempt to assist a clinician to arrive at a diagnosis with a reasonable degree of confidence. A more precise diagnosis usually requires further analysis, including electrophysiologic evaluation. In some cases, eventual placement of a given VT into a specific category may require further analysis as is done currently in some cases of so-called channelopathies.[11–14] Although it is possible that in the future, most, if not all arrhythmias can be categorized on genetic basis, the approach listed in **Table 1** is more practical currently.

The foregoing discussion of VT (see **Table 1**) assumes that the diagnosis of VT (versus SVT) already has been made. Reaching that conclusion has its own set of difficulties. For that the reader is referred to other sources.[15–18] The purpose of this article is to present some interesting cases and see where they fit into the bigger scheme (see **Table 1**).

CASE 1

A 76-year-old man presented following an episode of syncope. He carried a diagnosis of coronary artery disease since he suffered a non-Q-wave infarct 8 years earlier. Coronary angiogram showed a 50% narrowing in the mid left anterior descending (LAD) coronary artery and distal right coronary artery (RCA). An echocardiogram showed mild aortic valvular sclerosis and regurgitation with an overall left ventricular ejection fraction (LVEF) of 40%. The baseline ECG is shown (**Fig. 1**). The 12-lead ECG shows right bundle branch block (RBBB) and left axis deviation compatible with the diagnosis of bifascicular block. The rhythm is sinus tachycardia at a rate of 120 beats/min. Near the end of the tracing there is a narrow QRS complex and shorter PR compared with the preceding QRS. The possibilities include

- Spontaneous or catheter-induced premature ventricular complex from near the right bundle branch (RBB) well timed with the arrival of sinus impulse at the LV level[18]
- A supraventricular capture of the ventricle—unless associated with supranormal conduction, such capture should produce longer rather than shorter right bundle branch PR intervals
- His bundle extrasystole arising from below the site of intra-His block, which is the reason for RBBB block

The patient was studied at another location. A common type of atrioventricular (AV) nodal

University of Wisconsin School of Medicine and Public Health, Aurora Sinai, St Luke's Medical Center, 960 North 12th Street, Milwaukee, WI, USA
E-mail address: Laurel.landis@aurora.org

Card Electrophysiol Clin 2 (2010) 245–265
doi:10.1016/j.ccep.2010.01.026
1877-9182/10/$ – see front matter

Table 1
Clinical spectrum

Ventricular Tachycardia					
SHD		No SHD			
			PMVT/VF		
MMVT	PMVT/VF	MMVT	Normal QT	Long QT	Short QT
CAD	Ischemia	RVOT	Brugada	Congenital	Congenital
IDCM	HCM	ILV	2 varieties	(1–10)	Acquired
(Valve) HD		BBR	Banqungut[a]	Acquired	
ARVD			Pakkuri[a]	Drugs	
Naxos			Lai Tai[a]	Electrolytes	
Venetian			Catecholaminergic	Ischemia	
Postoperative			Shortly coupled	CNS	
			SIDS		
			Idiopathic		

Abbreviations: ARVD, arrhythmogenic right ventricular dysplasia; BBR, bundle branch reentry; CAD, coronary artery disease; CNS, central nervous system HCM, hypertrophic cardiomyopathy; IDCM, idiopathic dilated cardiomyopathy; ILV, idiopathic left ventricular; MMVT, monomorphic ventricular tachycardia; Naxos (region in Greece); PMVT/VF, polymorphic VT ventricular fibrillation; RVOT, right ventricular output track; SHD, structural heart disease; SIDS, Sudden infant death syndrome; Venetian (Veneto region in Italy) similar to ARVD with high genetic preponderance.

[a] Other names given to Brugada-like syndrome in the Far East.

reentry (atrioventricular nodal tachycardia (AVNRT)-slow fast) was induced, and the patient was scheduled to have a slow pathway ablation at a subsequent date.[19–21]

Another syncopal episode occurred soon after discharge, and the patient was transferred. During his admission, the patient admitted to several other occasions when he felt palpitations, light headedness, but no other bouts of syncope. During the current admission, a 12-lead ECG was recorded (**Fig. 2**, Case 1). An RBBB and left axis deviation LAD again were noted; however, the underlying rhythm was different. Although superficially it looked like atrial fibrillation with a rapid ventricular rate, there were periods of regularity with a cycle length of 240 milliseconds. Furthermore, there were three QRS complexes with what appeared to be incomplete RBBB.

During the conduct of electrophysiologic (EP) evaluation pacing at a basic cycle length of 460

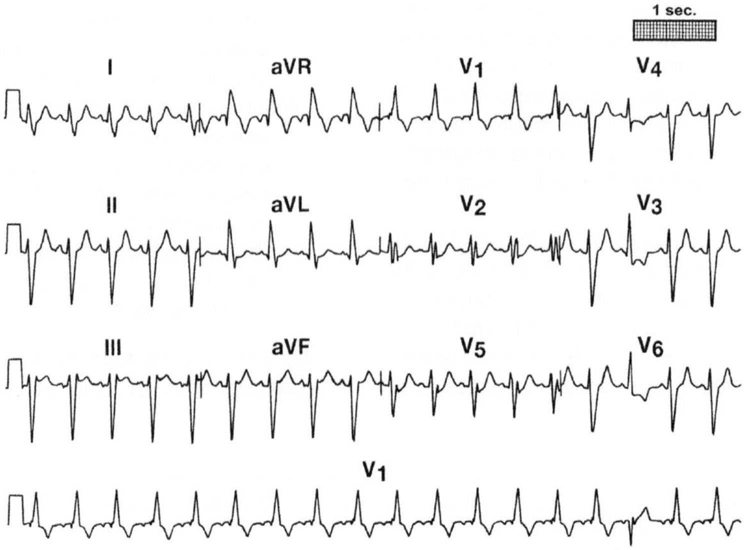

Fig. 1. Shows a 12-lead ECG; the leads are labeled. The RBBB and left anterior fascicular blocks are obvious. There is one narrow QRS, toward the end tracing.

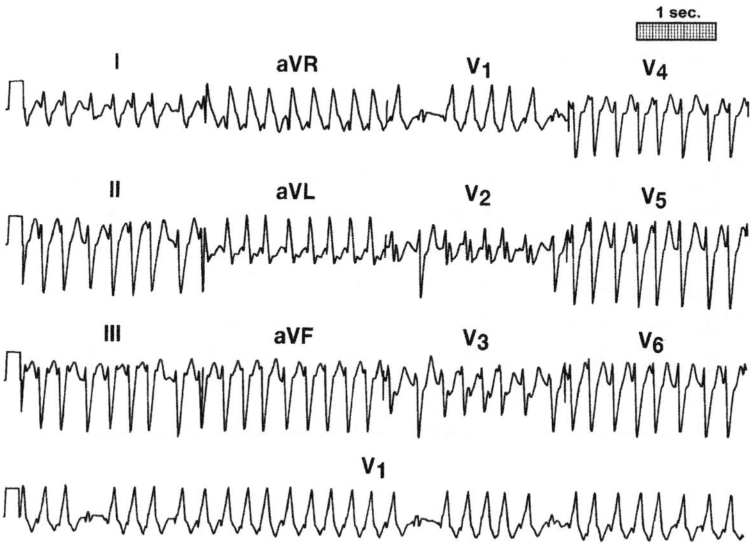

Fig. 2. 12-lead ECG. Shows atrial fibrillation, periods of rapid and regular RR, and some complexes slowing incomplete RBBB pattern while most of this ECG shows RBBB and LAD.

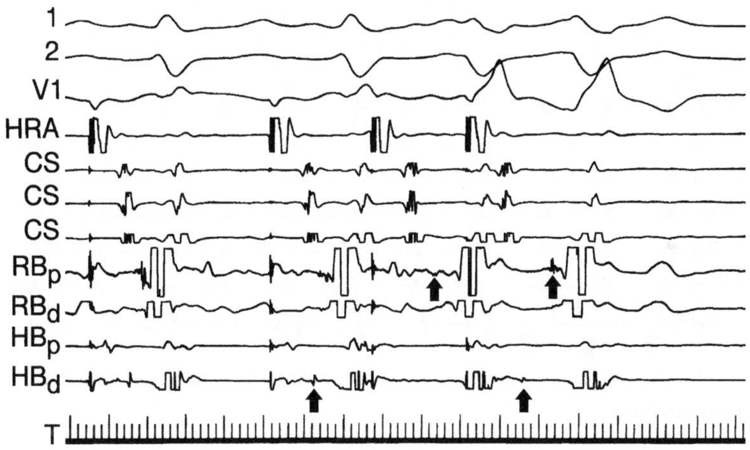

Fig. 3. Tracings, from top to bottom are: surface ECG 1, 2, V1, HRA (high right atrium); CS, coronary sinus; HB, His bundle; Pro. D, proximal, distal. Time at lines 100 and 10 milliseconds. Similar abbreviations are used throughout the text. Time line may at times be 50 and 20 rather than 100 and 10.

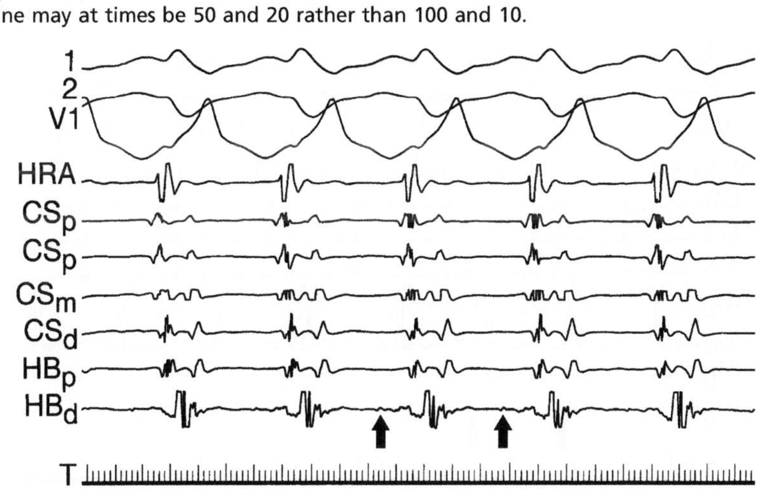

Fig. 4. See text for explanation.

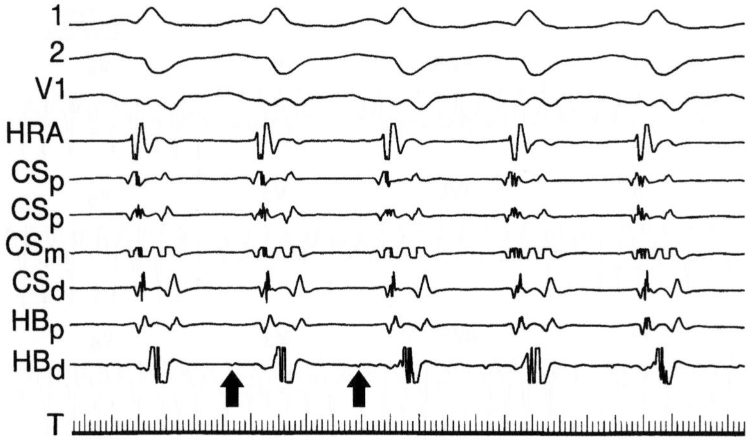

Fig. 5. See text for explanation.

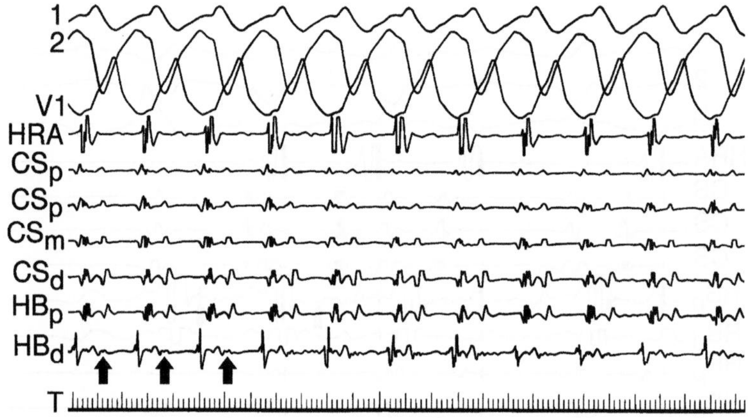

Fig. 6. See text for explanation.

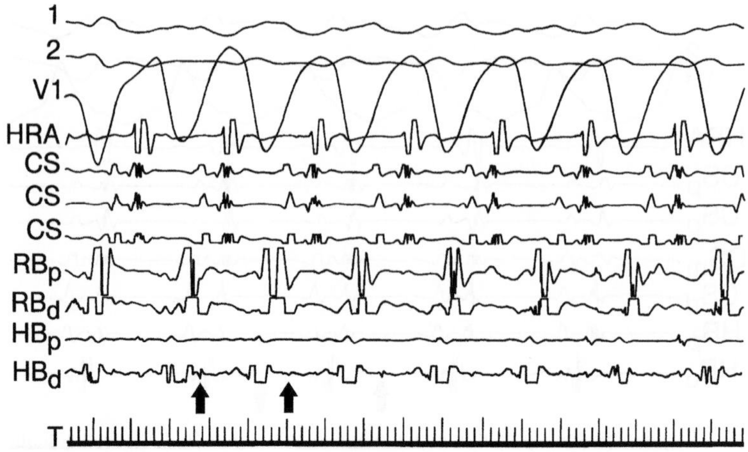

Fig. 7. See text for explanation.

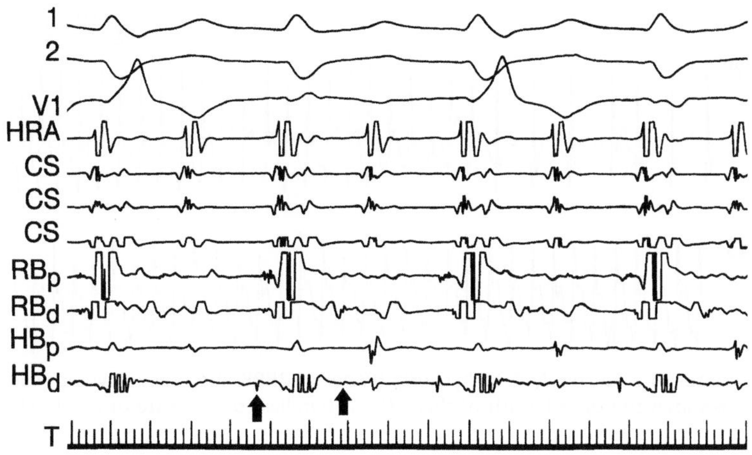

Fig. 8. See text for explanation.

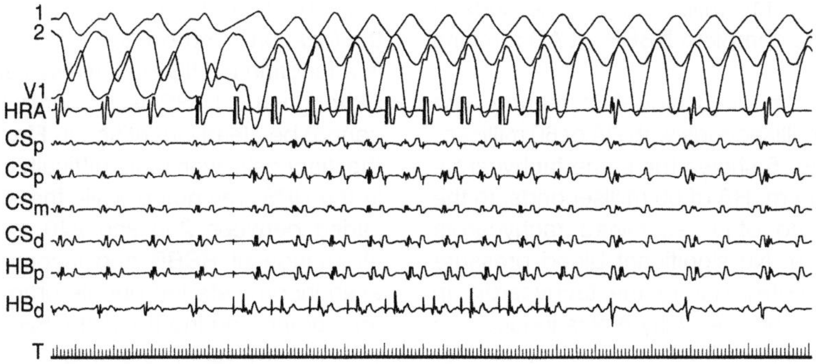

Fig. 9. See text for explanation.

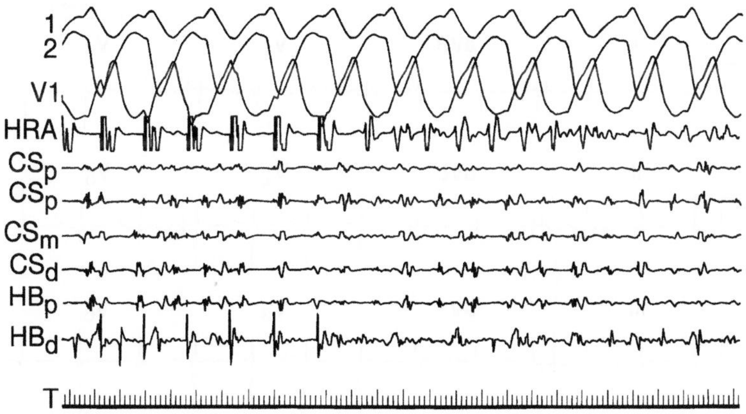

Fig. 10. See text for explanation.

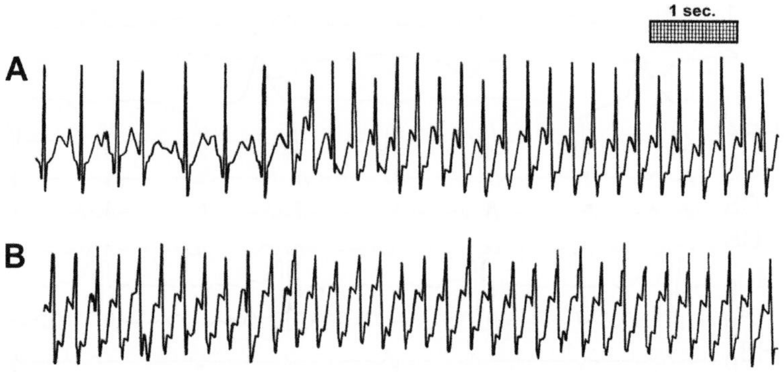

Fig. 11. Shows the onset of a narrow QRS tachycardia (*Panel A*) RBBB aberrancy develops soon after the tachycardia starts. *Panel B* shows the cycle length of this SVT—250 milliseconds. (Rate of 240 beats/min.)

milliseconds, two atrial premature stimuli are delivered at 260 and 240 milliseconds, respectively (**Fig. 3**). During the basic drive, the surface ECG shows incomplete RBBB and an HV of 60 milliseconds (HBd). With extra stimuli, the HV increases and now HIS bundle deflection (arrows) is clearly visible with HV = 110 milliseconds. The surface ECG shows more complete RBBB – LAD remains the same.

Further testing induced slow-fast reentry with RBBB with 440 milliseconds with HA of 60 milliseconds (**Fig. 4**). **Fig. 5** shows the same tachycardia with a LBBB pattern, HA of 60 milliseconds. In the baseline state, no other sustained tachycardia could be induced. No significant blood pressure (BP) drop was noted during the tachycardia in supine position. From the arrhythmias induced so far, it did not appear that an explanation for syncope was found. In this patient with syncope, low ejection fraction, some degree of valvular (aortic) sclerosis and prolonged HV interval, the AV nodal re-entry seemed like an incidental finding.

At this point, 2 μg of isoproterenol were infused, and tachycardia induction was retried. Three tracings are presented in **Figs. 6–8**. The cycle lengths (H-H, V-V) are 240, 230, and 210 milliseconds, respectively. The distal His (or proximal RB) potential can be identified with an HV interval of 80 milliseconds and H-A of 60 milliseconds. Note that the location of retrograde A in the diastolic period is a function of HIS-Purkinje system (HPS) delays. Although the H-RB is recognizable in **Fig. 7**, it cannot be clearly identified in **Fig. 6**. **Fig. 8** makes the diagnosis even more difficult, where a 2:1 block in the HPS was noted while the atrial cycle length varied between 230 and 240 milliseconds. With alternation of RBBB and incomplete RBBB and even incomplete left bundle branch block (LBBB) appearance during the last QRS, this tachycardia with a fairly rapid rate was clearly of supra-His origin. During attempted conversion of this tachycardia (**Fig. 9**), there was a conversion of the RBBB pattern tachycardia to LBBB pattern that was associated with 2:1 VA block, documenting

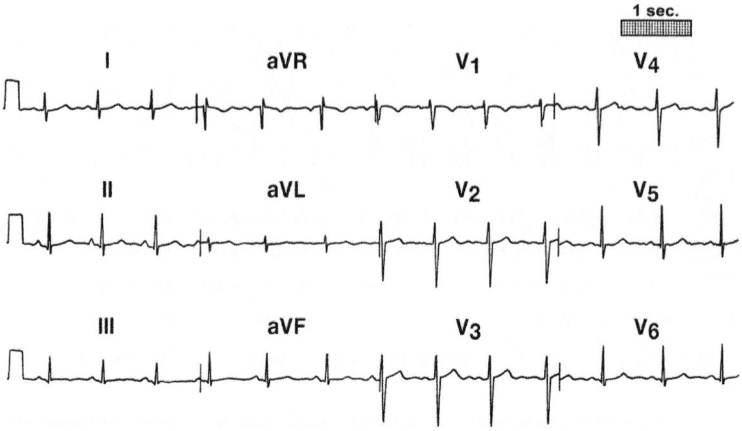

Fig. 12. Normal baseline ECG.

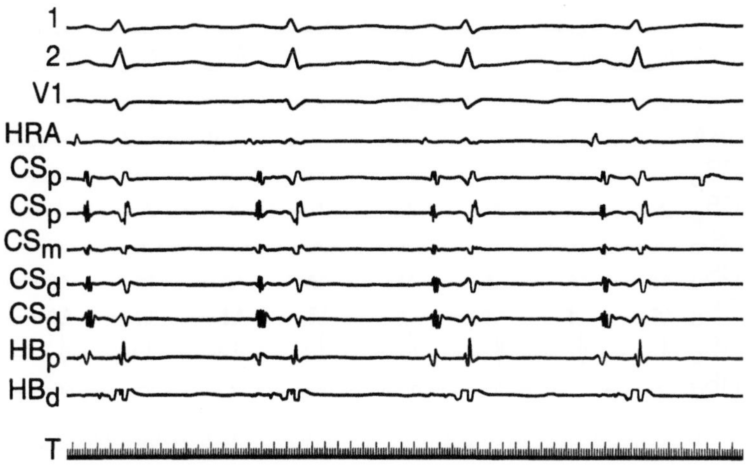

Fig. 13. Tracings are, from top to bottom, surface ECG lead I, II, and V1, intracardiac HRA (high right atrium), CS (coronary sinus), HB (His bundle) electrogram, p, m, d (proximal, middle, distal). Time line at 50 and 20 milliseconds. All intervals are normal, and His bundle potential can be clearly appreciated in the bottom tracing.

ventricular origin. HB electrogram showed movement (ie, the catheter toward the atrium and loss of His potential) so that the exact nature of this VT (ie, bundle branch re-entry [BBR] versus myocardial VT) was uncertain. Rapid S wave in V1 and similarity in the tachycardia to **Fig. 7** suggested BBR.[22–24]

Subsequent-to-slow AV nodal pathway ablation the tachycardia in **Fig. 6** remained inducible, and 1:1 VA relationship remained persistent. At this point, atrial overdrive and induction of atrial fibrillation were attempted (**Fig. 10**). It should be noted that during atrial pacing at a cycle length of 180 milliseconds and subsequent atrial fibrillation V-V cycle length were steady at 240 milliseconds, indicating ventricular origin, because changes in atrial rate do not influence the ventricular rate.

Persistent VT following ablation of slow AV nodal pathway suggested existence of VT, most likely caused by BBR, because the QRS retained identical morphology to what was noted during supraventricular conduction such as in atrial fibrillation and slow–fast AVNRT. BBR was further suggested by the fact that the RBBB represented conduction delay rather than block as noted in **Figs. 2, 3, 5, 7, 8** and **9**. Although the VT in **Fig. 7** with an LBBB pattern could not be proven as a BBR, it conceivably could represent reversal of the circuit shown in **Figs. 6** and **9**.

RBBB ablation was tried where distal RBB potential was recorded. Although it did not change

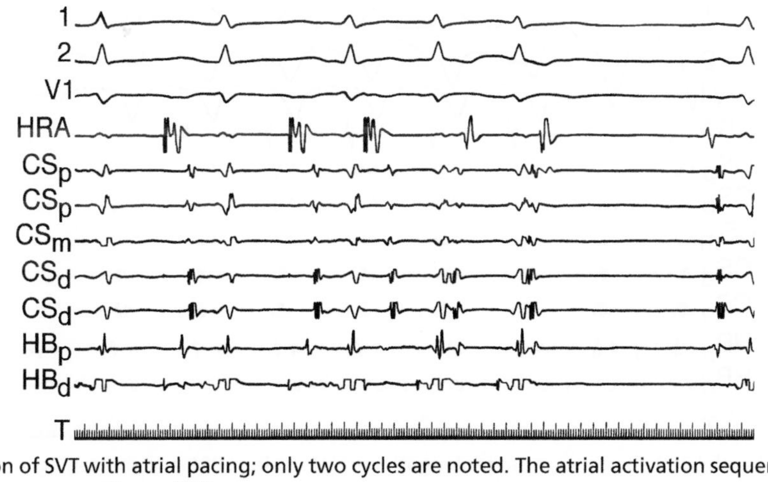

Fig. 14. Initiation of SVT with atrial pacing; only two cycles are noted. The atrial activation sequence suggests left posterolateral accessory pathway (AP).

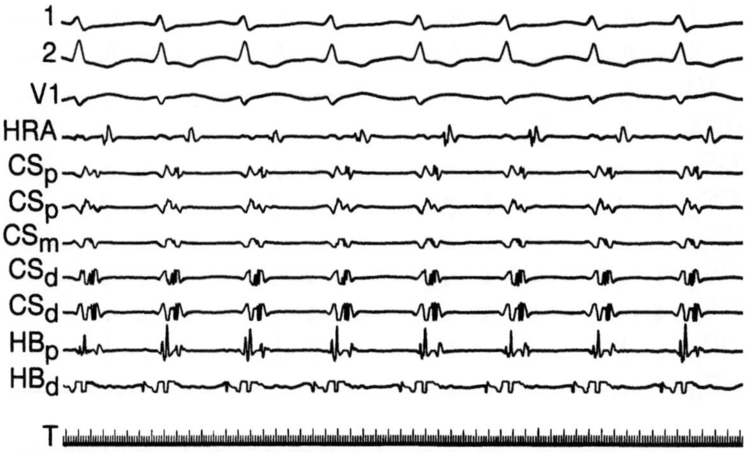

Fig. 15. Sustained orthodromic SVT CL 350 milliseconds.

the surface ECG, VT no longer could be induced. None of the other tachycardias could be induced, and AF eventually was initiated. Irregular VR with the same QRS morphology was noted. Coexistence of VT and atrial fibrillation also was suggested in **Fig. 2**.

This case can be summarized as follows

The history of palpitations and syncope suggested two sets of arrhythmias and possibly two mechanisms for those symptoms.

Although **Fig. 1** may be suggestive of possible intermittent AV block as a cause of syncope, **Fig. 3** raises the possibility of AF plus atrial flutter or VT.

Baseline AVNRT rate would be unlikely to produce syncope unless a significant BP drop was noted in supine position.

Post isoproterenol, the cycle length of AVNRT was sufficiently rapid to produce syncope. AVNRT at this rate, however, resulted in 2:1 HPS block.

The HV was prolonged at the baseline, and almost all the induced and spontaneous tachycardias had QRS morphologies that were similar to sinus rhythm ECG. The exceptions had either an incomplete RBBB or LBBB suggesting aberrant conduction (ie, rapid S in V1). (see **Figs. 4, 5, 6** and **7**)

Although myocardial VT could not be excluded with certainty, elimination of all VT morphologies with RB ablation was highly indicative of BBR.

The substrate in this case was most likely to be aortic valve pathology and

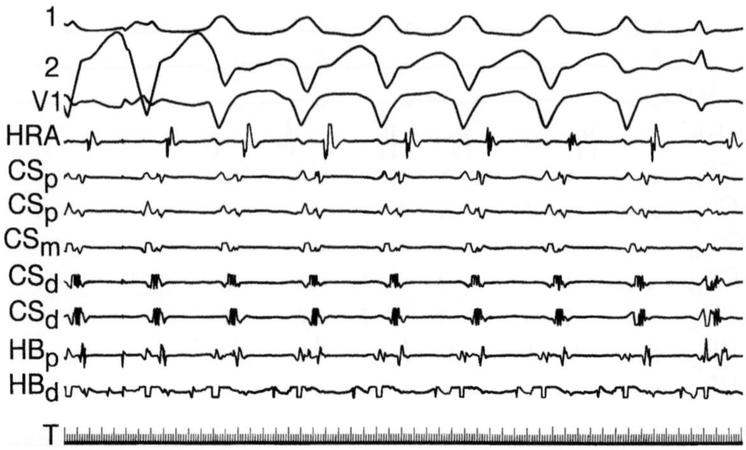

Fig. 16. Same SVT with LBBB aberrancy; note prolongation of VA during LBBB and shortening with normalization (last complex in the tracing).

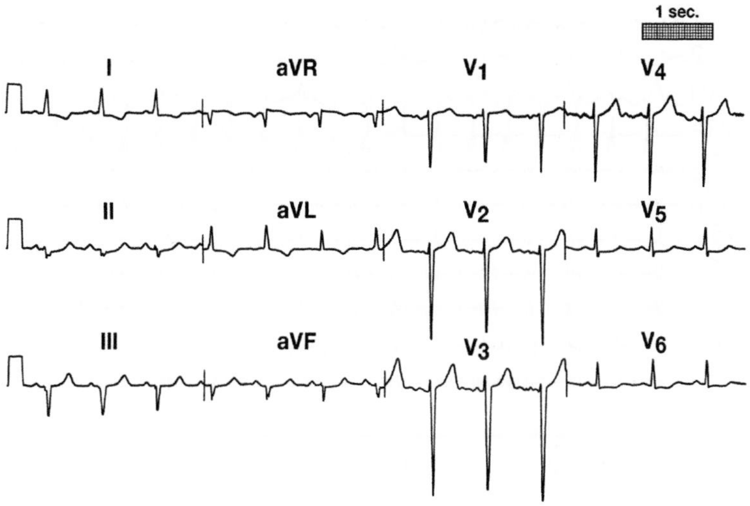

Fig. 17. The ECG now shows leftward axis shifts. Compare this with Fig. 2.

consequently HPS disease caused by this pathology.[22]

Conduction delay, rather than block (along with the HB) may have caused longitudinal dissociation within the His bundle. This may explain intermittent improvement of HPS conduction delay (see **Fig. 8**), allowing reversal of the circuit. Elimination of VT with ablation of RBB confirmed the diagnosis of BBR.

CASE 2

A 27-year-old woman with recurrent palpitations was referred for a documented SVT documented during ambulatory monitoring (**Fig. 11**). The tracing shows the onset of a narrow QRS tachycardia that changes with a widening of that QRS with a RBBB pattern. This arrhythmia was associated with reproduction of her symptoms. The baseline ECG showed normal sinus rhythm and normal ECG (**Fig. 12**). There was no evidence of ventricular pre-excitation. An electrophysiologic evaluation was performed with the intent to ablate the electrophysiologic substrate if one was found. The baseline tracings during sinus rhythm are shown (**Fig. 13**). The ECG tracings, from top to bottom, are surface ECG leads 1, 2, and V1, and the intracardiac tracings are right atrial electrograms (HRA) proximal, middle, and distal coronary sinus

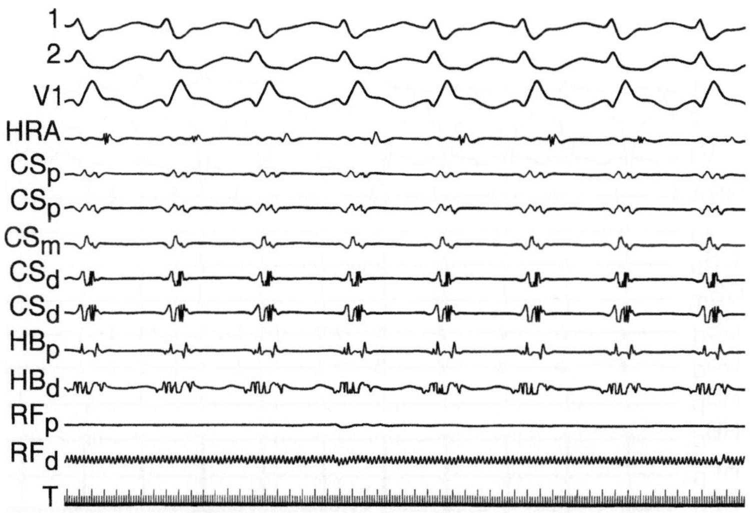

Fig. 18. Sustained tachycardia with a RBBB pattern and rightward axis. V1 suggests classical appearance of aberrant conduction intracardiac recording showing a 1:1 VA via the left side AP. A somewhat surprising aspect of this tracing is that it has no His bundle potential preceding the QRS (unlike Figs. 3–5). This is in fact VT.

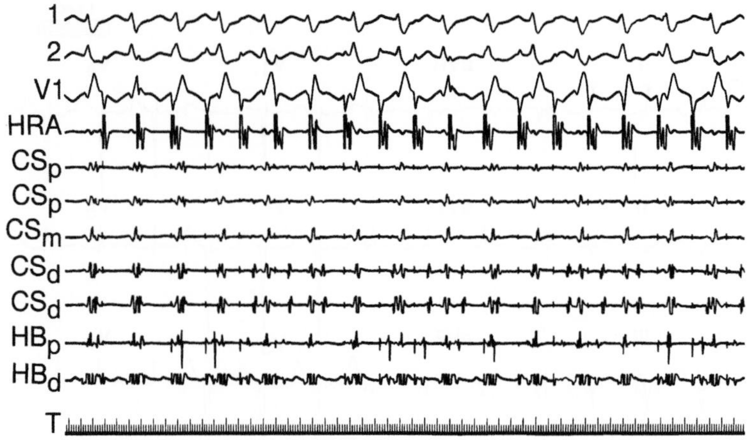

Fig. 19. Rapid atrial pacing has no effect on this tachycardia, again confirming its ventricular origin.

tracings (CSp, CSm, CSd), the proximal and distal His bundle (HBp and HBd) recordings; and timelines at 20 and 50 milliseconds (T). As can be noted, all of the intracardiac and surface activation times are within normal limits.

Atrial pacing at a basic drive and extra stimulus starts two atrial echo beats, with the second one blocking in the AV node (**Fig. 14**). The atrial activation sequence during the echo (or reciprocal) beats is eccentric, with the distal coronary sinus (left atrial) electrogram preceding others, suggesting a left posterolateral accessory pathway (AP) concealed anterogradely during sinus rhythm and right atrial pacing (see **Figs. 11 to 14**). Sustained narrow QRS tachycardia with a cycle length of 350 milliseconds is depicted in **Fig. 15**. Induction of the same orthodromic SVT with a left bundle brand block (LBBR) as shown in **Fig. 16**. The first two QRS complexes are the last of the right ventricular (RV) pacing sequence. Prolongation of ventricular (VA) interval is seen in **Fig. 16**, suggesting the left-sided AP. At this time, using radiofrequency (RF) energy application was attempted via a retrograde transaortic approach.

A few seconds after initiation of RF ablation, a slight change in the ECG was noted, and this is shown in **Fig. 17**. RF ablation stopped and the induction of SVT tried again. The next figure (**Fig. 18**) shows tachycardia with RBBB pattern with the intact AP still conducting 1:1 retrogradely. **Fig. 18** shows a classic RBBB pattern in V1 and

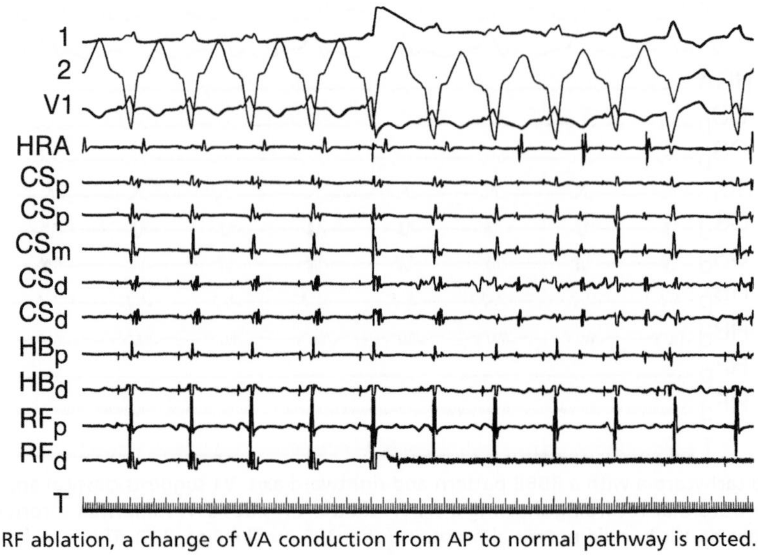

Fig. 20. During RF ablation, a change of VA conduction from AP to normal pathway is noted.

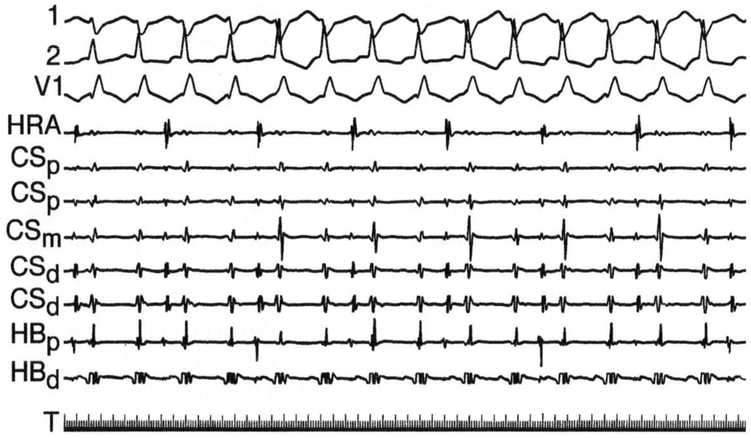

Fig. 21. Note the RB-RA VT with no VA conduction.

gives and initial impression of orthodromic SVT with an RBBB, not an unexpected finding in a patient with orthodromic SVT. On a closer examination, however, it can be appreciated that there is no His bundle potential preceding the QRS. The possibility of misplacement of electrode catheter recording the His bundle region was under consideration. When the tachycardia terminated, however, the underlying sinus recording showed that the catheter had not moved, and further leftward shift of QRS axis was noted. The tachycardia with an RBBB pattern and somewhat rightward axis did not change its rate with rapid atrial pacing (**Fig. 19**). Sinus rhythm with leftward axis was seen until it was recognized that the transaortic entry of the ablation catheter may have injured the left anterior fascicle (see **Fig. 17**).

The catheter was repositioned, and the ablation of AP was retried. Ventricular pacing with RF energy delivery is shown with **Fig. 20**. In less than a second, the VA conduction switched from AP to normal pathway. Subsequently during the waiting period, VT with a RBBB pathway was induced several times, and sinus rhythm showed continued evidence of trauma to the LBB. **Fig. 21** shows VT with right axis, and no VA conduction VT gradually subsided after all the catheters were removed.

Before ending the procedure, there was a temptation to ablate the fascicular VT, which could have been an unrecognized clinical VT. To ablate this VT would in all probability lead to a permanent left anterior hemiblock and possible LBBB. It was decided that no further ablation would be

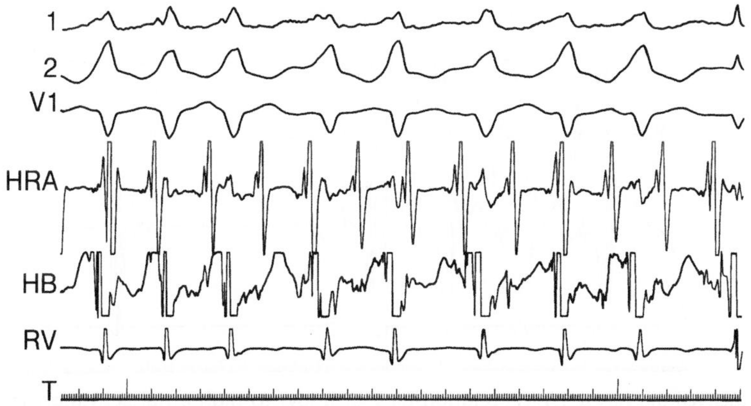

Fig. 22. The tracings are, from top to bottom, ECG leads 1, 2, V1. HRA (high right atrium), HB (His bundle), and RV (right ventricle) time (T) line at 100 and 10 milliseconds. Atrial fibrillation on the HRAs and RR variation (250 to 400 milliseconds) can be appreciated. The immediate diagnosis appeared to be atrial fibrillation with ventricular pre-excitation, most likely in the anteroseptal region.

performed, and allow the tissue recover from trauma. VT induction would be tried next day before discharge. The following day the ECG axis had normalized, and no SVT or VT could be induced.

To summarize this case

- It represents an example of traumatic (ie, iatrogenic) fascicular VT in a patient undergoing ablation for recurrent document SVT. Imagine if the patient had only the symptoms and no prior SVT documentation, and the tachycardia in **Fig. 17** was the first one induced after placement of all catheters.[25]
- The case also illustrates the value of careful observation of all surface and intercardiac ECG as the case proceeds.
- It is important to keep track of all the baseline data before any catheters are placed and continue monitoring. Iatrogenic events occur from all cardiac chambers that the catheters traverse, or ultimately reside. It can be a source of immediate and continued irritation leading to misinterpretation, hence misdiagnosis. When in doubt, take a little extra time to think it out before making a judgment with the possible undesirable consequences. When in doubt, remove the offending catheter or catheters to settle the issue.
- A subjunctional origin of tachycardia may mimic an SVT with aberration to a degree of perfection as seen in this case (see **Figs. 17, 19** and **21**), and His bundle electrogram remains valuable to distinguish

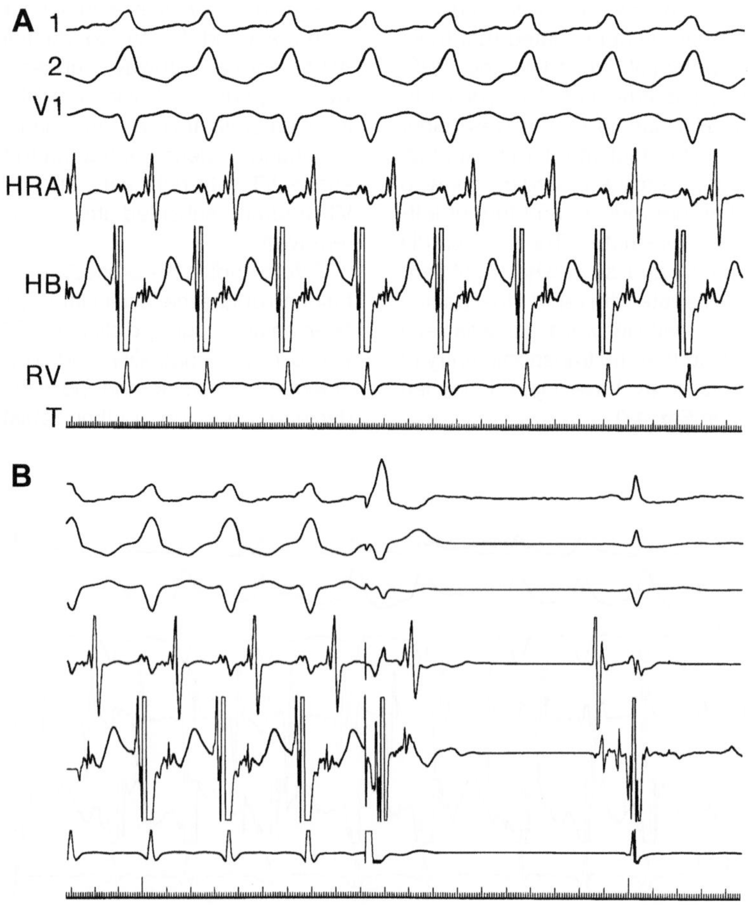

Fig. 23. Induced tachycardia has a 1:1 VA relationships with low to high atrial activation sequence. The cycle length is 330 milliseconds, and now the tachycardia is regular. A single ventricular extrastimulus terminated the tachycardia. There is a minimum of atrial pre-excitation, so whether the tachycardia is VT, AVJ, or atrial could not be clearly settled. It is clear, however, that the His bundle recording is stable, and there was no pre-excitation during sinus rhythm.

SVT from VT in patients with 1:1 AV relationships.

CASE 3

A 33-year-old physically active woman presented with a history of palpitations. While she was feeling skipped beats on and off, it had only been during the last year that she experienced episodes of continuous heart racing. She had noticed that strenuous physical exertion tended to trigger these and spontaneously stopped at rest. Several ECGs and at least one 24-hour Holter recording were unremarkable. It was decided on electrophysiology evaluation to determine the nature of arrhythmias if inducible and then direct therapy. Because of her athletic nature, she was not interested in trying any medication, particularly beta blockers.

During the initial placement of electrode catheters, she developed a wide QRS tachycardia, and when the catheters were connected, she seemed to be in atrial fibrillation (**Fig. 22**). The wide QRS tachycardia had an LBBB appearance with normal axis with irregular RR intervals and an overall rate of 200 beats/min. After waiting several minutes, the cardioversion was done to restore sinus rhythm, and it showed normal conduction intervals with no evidence of ventricular pre-excitation. To avoid catheter-induced atrial fibrillation, tachycardia induction was tried from the ventricle. The induced tachycardia is shown (**Fig. 23**). Wide QRS tachycardia has the same QRS morphology and axis but has 1:1 retrograde conduction. No identifiable His bundle potential is visible before the QRS, but this is clearly seen during sinus rhythm (see **Fig. 23**B). There is no evidence of ventricular pre-excitation, however. Up to this point, the differential diagnosis was between atrial tachycardia, AV re-entry, and VT, because the presence of an AP was a natural thought (see **Fig. 22**). When there was an opportunity to pace the atrium to dissociate it from the ventricle, the author and colleagues tried ventricular pacing instead to avoid reinduction of AF. A single ventricular extrastimulus introduced (see **Fig. 23**B) terminated the tachycardia, but there was also a slight pre-excitation of the atrium that did not help to exclude an AP.

Why think of AP in a patient who does not have any evidence of AP during sinus rhythm? There are several reasons why an AP may not manifest itself during sinus rhythm while manifesting during atrial fibrillation:

- The AP is located too far from the origin of impulse. This occurs mostly in patients who have left lateral AP, which was not the situation here.
- There is an intra-atrial block of a sinus impulse. In this situation, any impulse beyond the site of block, such as with AF, other atrial tachycardia, or pacing near the atrial insertion of the AP, unmasks AP.
- Under certain circumstances, such as with adrenergic stimulation, AP may become visible. In essence, the diagnosis of true so-called concealed AP could not be made so far.

Termination of tachycardia with ventricular extrastimulus that conducted to the atrium was not helpful; continuation of the tachycardia where ventricular extrastimulus blocks in the AV junction (**Fig. 24**) would suggest VT as the diagnosis. Fortuitously, a spontaneous atrial premature complex also occurred (see **Fig. 24**) without influencing

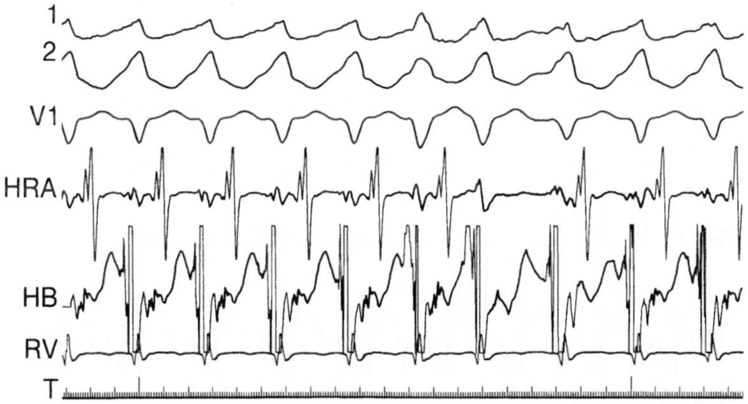

Fig. 24. A ventricular extrastimulus blocks in the AV junction. The tachycardia continues. The prior A is premature and has no effect on the subsequent QRS, indicating the independence of VT from atrial events. The A-V-V-A sequence in bottom tracing supports VT as the diagnosis.

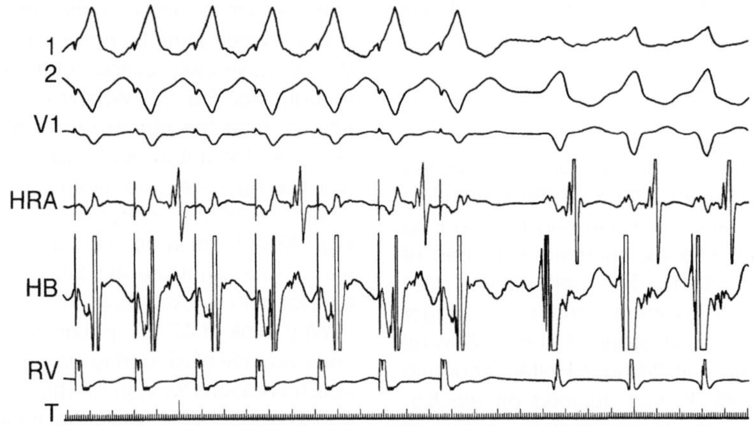

Fig. 25. VT is initiated by ventricular pacing during which a 2:1VA block is noted but the tachycardia is initiated. This and the previous figure show the sequence of A-V-V-A supporting the diagnosis of VT.

the timing of next QRS, suggesting VT as an additional diagnosis. Ventricular (V) pacing without the ventricular impulse reaching the atria (ie, [A-V-V-A] sequence shown in **Figs. 23, 25** and **26**) was fairly conclusive of VT as the mechanism. A convincing VT diagnosis can be made at this point.

A small amount of isoproterenol made the VT incessant very much in line from what may have been suggested from the clinical presentation. Because the ventricular origin is quite certain at this point, atrial pacing was tried to exclude possible coexistence of AP, a question asked at the very beginning of the case. Isolated and multiple atrial stimuli were applied and had no influence on the tachycardia (**Fig. 27**), and overdrive pacing captured the ventricle via the normal pathway with immediate resumption of VT at the cessation of pacing (**Fig. 28**). Consequently the diagnosis of RV VT in the absence of SHD[26,27] was made, and VT ablation was planned after excluding arrhythmogenic RV dysplasia with cardiac magnetic resonance imaging (MRI).

This case provides an opportunity to discuss some unique aspects of VT:

A young, otherwise healthy individual presenting with a recurrent symptoms suggestive of arrhythmia but have no prior documentation may present a diagnostic dilemma despite the help of invasive electophysiologic evaluation.

Coexistence of AF and a wide QRS tachycardia with irregular R-R intervals may at times represent two independent arrhythmias. AF in this case was neither suspected nor deliberately induced but did nonetheless create an undesirable situation and hampered electrophysiologic evaluation, necessitating direct current cardioversion.

In patients with wide QRS tachycardia with 1:1 AV relation, an identifiable His bundle deflection helps to decipher aberrant conduction from other causes. However, the very first time when a catheter could

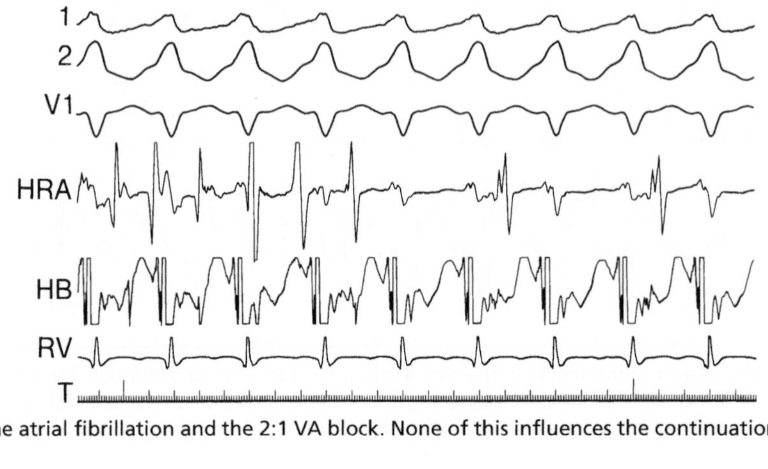

Fig. 26. Note the atrial fibrillation and the 2:1 VA block. None of this influences the continuation of tachycardia.

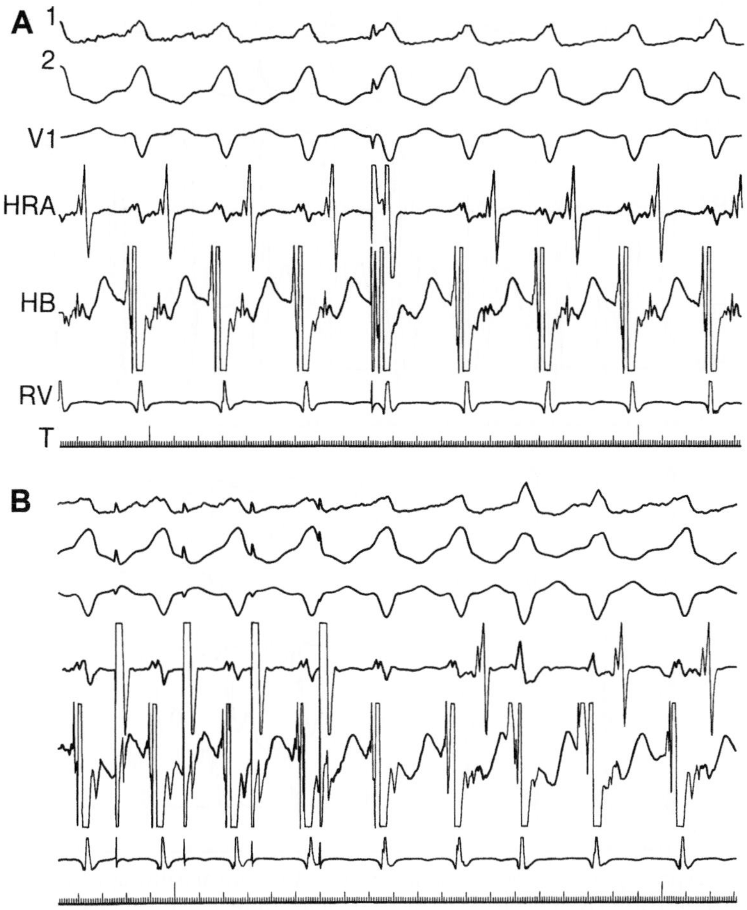

Fig. 27. *Panel A* shows a single, and *Panel B* is a series of atrial premature complexes without any effect on the cycle length of the VT.

be placed across the AV junction to record the His bundle electrogram, the patient had AF with irregular RR intervals. The inability to record the His potential could be due to many reasons, including an unsatisfactory catheter position.

Once the AF is terminated and a satisfactory catheter position is obtained, a periodic attention to a reference sinus (see **Fig. 23**) or other supraventricular-conducted complexes is important to confidently interpret tracings, because the catheter may move with change in rhythm.

To avoid inadvertent initiation of AF, atrial pacing was avoided, and ventricular stimulation was accomplished instead to demonstrate independence of ventricular event from atrial primary (as opposed to secondary) nature of the ventricular event. This gave sufficient diagnostic information to achieve clarity on other aspects of the case with atrial stimulation protocols.

A combination of LBBB and left axis morphology leads one to consider ARVD that is less likely with normal or right axis.[4] Even with the latter, ARVD should be excluded (preferably with cardiac MRI) before RV ablation for VT is done.

CASE 4

A 48-year-old man, otherwise in good health, suffered a syncopal episode and was admitted through the emergency room. He admitted prior light-headed spells and concomitant sensation of heart fluttering. His overall physical examination was unremarkable except for the cardiac findings of an ejection systolic murmur radiating to the neck. Baseline ECG (**Fig. 29**) showed sinus

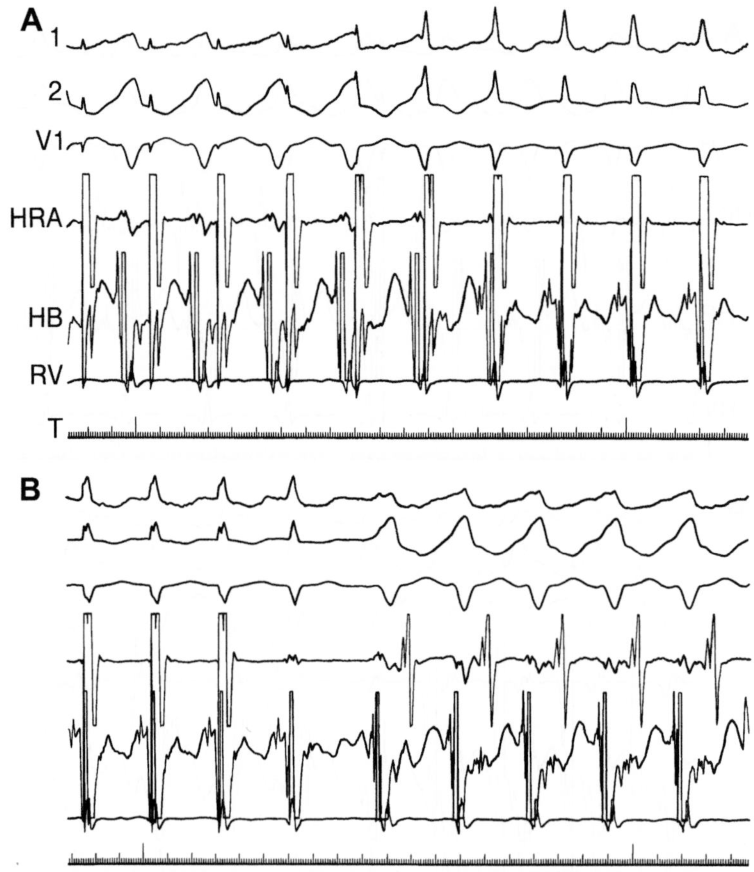

Fig. 28. Overdrive atrial pacing shows good AV conduction over the normal pathway and good His bundle potential (*Panel A*). When atrial pacing is stopped (*Panel B*), VT resumes. Note the first complex at cessation of pacing is ventricular in origin.

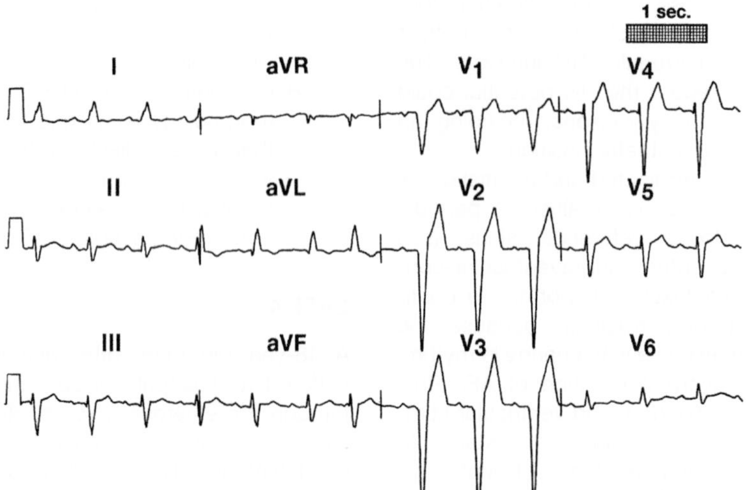

Fig. 29. 12-lead ECG shows a complete left bundle branch block (LBBB) pattern and leftward axis.

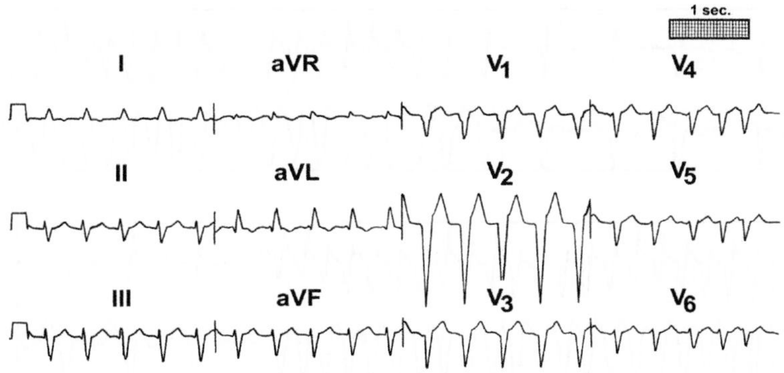

Fig. 30. 12-lead ECG of tachycardia, QRS morphology is quite similar to **Fig. 1**. Rate of the tachycardia is around 125/min. There is some acceleration of the rate at the end of tracing the exact nature of which is not clear but has the same QRS morphology.

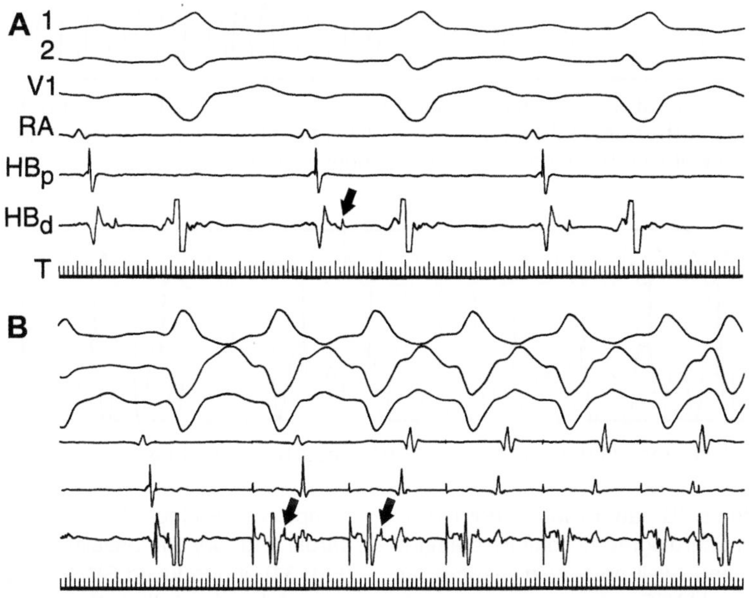

Fig. 31. Baseline EP and ECG tracing *Panel A* shows sinus rhythm with a long HV of 160 milliseconds. The H is depicted with arrows here and elsewhere in the figures. During RV pacing, the retrograde His bundle can be seen at the end of the paced QRS (retrograde RBBB), and there is short HA. A 1:1 VA conduction is noted during the last four complexes.

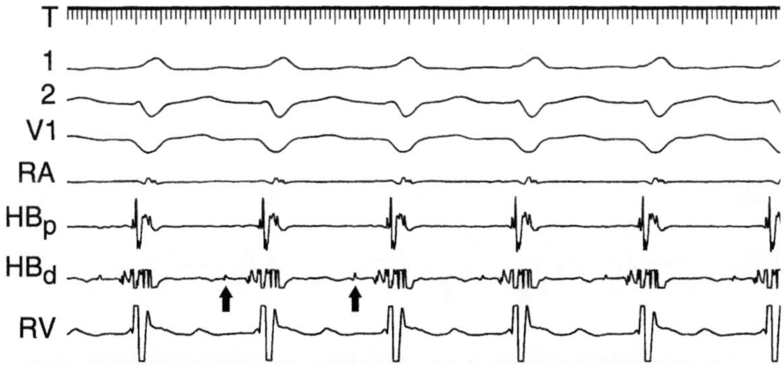

Fig. 32. Sustained AVNRT is depicted. The H-A is shorter than HV, and the cycle length of tachycardia is 510 milliseconds. This tachycardia did not produce any symptoms.

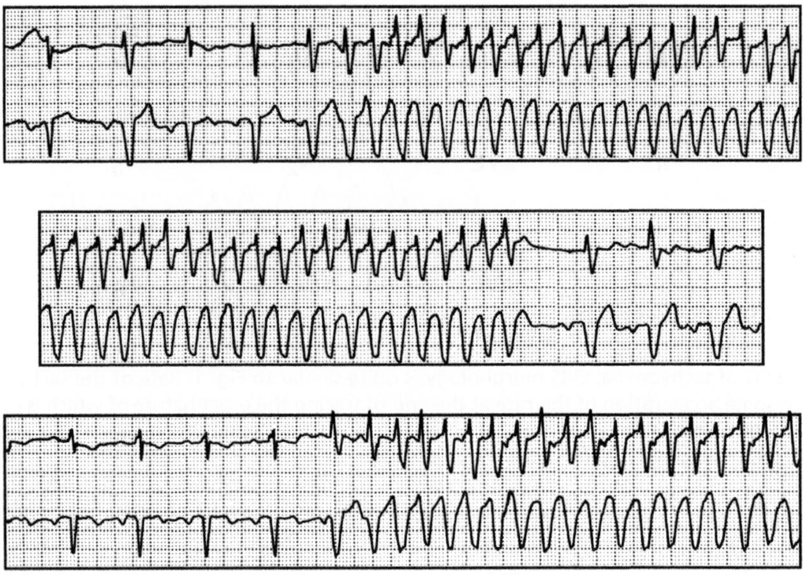

Fig. 33. Spontaneous runs of wide QRS tachycardia are seen. Please note the baseline ECG shows incomplete to complete LBBB pattern. The tachycardia morphology is similar to sinus rhythm in the middle panel, and PR before the first beat of tachycardia is shorter even though the sinus is on time.

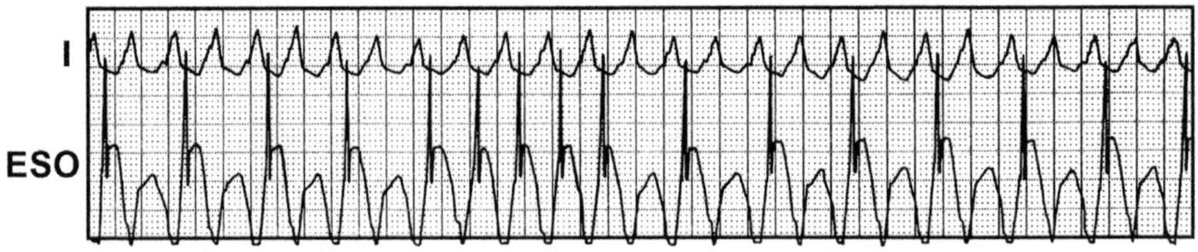

Fig. 34. Esophageal electrogram shows a 2:1 and 1:1 VA conduction indicating VT as the diagnosis.

rhythm, complete LBBB pattern with a borderline left axis (-30). Echocardiography confirmed a tight aortic stenosis and well-preserved ventricular function with normal LVEF.

A valve replacement was scheduled, and the patient underwent preoperative evaluation for possible arrhythmic etiology to explain his symptoms. Surface 12-lead ECG of the tachycardia (**Fig. 30**) and baseline intracardiac tracings (**Fig. 31**) and induced SVT (**Fig. 32**) are shown. It was determined that the induced tachycardia was slow–fast AVNRT. In view of the fact the patient had a prolonged PR mostly due to prolonged HV (160 milliseconds), possibility of BBR

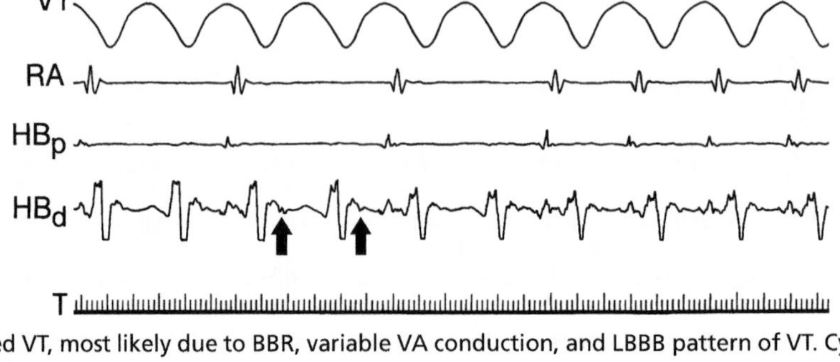

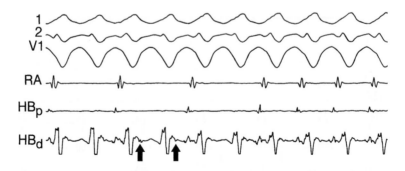

Fig. 35. Sustained VT, most likely due to BBR, variable VA conduction, and LBBB pattern of VT. Cycle length of VT is 300 milliseconds.

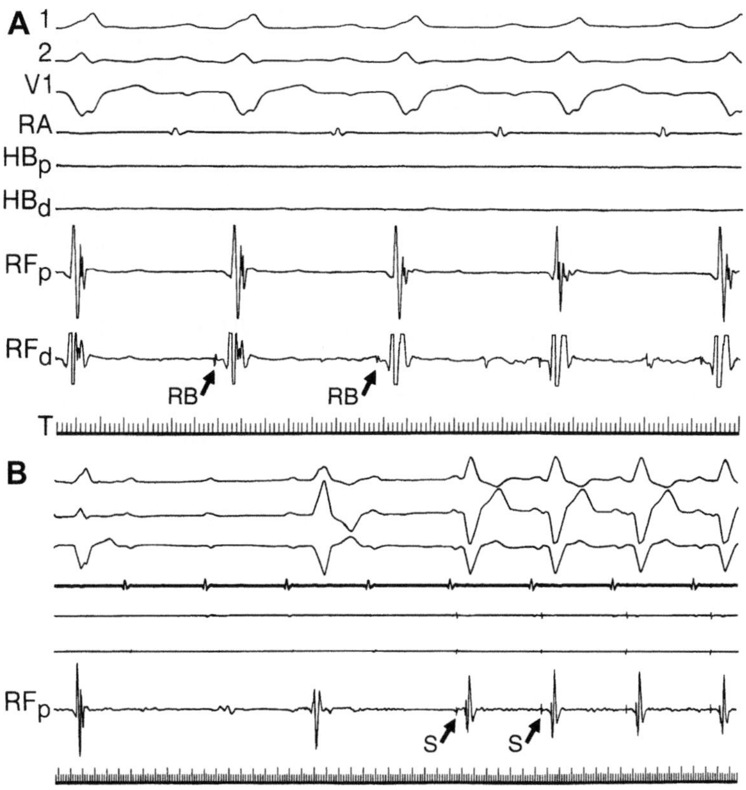

Fig. 36. Recording of distal RB and temporary pacing after creation of complete AV block after ablation of RBB (*Panels A and B*).

was entertained but could not be induced, and the patient underwent slow AV nodal pattern ablation and returned to his room. Aortic valve surgery was performed the next day.

The initial postoperative recovery was uneventful. On the third postoperative day, the patient developed several nonsustained and some sustained runs of wide QRS tachycardia (**Fig. 33**). It showed on surface ECG lead 1 and MCL1 (modified chest lead V1). The sinus rhythm was associated with rate-related LBB. The wide QRS tachycardia has a configuration of a LBBB pattern similar to that seen during sinus rhythm (last three sinus complexes in the middle panel). All three panels—top, middle and bottom—are continuous. It should be further noted that at the onset of tachycardia the PR of the first complex shortens and that the first QRS complex and the rest of the tachycardic complexes are similar. This tachycardia has a much shorter cycle length than the ones previously recorded, and it reproduced the patient's symptom of presyncope even in a supine position. VT instead of AVNRT was suspected, but because of inability to identify the P wave, VT or SVT could not be diagnosed definitively. Because the episodes were quite frequent, and the diagnosis was critical, a bedside esophageal (eso) electrogram was tried (**Fig. 34**) and correct diagnosis made. The figure depicts a variable VA block during the tachycardia on the esophageal tracing (see **Fig. 34**).

A repeat electrophysiological evaluation was done with the expectation that BBR was the most likely culprit and was facilitated by the recent valve surgery and would be readily inducible.[22] Because the patient had a recent prosthetic valve, LBB ablation was not feasible, and RBB ablation was planned instead with a pacemaker to follow, as AV block was anticipated. Sustained VT with an LBBB pattern with longer HV with variable VA block (**Fig. 35**) was induced. Even though the His bundle (arrows) recording was difficult to identify, a high index of clinical suspicion suggested BBR, and RBB ablation was accomplished (**Fig. 36**). BBR was suggested by

A combination of aortic valvular disease and normal LVEF

A prolonged HV interval during sinus rhythm

LBB delay rather than block in the anterograde direction (rate-related LBBB seen in **Fig. 34**)

Retrograde RBBB and anterograde LBBB (see **Fig. 31**) The top panel shows a long HV with a LBBB during sinus rhythm.

The long HV either represents a prolonged intra-His or RBB conduction delay or both. There is also evidence of retrograde RBBB or delay during baseline ventricular pacing as evidenced by recognizable His bundle potential following the local ventricular electrogram. In short, there was evidence of extensive HPS disease in anterograde and retrograde direction, an essential prerequisite for BBR. At the same time, normal LVEF limits the scenarios for myocardial VT:

Similarity of QRS complex morphology between sinus and VT complexes coexisting with intermittent VA block narrows it down to BBR as the most likely diagnosis for the more rapid tachycardia

The final proof for BBR when RB ablation eliminates all the inducible VT.

Some interesting aspects of this case are as follows

It is always critical to address the patient's relevant arrhythmia. The patient came for a specific problem (ie, syncope in cases 2 and 4), and until that is figured out, management is not complete. Both of these cases had induced arrhythmia, which in some patients will be sufficient to explain the symptoms, but was not the case here. There were sufficient clues to indicate the possibility of coexisting, more life-threatening arrhythmia, and induction of AVNRT led to a false sense of possible successful outcome, necessitating a second EP study.

Rapid 1:1 VA is uncommon in patients with VT, but clearly possible, as all of these cases demonstrate. In settings like these, the driving (primary) arrhythmia SVT versus VT determination becomes difficult, and a dissociation of atrial activity from ventricular activity becomes crucial.

In the case of a normal left ventricular function, BBR can occur in patients with valvular disease in a high proportion of cases.[23,24] Regardless, however, the presence of prolonged HPS time (HV) intervals should alert one to seriously consider BBR as the mechanism of wide QRS tachycardia, in any setting.

Although many patients with dilated cardiomyopathy have fairly low LVEF, and a cardioverter–defibrillator (CD) is often implanted, one might choose CD implant over bundle branch ablation. This is, however, not an option in patients with BBR and preserved LVEF, because bundle branch ablation and not the CD is the appropriate treatment.

ACKNOWLEDGMENTS

The author acknowledges the assistance of Laurel J. Landis, Brian P. Miller, Indrajit Choudhuri, MD in the preparation of this manuscript.

REFERENCES

1. Josephson ME, Waxman HL, Cain ME, et al. Ventricular activation during ventricular endocardial pacing, II: role of pace-mapping to localize origin of ventricular tachycardia. Am J Cardiol 1982;50:11–22.
2. Mason JW. Electrophysiology study versus electrocardiographic monitoring investigators: a comparison of electrophysiologic testing with Holter monitoring to predict antiarrhythmic drug efficacy for ventricular tachycarrthythmias. N Engl J Med 1993;329:445.
3. De Bakker JMT, Van Capelle FJL, Janse MJ, et al. Reentry as a cause of ventricular tachycardia in patients with chronic ischemic heart disease: Electrophysiologic and anatomic correlation. Circulation 1988;77:589–606.
4. Peters S, Peters H, Thierfelder L. Risk stratification of sudden cardiac death and malignant ventricular arrhythmias in right ventricular dysplasia/cardiomyopathy. Int J Cardiol 1999;71:243–50.
5. Brugada J, Brugada R, Brugada P. right bundle-branch block and ST-segment elevation in leads V1 through V3: a marker for sudden death in patients without demonstrable structural heart disease. Circulation 1998;897:457–60.
6. Stevenson WG, Friedman PL, Sager PT, et al. Exploring postinfarction reentrant ventricular tachycardia with entrainment mapping. J Am Coll Cardiol 1997;29:1180–9.
7. Blanck Z, Dhala A, Deshpande S, et al. Bundle branch reentrant ventricular tachycardia: cumulative experience in 48 patients. J Cardiovasc Electrophysiol 1993;4:253.
8. Antzelevitch C, Brugada P, Brugada J, et al. Brugada syndrome: 1992–2002: a historical perspective. J Am Coll Cardiol 2003;41:1665–71.
9. Akhtar M. Clinical spectrum of ventricular tachycardia. Circulation 1990;82:1561–73.

10. Janse MJ, Wit AL. Electrophysiological mechanisms of ventricular arrhythmias resulting from myocardial ischemia and infarction. Physiol Rev 1989;69: 1049–169.
11. Lahat H, Pras E, Olender T, et al. A missense mutation n a highly conserved region of CASQ2 is associated with autosomal recessive catecholamine-induced polymorphic ventricular tachycardia in Bedouin families from Israel. Am J Hum Genet 2001;69:1378–84.
12. Brugada P, Brugada R, Anztzelevitch C, et al. The Brugada syndrome. In: Zipes D, Jalife J, editors. Cardiac electrophysiology from cell to bedside. Philadelphia: WB Saunders. 2004. p. 625–32.
13. Schwartz PJ, Periti M, Malliani A. The long QT syndrome. Am Heart J 1975;89:378–90.
14. Schwartz PJ, Moss AJ, Vincent GM, et al. Diagnostic criteria for the long QT syndrome: an update. Circulation 1993;88:782–4.
15. Akhtar M, Shenasa M, Jazayeri M, et al. Wide QRS complex tachycardia. Reappraisal of a common clinical problem. Ann Intern Med 1988;109:905–12.
16. Wellens HJJ, Bar FWHM, Lie KI. The value of the electrocardiogram in the differential diagnosis of a tachycardia with a widened QRS complex. Am J Med 1978;64:27–33.
17. Miller JM. The many manifestations of ventricular tachycardia. J Cardiovasc Electrophysiol 1992;3:88–107.
18. Steinman RT, Herrera C, Schuger CD, et al. Wide QRS tachycardia in the conscious adult. Ventricular tachycardia is the most frequent cause. JAMA 1989; 261:1013–6.
19. Jackman WM, Beckman KJ, McClelland JH, et al. Treatment of supraventricular tachycardia due to atrioventricular nodal reentry by radiofrequency catheter ablation of slow-pathway conduction. N Engl J Med 1992;327:313–8.
20. Haissaguerre M, Gaita F, Fischer B, et al. Elimination of atrioventricular nodal reentrant tachycardia using discrete slow potentials to guide application of radiofrequency energy. Circulation 1992;85: 2162–75.
21. Jazayeri MR, Hempe SL, Sra JS, et al. Selective transcatheter ablation of the fast and slow pathways using radiofrequency energy in patients with atrioventricular nodal reentrant tachycardia. Circulation 1992;85:1318–28.
22. Narasimhan C, Jazayeri MR, Sra J, et al. Ventricular tachycardia in valvular heart disease. Circulation 1997;96:4307–13.
23. Blanck Z, Jazayeri M, Akhtar M. Facilitation of sustained bundle branch reentry by atrial fibrillation. J Cardiovasc Electrophysiol 1996;7:348–52.
24. Akhtar M, Damato AN, Batsford WP, et al. Demonstration of re-entry within the His-Purkinje system in man. Circulation 1974;50:1150.
25. Akhtar M, Damato AN, Gilbert-Leeds CJ, et al. Induction of iatrogenic electrocardiographic patterns during electrophysiologic studies. Circulation 1977;56:60.
26. Hair TE Jr, Eagen JT, Orgain ES. Paroxysmal ventricular tachycardia in the absence of demonstrable heart disease. Am J Cardiol 1962;9:209–14.
27. Lerman BB, Stein KM, Markowitz SM, et al. Recent advances in right ventricular outflow tract tachycardia. Card Electrophysiol Rev 1999;3: 210–4.

Approach to Cardiac Device Malfunction

Byron K. Lee, MD

KEYWORDS

• Cardiac device • Malfunction • Reprogramming
• Technical assistance

The evaluation of a patient with a new complaint related to his or her implanted cardiac device should always begin with taking a careful history. This point cannot be overemphasized. Too frequently on interrogation, clinicians find suboptimal settings and make corresponding programming changes, but fail to make the appropriate change to alleviate the patient's main presenting symptom.

After a careful history, doing a brief physical examination is frequently helpful. Looking at the device pocket is necessary if the patient complains of pain or discomfort in that region. Listening to the heart and lungs is important if the patient complains of palpitations or shortness of breath.

Next is the actual interrogation of the device. The new devices have many self-diagnostic features that will alert the clinician during interrogation of new problems such as a sudden increase in lead impedance or threshold. The device log and rate histograms can also be helpful in alerting one to any new arrhythmias that the patient may be experiencing. Although many of the new devices perform automatic threshold and sensitivity checks, it is important to be able to do these processes manually. Threshold and sensitivity issues may occur only transiently, and the last recorded automatic check may be erroneous.

Once the taking of history, physical examination, and interrogation of the device are finished, a plan needs to be formulated and executed. Frequently, this only involves a simple reprogramming of the device. Other times it may require further testing, such as a chest X-ray for a patient with a new increase in lead threshold possibly caused by lead dislodgment or a stress test for a patient with new frequent premature ventricular contractions. When the intervention is reprogramming of the device, one should consider asking patients to return to the device clinic soon after. Reprogramming for nonspecific symptoms such as palpitations may require some degree of trial and error. Sometimes the patients feel worse after reprogramming, and a change back to the original settings may be required.

Finally, all clinicians should acknowledge that the current implantable cardiac devices are immensely complex. A single person cannot know all the features of every device from every manufacturer. Therefore, it is crucial for clinicians to be comfortable with calling on the device company's representative or its technical services for help. The possibility exists that the patient's symptoms are caused by a software glitch that was purposely not well advertised.

In summary, dealing with cardiac device malfunctions can be fun. Most of the time, the cause of the patient's new symptom can be discovered and alleviated. However, the clinician needs to approach the patient in a step-by-step manner and humbly ask for technical assistance when necessary.

UCSF Medical Center, Cardiac Electrophysiology and Arrhythmia Service, 500 Parnassus Avenue, Box 1354, San Francisco, CA 94143-1354, USA
E-mail address: leeb@medicine.ucsf.edu

Card Electrophysiol Clin 2 (2010) 267
doi:10.1016/j.ccep.2010.01.012
1877-9182/10/$ – see front matter

Right Atrial Isolation After Maze Procedure Discovered at the Time of Pacemaker Implantation

José Dizon, MD[a,*], Daniel Wang, MD[a],
Michael Argenziano, MD[b]

KEYWORDS

• Atrial fibrillation • Pacemaker • Maze procedure

Ablation procedures for atrial fibrillation have resulted in clinical benefit for many patients.[1,2] They have also generated interesting clinical scenarios, intended or not, as a result of the ablation lesions.[3–5] This article describes the case of a gentleman who required a permanent pacemaker after mitral valve replacement and a modified maze procedure, with an unusual observation after right atrial lead insertion.

CASE REPORT

The patient is a 56-year-old man with a history of mitral regurgitation and paroxysmal atrial fibrillation (AF). He had a mitral valve repair in 2004 and 2 previous attempts at catheter ablation for AF at an outside institution. These procedures had failed, and he was maintained on metoprolol, 100 mg twice a day, as well as dofetilide, 250 μg twice a day. Because of recurrent severe mitral regurgitation and paroxysmal AF with rapid ventricular rates, he was referred to the authors' institution for mitral valve replacement and intraoperative maze procedure. The maze procedure consisted of a radiofrequency box lesion around the pulmonary veins plus a connecting lesion from the box to the mitral annulus. In the right atrium, there was a lateral incision between the venae cavae with connecting radiofrequency lesions to the tricuspid annulus from the superior and inferior aspects of the intercaval line. The procedure occurred without immediate complications, but in the early postoperative course it was noted that the patient would alternate between rapid AF at more than 140 beats per minutes (bpm) and a junctional rhythm at 35 bpm (**Fig. 1**). A dual-chamber pacemaker was deemed appropriate for presumed tachy-brady syndrome. The implant occurred while the patient was in apparent rapid AF. During implant of the atrial lead, which was positioned in the high lateral right atrium, it was noted that the atrial electrogram had a regular high-amplitude signal with a smaller signal that corresponded to the simultaneous signal on the ventricular channel (**Fig. 2**). This pattern persisted despite moving the atrial lead more inferior or septal. Pacing and sensing thresholds and impedance measurement were otherwise normal for the atrial lead. Atrial pacing at rapid rates failed to affect the ventricular signal in any way.

CLINICAL QUESTION

Given these findings, what is the electrophysiologic explanation and how would one program the pacemaker?

[a] Division of Cardiology, Columbia University, 630 West, 168th Street, New York, NY 10032, USA
[b] Division of Cardiothoracic Surgery, Columbia University, 177 Fort Washington Avenue, New York, NY 10032, USA
* Corresponding author.
E-mail address: jmd11@columbia.edu

Card Electrophysiol Clin 2 (2010) 269–271
doi:10.1016/j.ccep.2010.01.015
1877-9182/10/$ – see front matter

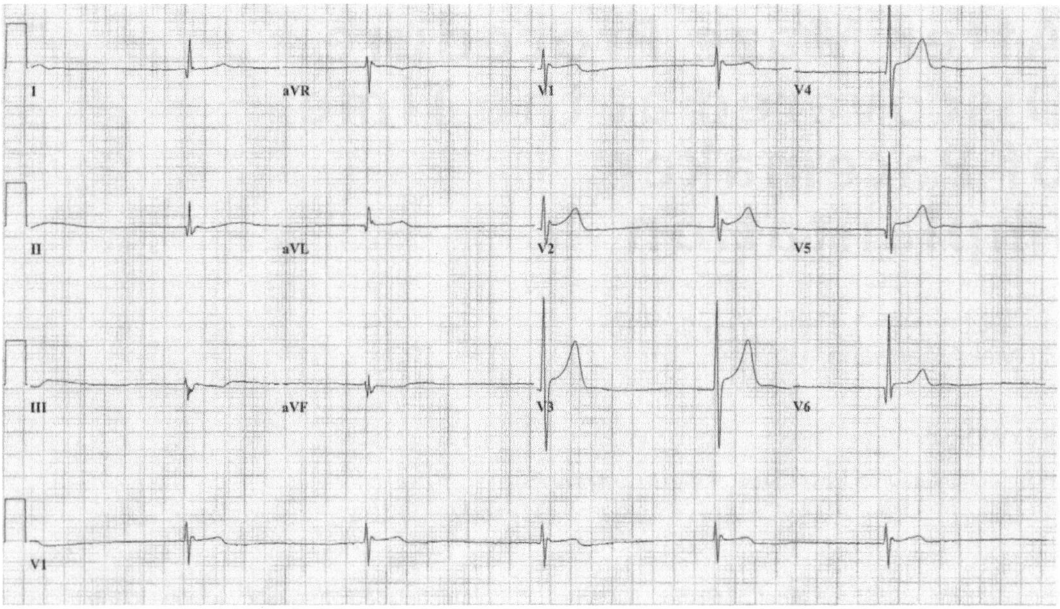

Fig. 1. A 12-lead electrocardiogram showing slow junctional rhythm after spontaneous termination of atrial fibrillation.

DISCUSSION

This case demonstrates an unusual result after the maze procedure with probable contributions from prior catheter ablation. Although catheter and operative procedures for AF are designed to isolate the pulmonary veins and prevent macroreentrant atrial tachycardias, the unintended effect can be proarrhythmia or, in this case, isolation of other structures. The right atrium was in sinus rhythm but was dissociated from the left atrium and, in addition, was isolated from the atrioventricular (AV) node. The small signals in the right atrial channel were from far-field sensing of the ventricular signal. Because of the inability

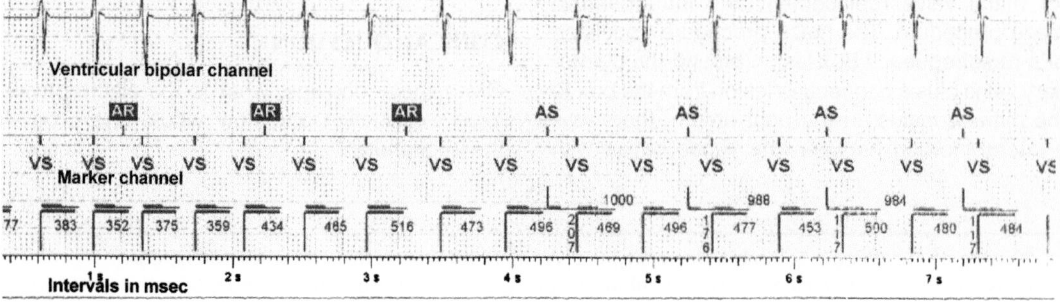

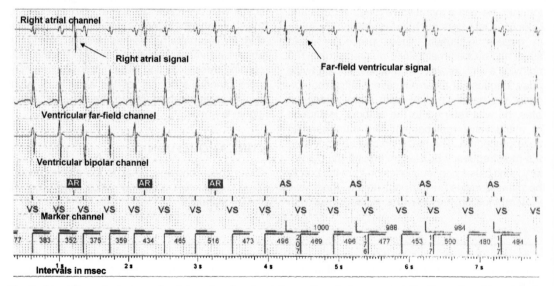

Fig. 2. Recording using pacemaker telemetry showing intracardiac electrograms at the time of rapid ventricular rates during pacemaker implant. Note the regular high amplitude signals representing sinus rhythm in the right atrial channel, with smaller signals corresponding to far-field ventricular sensing. The right atrium is electrically dissociated from the rest of the heart.

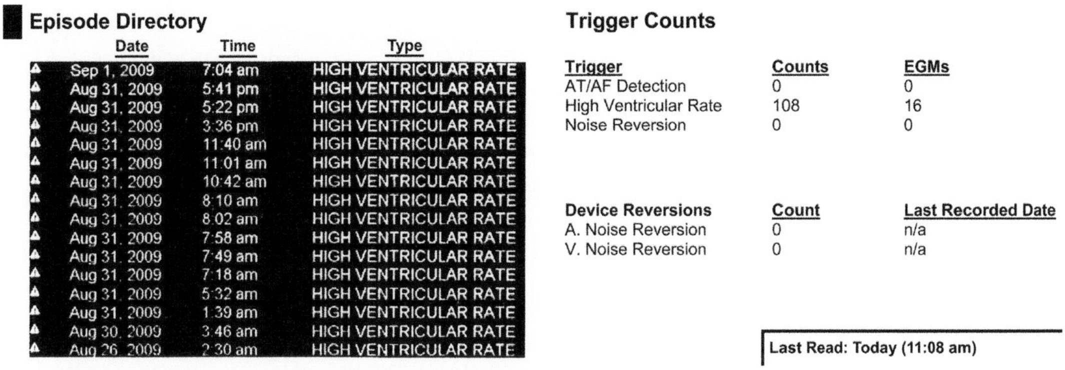

Episode Directory

Date	Time	Type
Sep 1, 2009	7:04 am	HIGH VENTRICULAR RATE
Aug 31, 2009	5:41 pm	HIGH VENTRICULAR RATE
Aug 31, 2009	5:22 pm	HIGH VENTRICULAR RATE
Aug 31, 2009	3:36 pm	HIGH VENTRICULAR RATE
Aug 31, 2009	11:40 am	HIGH VENTRICULAR RATE
Aug 31, 2009	11:01 am	HIGH VENTRICULAR RATE
Aug 31, 2009	10:42 am	HIGH VENTRICULAR RATE
Aug 31, 2009	8:10 am	HIGH VENTRICULAR RATE
Aug 31, 2009	8:02 am	HIGH VENTRICULAR RATE
Aug 31, 2009	7:58 am	HIGH VENTRICULAR RATE
Aug 31, 2009	7:49 am	HIGH VENTRICULAR RATE
Aug 31, 2009	7:18 am	HIGH VENTRICULAR RATE
Aug 31, 2009	5:32 am	HIGH VENTRICULAR RATE
Aug 31, 2009	1:39 am	HIGH VENTRICULAR RATE
Aug 30, 2009	3:46 am	HIGH VENTRICULAR RATE
Aug 26, 2009	2:30 am	HIGH VENTRICULAR RATE

Trigger Counts

Trigger	Counts	EGMs
AT/AF Detection	0	0
High Ventricular Rate	108	16
Noise Reversion	0	0

Device Reversions	Count	Last Recorded Date
A. Noise Reversion	0	n/a
V. Noise Reversion	0	n/a

Last Read: Today (11:08 am)

Fig. 3. Pacemaker log taken days after implant showing multiple high-ventricular-rate episodes. Despite this, the atrial tachycardia/AF detection counts are zero, indicating inability of the device to detect AF and mode switch.

to sense the left atrium, the device is incapable of mode switching, as evidenced by a device log days after the procedure (**Fig. 3**, note multiple ventricular high-rate episodes from rapid AF, without atrial tachycardia or AF counts). Hence programming to dual-lead pacemaker that paces and senses in atrium and ventricle (DDD) mode is inappropriate because it will result in inappropriate right atrial pacing during AF. However, when the left atrial arrhythmia terminates, sinus rhythm in the right atrium is incapable of conducting to the ventricle and a junctional rhythm ensues, and so a dual-chamber mode is still desirable. Therefore the dual-chamber pacing and sensing, but inhibited (DDI) mode was selected as the best option. In this mode, when the patient is in AF, the atrial and ventricular outputs will be inhibited by conducted ventricular responses that are higher than the programmed lower rate limit. When the patient is not in AF, the device will track sinus activity in the right atrium and pace the ventricle, or AV sequentially pace if the sinus rate is less than the programmed lower rate limit. On follow-up after 2 months thus far, the patient is relatively asymptomatic, with approximately 75% AV pacing and 25% high ventricular rates by the pacemaker event logs. The latter are mitigated by the use of metoprolol, 100 mg by mouth twice a day.

This case highlights the potential effects of multiple ablation lesions within the atria as well as the need to modify pacemaker programming based on presenting electrophysiologic and clinical scenarios.

REFERENCES

1. Prasad SM, Maniar HS, Camillo CJ, et al. The Cox maze III procedure for atrial fibrillation: long-term efficacy in patients undergoing lone versus concomitant procedures. J Thorac Cardiovasc Surg 2003;126(6):1822–8.
2. Pappone C, Rosiano S, Oreto G, et al. Circumferential radiofrequency ablation of pulmonary vein ostia: a new anatomic approach for curing atrial fibrillation. Circulation 2000;102(21):2619–28.
3. Morady F, Oral H, Chugh A. Diagnosis and ablation of atypical atrial tachycardia and flutter complicating atrial fibrillation ablation. Heart Rhythm 2009;6(Suppl 8):S29–32.
4. Wazni OM, Saliba W, Fahmy T, et al. Atrial arrhythmias after surgical maze: findings during catheter ablation. J Am Coll Cardiol 2006;48(7):1405–9.
5. Albage A, Lindblom D, Insulander P, et al. Electrophysiological evaluation of the sinus node and the cardiac conduction system following the maze procedure for atrial fibrillation. Pacing Clin Electrophysiol 2004;27(2):194–203.

The Path Less Taken

Prashant D. Bhave, MD[a,*], Byron K. Lee, MD[b]

KEYWORDS

• Pacemaker • Lead • Malposition • Complications • ASD

CASE REPORT

An 85-year-old man presented to the cardiology clinic for follow-up. He received a dual-chamber pacemaker at another institution about 5 years ago for symptomatic bradycardia. The patient was subsequently lost to follow-up for several years. He reports no significant recent changes in his health. He does recall a syncopal episode 2 years ago, which occurred in the setting of excessive alcohol use. He has not had any repeat syncopal episodes.

Interrogation of the patient's device reveals a St Jude Medical (St Paul, MN, USA) Identity XLDR dual-chamber pacemaker. Both the atrial and ventricular leads have adequate sensed amplitudes and normal capture thresholds; lead impedances are also within normal limits. The device is programmed to dual-chamber adaptive-rate (DDDR) mode with backup ventricular rate set at 50 beats per minute. Ninety-five percent of QRS complexes are v-paced. The electrocardiogram (ECG) is shown in **Fig. 1**.

CLINICAL QUESTION

Is there anything unusual about the patient's ECG that warrants further investigation?

DISCUSSION

In a dual-chamber pacing system, the leads are typically placed in the right atrium and the right ventricle. The resultant ventricular-paced QRS complex almost always has left bundle branch block morphology. This patient's ECG shows a paced QRS complex, which has right bundle branch block morphology. This should immediately raise suspicion that the ventricular lead is malpositioned and may actually be in the coronary sinus or left ventricle. Leads can enter the left ventricle via septal perforation, via migration across an atrial or ventricular septal defect, or if a retrograde arterial path is accidentally taken. It should be noted that a safe right ventricular pacing position can sometimes produce a right bundle branch block pattern in the precordial leads (usually V1 and V2), particularly if the lead tip is against the septum.[1] Nonetheless, further investigation is prudent. Chest radiography and transthoracic echocardiography are the best initial tests to evaluate lead position in this scenario.

The chest radiograph (**Fig. 2**) shows the ventricular lead following a posterior trajectory, raising concern that the lead is not in the right ventricle. A transthoracic echocardiogram (**Fig. 3**) clearly shows the ventricular pacing lead crossing the interatrial septum into the left atrium, passing through the mitral valve, and entering the left ventricle.

PACEMAKER LEAD IN THE LEFT VENTRICLE

Whether the result of initial misplacement or migration, pacemaker lead implantation in the left ventricle is a known complication of pacemaker insertion. The patient's ventricular pacemaker lead had crossed an atrial septal defect and lodged in his left ventricle. The pacemaker is functioning properly, but there are some interesting management decisions that must be made.

The first is the question of whether or not to remove the left ventricular lead. The pacer lead is

[a] Department of Cardiology, University of California San Francisco Medical Center, 505 Parnassus Avenue, M1186, San Francisco, CA 94121, USA
[b] Department of Cardiology, University of California San Francisco Medical Center, Electrophysiology Service, 500 Parnassus Avenue, San Francisco, CA 94143-1354, USA
* Corresponding author.
E-mail address: prashant.bhave@ucsf.edu

Card Electrophysiol Clin 2 (2010) 273–275
doi:10.1016/j.ccep.2010.01.014
1877-9182/10/$ – see front matter

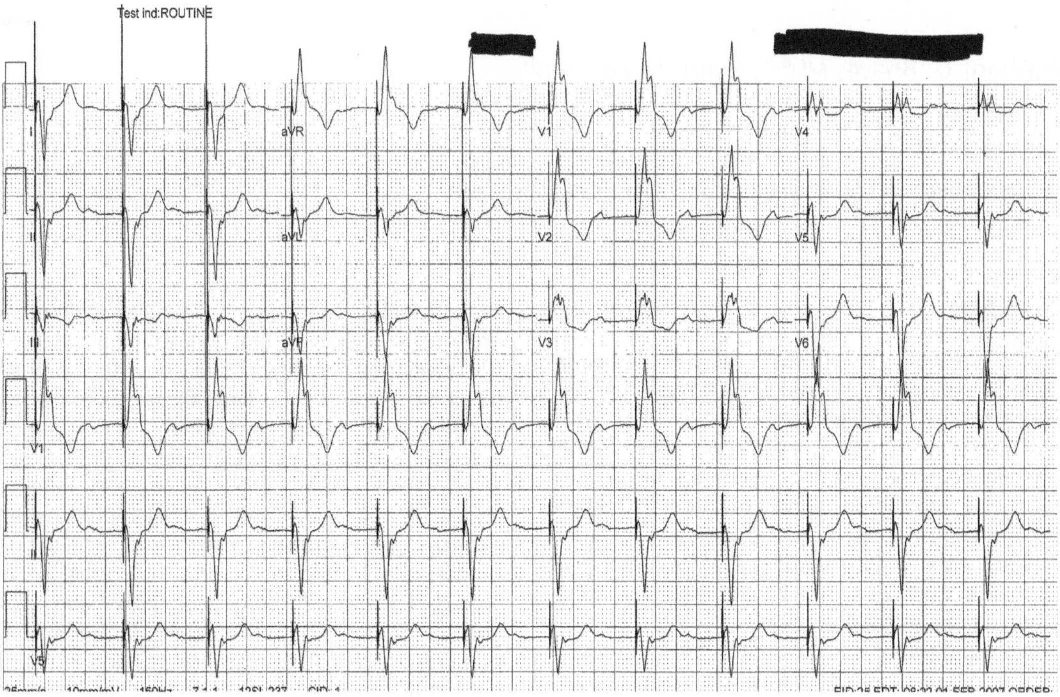

Fig. 1. ECG.

a potential source of arterial thromboembolism. There is a consensus in the literature that a left ventricular lead should be removed percutaneously if the diagnosis is made shortly after implantation. There are case reports of successful percutaneous left ventricular lead extraction up to 10 months after implantation.[2] This patient's device was placed several years earlier. The chronicity of the left ventricular lead increases the risk of perforation or thromboembolism during percutaneous extraction. Surgical removal of the left ventricular lead, which would involve a thoracotomy, could be considered. The patient made the decision not to pursue percutaneous extraction or surgical lead removal.

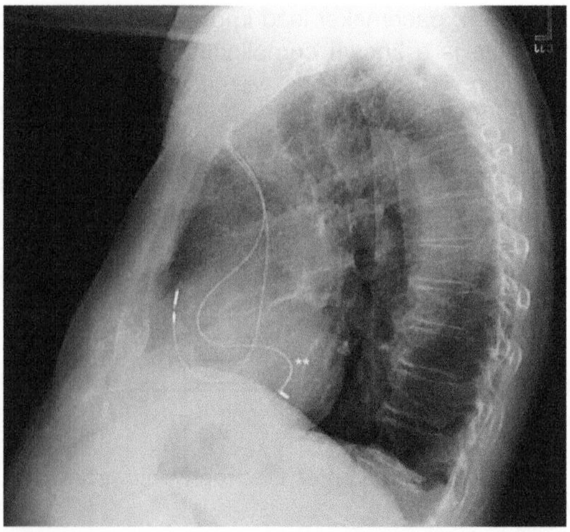

Fig. 2. Lateral chest radiograph. The ventricular lead (**) follows a posterior trajectory, suggesting that it does not terminate in the right ventricle.

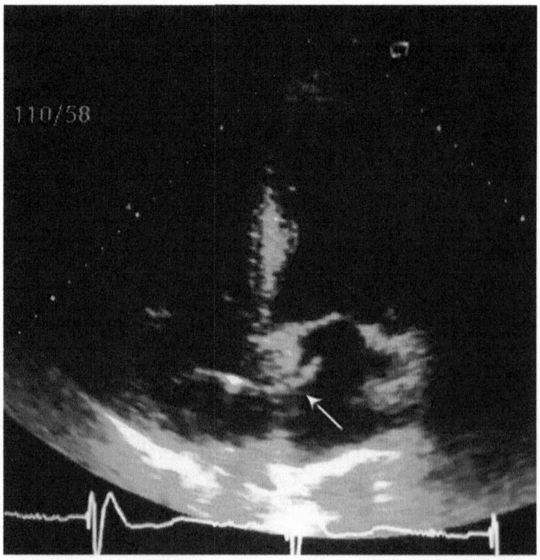

Fig. 3. Transthoracic echocardiogram. The transvenous pacing lead (*arrow*) is seen to cross an atrial septal defect in this apical 4-chamber view.

Next, we had to decide whether or not to recommend anticoagulation. There are numerous case reports of embolic stroke in patients with a pacemaker lead in the left ventricle who were not taking warfarin. Small case series of patients who had endocardial left ventricular leads placed intentionally (to achieve biventricular pacing) have shown a low incidence of thromboembolism when the patients are administered warfarin as anticoagulant.[3] Similarly, a large case series of patients with left ventricular assist devices (LVAD) showed a 3% long-term stroke risk in patients taking warfarin.[4–8] Of note, a significant percentage of the LVAD patients who suffered a stroke had a subtherapeutic international normalized ratio. Our patient started taking warfarin and has had no manifest thromboembolic events in 3 years of follow-up.

SUMMARY

This case illustrates the importance of obtaining and carefully analyzing a paced ECG immediately after pacemaker implantation. Early recognition of a malpositioned lead in the left ventricle would allow correction before the lead becomes difficult to remove. Chest radiography and echocardiography are simple tests that can help confirm appropriate lead placement.

REFERENCES

1. Erdogan O, Aksu F. Right bundle branch block pattern during right ventricular permanent pacing: Is it safe or not? Indian Pacing Electrophysiol J 2007;7(3):187–91.
2. Trohman RG, Wilkoff BL, Byrne T, et al. Successful percutaneous extraction of a chronic left ventricular pacing lead. Pacing Clin Electrophysiol 1991;14(10):1448–51.
3. Leclercq F, Hager FX, Macia JC, et al. Left ventricular lead insertion using a modified transseptal catheterization technique: a totally endocardial approach for permanent biventricular pacing in end-stage heart failure. Pacing Clin Electrophysiol 1999;22(11):1570–5.
4. Boyle AJ, Russell SD, Teuteberg JJ, et al. Low thromboembolism and pump thrombosis with the HeartMate II left ventricular assist device: analysis of outpatient anti-coagulation. J Heart Lung Transplant 2009;28(9):881–7.
5. de Cock CC, van Campen CM, Kamp O, et al. Successful percutaneous extraction of an inadvertently placed left ventricular pacing lead. Europace 2003;5(2):195–7.
6. McManus DD, Mattei ML, Rose K, et al. Inadvertent lead placement in the left ventricle: a case report and brief review. Indian Pacing Electrophysiol J 2009;9(4):224–8.
7. Pasquie JL, Massin F, Macia JC, et al. Long-term follow-up of biventricular pacing using a totally endocardial approach in patients with end-stage cardiac failure. Pacing Clin Electrophysiol 2007;30(Suppl 1):S31–3.
8. Van Gelder BM, Bracke FA, Oto A, et al. Diagnosis and management of inadvertently placed pacing and ICD leads in the left ventricle: a multicenter experience and review of the literature. Pacing Clin Electrophysiol 2000;23(5):877–83.

Ventricular Tachycardia After Implantable Cardioverter-Defibrillator Placement

Duy Thai Nguyen, MD, Zian H. Tseng, MD, MAS, Byron K. Lee, MD, Nitish Badhwar, MD*

KEYWORDS

• Catheter ablation • Implantable converter-defibrillator
• Ventricular tachycardia • Proarrhythmia

A 57-year-old woman, with a history of nonischemic cardiomyopathy secondary to mitral regurgitation, had undergone implantation of a Medtronic Concerto biventricular pacemaker-defibrillator (Medtronic, Minneapolis, MN, USA) 2 years previously. Recently, she had received several defibrillator shocks for ventricular tachycardia (VT). She was admitted and underwent noninvasive electrophysiologic (EP) testing to optimize her defibrillator settings. However, during the study, antitachycardia pacing only appeared to accelerate and sustain her left bundle branch block (LBBB)-morphology VT (**Fig. 1**). Multiple shocks from her implantable cardioverter defibrillator (ICD) failed to terminate the VT, and she required external defibrillation. Further electrical instability led to more than 20 ICD discharges. Despite treatment with intravenous amiodarone, lidocaine, and procainamide, as well as an ablation procedure, the patient continued to have episodes of symptomatic VT. She was therefore referred to our center for repeat EP study and possible ablation.

CLINICAL QUESTION

Where is the VT originating? (see **Fig. 1**.)

EP STUDY AND CLINICAL COURSE

In the EP study, multipolar catheters were placed in the right atrium, His-bundle region, right ventricle (RV), and coronary sinus. At baseline, the patient was initially biventricular pacing (BVP) at a cycle length of 1000 ms, with normal atrial-His and His-ventricular intervals. Multiple episodes of nonsustained VT occurred spontaneously. After the patient's BVP was turned off, and she was in her native rhythm, VT no longer occurred spontaneously; however, it was still easily inducible with minimal ventricular overdrive pacing at 800 ms from the RV catheter.

Both spontaneous VT and inducible VT, with tachycardia cycle lengths of 300 to 350 ms, were similar to the patient's clinical VT (**Fig. 2**A) and were unstable, requiring defibrillation. Electroanatomic mapping of the RV in sinus rhythm did not reveal significant low-voltage areas to suggest scar, although voltage at the apex was lower than the rest of the RV (**Fig. 3**). The earliest activation during VT was at the site of the ICD lead distal electrode, with a local electrogram noted 30 ms before the QRS onset. Pacing near the ICD

Disclosure: Dr Nguyen has received grants to attend educational events sponsored by Medtronic, St Jude Medical, and Boston Scientific.
Cardiac Electrophysiology, Division of Cardiology, University of California, 500 Parnassus Avenue, MU East 4, Box 1354, San Francisco, CA 94143, USA
* Corresponding author.
E-mail address: badhwar@medicine.ucsf.edu

Card Electrophysiol Clin 2 (2010) 277–280
doi:10.1016/j.ccep.2010.01.013

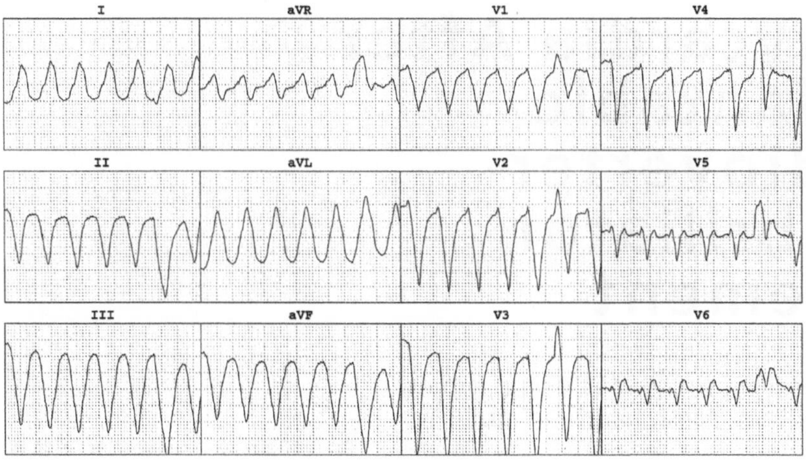

Fig. 1. Twelve-lead electrocardiogram of a patient presenting VT.

lead tip produced a 12-lead electrocardiogram morphology similar to the clinical VT (see **Fig. 2**B). Ablation was targeted to the RV apex near the ICD lead tip (see **Fig. 3**). Post ablation, VT was no longer inducible with ventricular overdrive pacing or triple extrastimuli. The lead impedance, capture, and sensing thresholds were all stable.

Because the patient was stable from a heart failure standpoint, with a New York Heart Association Class I status, and because her native QRS was narrower than her biventricular-paced QRS, we decided to turn off BVP, because evidence suggested that pacing (particularly pacing from the RV lead) was a contributor to her VT storm. With these interventions, the patient's antiarrhythmics were

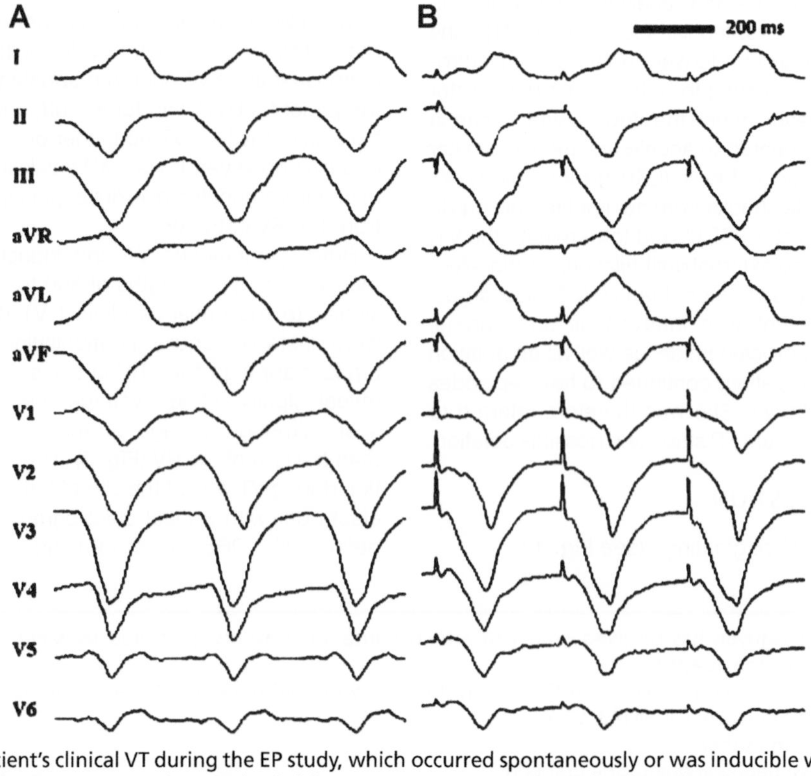

Fig. 2. (*A*) Patient's clinical VT during the EP study, which occurred spontaneously or was inducible with only brief pacing from the RV apex, near her ICD lead. (*B*) Pacemap near patient's ICD lead produced an LBBB-morphology, superior axis configuration similar to her VT.

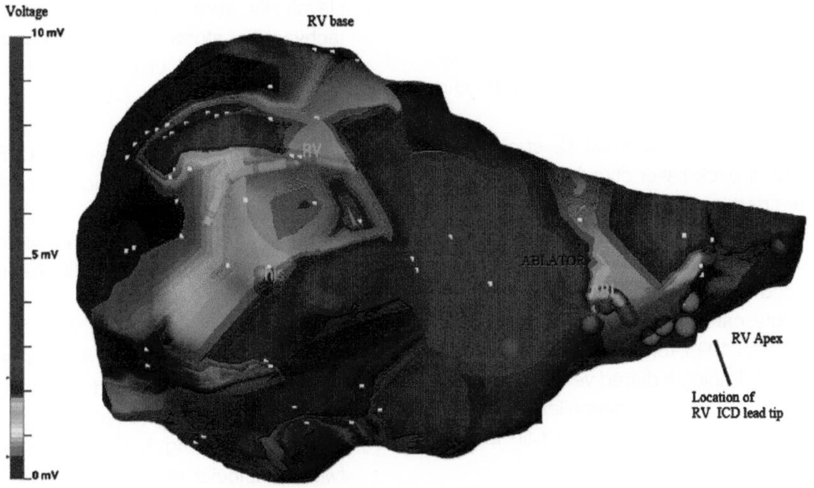

Fig. 3. Right anterior oblique view of a 3-dimensional electroanatomic map (EnSite System, St Jude Medical, Inc, MN, USA) showing successful sites of ablation in the RV apex in the region of the ICD lead tip (*red ablation dots* below the ablator). Note that the RV catheter (RV, in *blue*) has been pulled back to the RV base to facilitate ablation. The His catheter is in its traditional position.

weaned, and she has remained free of VT for more than 4 months.

DISCUSSION

Proarrhythmia from an endocardial ICD lead is a rare but serious complication. Lee and colleagues[1] reported that arrhythmias caused by the presence of an ICD constituted less than 1% of their referrals for VT ablation. Endocardial leads can cause arrhythmias by a variety of mechanisms. Proarrhythmia caused by pacing from an ICD lead is well described in the literature,[2–5] whereby RV pacing inappropriately initiates tachyarrhythmias. Furthermore, in a prospective series of patients who received BVP defibrillators, Nayak and colleagues[6] found that 8 of 191 (4%) patients developed VT storm that was attributable to left ventricular (LV) pacing. This development most likely reflects the unique nature of these investigators' tertiary care center, because such a high incidence has not been reported elsewhere. A possible explanation for the proarrhythmic effects of BVP is that by reversing normal activation, BVP may prolong the QT interval and increase transmural dispersion of repolarization.[7] Other potential mechanisms for proarrhythmia caused by the presence of an endocardial lead include acceleration of stable arrhythmias by antitachycardia pacing and loss of ventricular pacing post defibrillation.[8] Mechanical causes, such as retained fragments of leads or redundant leads, can cause myocardial irritation and arrhythmias.[9,10]

Arrhythmias due to mechanical causes are readily apparent and can be quickly rectified soon after implantation. Proarrhythmia caused by pacing usually occurs soon after the implantation of endocardial leads but can present months to years later, as seen with our patient. More chronic lead proarrhythmia may be caused by long-term development of microscopic fibrosis around the lead tip; such fibrosis can lead to nonuniform anisotropy and reentry, which are substrates for VT.[11]

Disabling pacing can be both diagnostic and therapeutic. Antiarrhythmics have had limited success, but this may be due to reporting bias in the literature, because it is possible that only those failing antiarrhythmics have further investigation into their arrhythmias. Other cases, including our own, have required ablation. Extraction or repositioning of the lead may be necessary.[1]

With regard to our patient, we are monitoring her LV function and heart failure symptoms. If these symptoms worsen, we may have to resume BVP or reposition the RV lead if VT recurs with BVP.

In summary, although implantation of an endocardial ICD is meant to protect against ventricular arrhythmias, in some cases it can be paradoxically proarrhythmic. Recognition of this device complication, although rare, is important because it is potentially reversible and can be treated by managing the device in lieu of, or in addition to, antiarrhythmics and catheter ablation of VT.

REFERENCES

1. Lee JC, Epstein LM, Huffer LL, et al. ICD lead proarrhythmia cured by lead extraction. Heart Rhythm 2009;6(5):613–8.
2. Himmrich E, Przibille O, Zellerhoff C, et al. Proarrhythmic effect of pacemaker stimulation in patients with implanted cardioverter-defibrillators. Circulation 2003;108(2):192–7.
3. Roelke M, O'Nunain S, Osswald S, et al. Ventricular pacing induced ventricular tachycardia in patients with implantable cardioverter defibrillators. Pacing Clin Electrophysiol 1995;18(3 Pt 1):486–91.
4. Vlay LC, Vlay SC. Pacing induced ventricular fibrillation in internal cardioverter defibrillator patients: a new form of proarrhythmia. Pacing Clin Electrophysiol 1997;20(1 Pt 1):132–3.
5. Reithmann C, Hahnefeld A, Oversohl N, et al. Reinitiation of ventricular macroreentry within the His-Purkinje system by back-up ventricular pacing—a mechanism of ventricular tachycardia storm. Pacing Clin Electrophysiol 2007;30(2):225–35.
6. Nayak HM, Verdino RJ, Russo AM, et al. Ventricular tachycardia storm after initiation of biventricular pacing: incidence, clinical characteristics, management, and outcome. J Cardiovasc Electrophysiol 2008;19(7):708–15.
7. Fish JM, Brugada J, Antzelevitch C. Potential proarrhythmic effects of biventricular pacing. J Am Coll Cardiol 2005;46(12):2340–7.
8. Pinski SL, Fahy GJ. The proarrhythmic potential of implantable cardioverter-defibrillators. Circulation 1995;92(6):1651–64.
9. Lickfett L, Wolpert C, Jung W, et al. Inappropriate implantable defibrillator discharge caused by a retained pacemaker lead fragment. J Interv Card Electrophysiol 1999;3(2):163–7.
10. Lindsay AC, Wong T, Segal O, et al. An unusual twist: ventricular tachycardia induced by a loop in a right ventricular pacing wire. QJM 2006;99(5):347–8.
11. de Bakker JM, van Rijen HM. Continuous and discontinuous propagation in heart muscle. J Cardiovasc Electrophysiol 2006;17(5):567–73.

Late Recognition of Malignant Vasovagal Syncope

Rima Arnaout, MD[a,*], Anne Thorson, MD[b]

KEYWORDS

• Vasovagal • Syncope • Malignant
• Neurocardiogenic • Pacemaker

CLINICAL PRESENTATION

A 21-year-old female with a history of seizures since the age of 5 years presented for long-term electroencephalographic (EEG) monitoring. Her episodes are characterized by a sudden feeling of doom, nausea, and tunnel vision, followed by altered mental status, convulsions, and cyanosis. These episodes often occur in the morning or are triggered by the sight of blood. Once, while getting her ears pierced, she had a 4-minute episode. Afterwards she is anxious but oriented and back to baseline within minutes.

She has no other medical problems and no allergies. She had an uncomplicated birth and no history of meningitis or head trauma. She currently attends college and has no history of alcohol, tobacco, or drug use. She has no family history of seizure but her maternal great-grandmother and aunts were known to faint easily. The patient had an EEG during childhood and was told she had complex partial seizures. She also had brain magnetic resonance imaging (MRI) at an outside hospital in February 2009, which was normal.

Her episodes recur once or twice a year despite several antiepileptic medications. She was therefore admitted for EEG monitoring to better characterize and treat her condition.

On the day of testing, the patient was fitted with standard international 10–20 electrode placement supplemented with surface sphenoidal, T1, and T2 electrodes as well as a single electrocardiogram chest electrode. A video sitter also observed her in real time. Her initial vitals were normal. When the nurse attempted to place a peripheral intravenous line, the patient became nervous and began having pauses on her ECG lead before developing asystole for 45 seconds. After 5 seconds of asystole, the patient lost consciousness and had a 5-second burst of high voltage slowing on EEG associated with some erratic jerking of the extremities and upward deviation of the eyes. When the patient's heart rate returned, she had an additional episode of jerking for 5 to 10 seconds before regaining consciousness, frightened. Within minutes, she was back to baseline with heart rate in the 60s. Throughout this episode, EEG monitoring noted no epileptiform activity. (A video of this patient can be accessed online at http://www.cardiacep.theclinics.com/.)

The patient was then referred to cardiology for neurocardiogenic syncope. She received a dual-chamber pacemaker and had an uncomplicated recovery.

CLINICAL QUESTION

Is it appropriate for this patient to get a pacemaker for treatment of neurocardiogenic syncope?

DISCUSSION

This patient had neurocardiogenic syncope misdiagnosed as epilepsy for many years. In one study of 1506 patients, Josephson and colleagues found that 12.9% of those referred

[a] Cardiology Division, University of California, 505 Parnassus Avenue, Box 0214, Moffit 1180D, San Francisco, CA 94143-0214, USA
[b] Cardiology Division, University of California, 505 Parnassus Avenue, Box 0214, Moffit 314A, San Francisco, CA 94143-0214, USA
* Corresponding author.
E-mail address: rima.arnaout@ucsf.edu

Card Electrophysiol Clin 2 (2010) 281–283
doi:10.1016/j.ccep.2010.01.019
1877-9182/10/$ – see front matter

to epilepsy clinics actually had severe neurocardiogenic syncope.[1] Fitzpatrick and colleagues[2] estimate that 16% of those with recurrent syncope have what is called malignant vasovagal syndrome. The 2006 American College of Cardiology Foundation/American Heart Association guidelines on syncope define severe syncope that occurs suddenly and causes injury as malignant.[3] Other groups have defined malignant vasovagal syncope as syncope with bradycardia or asystole. By either definition, our patient would be diagnosed with malignant vasovagal syncope.

Patients with malignant vasovagal syncope present a dilemma for the cardiologist. Treatments for this disorder have varied and include trigger avoidance, preemption with isometric exercises, or tilt-table training, as well as several pharmacologic therapies. Cardiac pacing also seems to be a logical therapy.

The Vasovagal Syncope International Study (VASIS) investigators established subclassifications of vasovagal syncope based on patients' reaction to tilt-table testing.[4] Patients with VASIS type 3 syncope had a predominantly vasodepressor response, whereas type 2 patients exhibited marked bradycardia without asystole (type 2A) or with asystole (type 2B). Type 1 patients showed a mixed response. It was postulated that cardiac pacing may best help avert syncope in those patients who have a type 2B response.

Initial retrospective studies suggested a benefit with cardiac pacing for vasovagal syncope.[5–7] In one study of 37 patients, for example, 89% had symptomatic improvement regardless of their VASIS classification.[5] Randomized studies also suggested benefit.[8–10] In the Vasovagal Pacemaker Study (VPS) study, 54 patients with recurrent syncope and bradycardia on tilt-table test were randomized to receive a pacemaker or not to receive a pacemaker. The pacemaker group had an 85.4% reduction in the risk of syncope.[9]

Blinded randomized studies seemed appropriate to confirm these initial findings. Both the VPS II and Vasovagal Syncope and Pacing Trial (SYNPACE) trials randomized patients with recurrent syncope, confirmed by tilt testing, by giving them all pacemakers and enabling pacing only in the experimental group in a double-blinded fashion.[11,12] Both found no benefit of pacing for vasovagal syncope. A meta-analysis by Sud and colleagues[13] confirmed that in nonblinded studies, pacing was found to benefit, whereas it did not help when patients were blinded to the therapy. This raised concern for an expectation effect biasing patients and providers to assume pacing would help.

Although these most recent trials would seem to have ended the use of pacers for neurocardiogenic syncope, controversy continues. One reason is the doubt that diagnosis and classification of syncope by tilt-table testing, on which the previous studies were based, is a reliable way to judge spontaneous events. The International Study on Syncope of Uncertain Etiology (ISSUE) investigators used implantable loop recorders (ILRs) to detect neurally mediated syncope. They found that the results of tilt testing did not reliably correlate with the severity, mechanism, or outcome of spontaneous events as detected by ILR.[14,15] Our patient was noted to have a significant asystolic pause in the setting of a spontaneous syncopal event rather than provocation by tilt testing. This helped strengthen the argument to give her a pacemaker despite the debate. The ISSUE investigators have a third trial underway, which now aims to use ILR as an inclusion criterion for randomized, double-blinded comparison of pacing versus no pacing for neurocardiogenic syncope.[16] The results are expected in 2010.

Although vasovagal pauses have not been observed to pose a risk for asystolic death, few patients have been recorded to have pauses as long as those of our patient. Although the trials mentioned earlier include patients with malignant vasovagal syncope, large-scale studies focusing exclusively on cases as dramatic as hers have not been published. With almost a minute-long pause, our patient was given a pacemaker as much to avoid syncope as to avoid terminal asystole. To date, she has not had recurrent symptoms. However, it has just been a few months since device implantation; time will tell if the pacemaker will alleviate or mitigate her syncope.

APPENDIX: VIDEO

A video associated with this article can be found in the online version, at doi 10.1016/j.ccep.2010.01.019.

REFERENCES

1. Josephson C, Rahey S, Sadler R. Neurocardiogenic syncope: frequency and consequences of its misdiagnosis as epilepsy. Can J Neurol Sci 2007;34(2):221–4.
2. Fitzpatrick A, Theodorakis G, Vardas P, et al. The incidence of malignant vasovagal syndrome in patients with recurrent syncope. Eur Heart J 1991;12:389–94.
3. Strickberger S, Benson D, Biaggioni I, et al. AHA/ACCF scientific statement on the evaluation of syncope. J Am Coll Cardiol 2006;47(2):473–84.

4. Sutton R, Bloomfield D. Indications, methodology, and classification of results of tilt table testing. Am J Cardiol 1999;84:10–9.
5. Peterson M, Chamberlain-Webber R, Fitzpatrick A, et al. Permanent pacing for cardioinhibitory malignant vasovagal syndrome. Br Heart J 1994;71:274–81.
6. Benditt D, Sutton R, Gammage M, et al. Clinical experience with Thera DR rate-drop response pacing algorithm in carotid sinus syndrome and vasovagal syncope. The International Rate-Drop Investigators Group. Pacing Clin Electrophysiol 1997;20:832–9.
7. Sheldon R, Koshman M, Wilson W, et al. Effect of dual-chamber pacing with automatic rate-drop sensing on recurrent neurally medicated syncope. Am J Cardiol 1998;81:158–62.
8. Ammirati F, Collvicchi F, Santini M. Permanent cardiac pacing versus medical treatment for the prevention of recurrent vasovagal syncope: a multicenter, randomized, controlled trial. Circulation 2001;104(1):52–7.
9. Connolly S, Sheldon R, Roberts R, et al. The North American Vasovagal Pacemaker Study (VPS). A randomised trial of permanent cardiac pacing or the prevention of vasovagal syncope. J Am Coll Cardiol 1999;33:16–20.
10. Sutton R, Brignole M, Menozzi C, et al. Dual-chamber pacing in the treatment of neurally mediated tilt-positive cardioinhibitory syncope; pacemaker versus no therapy – a multicoated randomised study. The Vasovagal Syncope International Study (VASIS) Investigators. Circulation 2000;102:294–9.
11. Connolly S, Sheldon R, Thorpe K, et al. Pacemaker therapy for prevention of syncope in patients with recurrent severe vasovagal syncope: Second Vasovagal Pacemaker Study (VPS II): a randomized trial. JAMA 2003;289(17):2224–9.
12. Raviele A, Giada F, Menozzi C, et al. A randomized, double-blind, placebo-controlled study of permanent cardiac pacing for the treatment of recurrent tilt-induced vasovagal syncope. The Vasovagal Syncope and Pacing Trial (SYNPACE). Eur Heart J 2004;25(19):1741–8.
13. Sud S, Massel D, Klein G, et al. The expectation effect and cardiac pacing for refractory vasovagal syncope. Am J Med 2007;120(1):54–62.
14. Brignole M, Sutton R, Menozzi C, et al. Lack of correlation between the responses to tilt testing and adenosine triphosphate test and the mechanism of spontaneous neurally mediated syncope. International Study on Syncope of Uncertain Etiology 2 (ISSUE 2) Group. Eur Heart J 2006;27(18):2232–9.
15. Brignole M, Sutton R, Menozzi C, et al. Early application of an implantable loop recorder allows effective specific therapy in patients with recurrent suspected neurally mediated syncope. International Study on Syncope of Uncertain Etiology 2 (ISSUE 2) group. Eur Heart J 2006;27(9):1085–92.
16. Brignole M. International Study on Syncope of Uncertain Etiology 3 (ISSUE 3): pacemaker therapy for patients with asystolic neurally-mediated syncope: rationale and study design. Europace 2007;9(1):25–30.

An Unusual Case of Pacemaker Malfunction

Jonathan C. Hsu, MD[a,*], Nora Goldschlager, MD[b]

KEYWORDS

• Lead dislodgement • Pacemaker • Pacing system
• Ventricular lead

BRIEF PRESENTATION OF CLINICAL PROBLEM

A 66-year-old man with a St Jude Zephyr dual-chamber pacing system for symptomatic Mobitz type II second-degree atrioventricular (AV) block was sent for evaluation in the pacemaker clinic because of episodes of light-headedness and syncope occurring on the day of evaluation. He reported similar episodes of light-headedness and syncope in the past, which were completely alleviated after the original pacing system was implanted. He had seen his primary care physician in the urgent care clinic, who obtained a 12-lead electrocardiogram and referred him to the pacemaker clinic because of concern for pacemaker malfunction. Previous programmed parameters of the pacing system were on file and revealed that the mode of function on his last visit was set to DDD with a base rate of 55 bpm, a paced AV delay of 225 milliseconds and a sensed AV delay of 225 milliseconds.

Several 12-lead electrocardiograms obtained during his visit to the pacemaker clinic revealed paced and spontaneous rhythms (tracings 1 and 2 in **Fig. 1**).

CLINICAL QUESTION

What type of pacemaker problem do the tracings suggest and what simple in-office interrogation data and diagnostic tests can confirm this diagnosis?

DISCUSSION OF CORRECT INTERPRETATION

The lack of appropriate ventricular pacing stimuli in tracing 1 and the lack of ventricular capture in tracing 2 suggest ventricular lead dislodgement. Interrogation of the device was performed. The trend of the ventricular lead impedance, an automatic measure performed at weekly intervals, revealed a sudden drop in impedance of the ventricular lead from baseline (**Fig. 2**). There was also an abrupt decrease in the trended R wave amplitude occurring at around the same date (**Fig. 3**). Because of the suspicion of ventricular lead dislodgement as the presumed explanation for the 12-lead electrocardiograms, the mode of function was programmed to VOO at a lower rate of 90 ppm; in this mode, the intracardiac atrial and ventricular electrograms revealed near-simultaneous atrial and ventricular signals

Author disclosures/potential conflicts of interest: Dr Goldschlager discloses honoraria from St Jude Medical and Medtronic.

[a] Division of Cardiology, Department of Medicine, University of California, San Francisco, 505 Parnassus Avenue, M1181, San Francisco, CA 94143, USA
[b] Division of Cardiology, San Francisco General Hospital, Department of Medicine, University of California, San Francisco, 1001 Potrero Avenue, 5G1, UCSF Box 0846, San Francisco, CA 94110, USA
* Corresponding author.
E-mail address: jhsu@medicine.ucsf.edu

Card Electrophysiol Clin 2 (2010) 285–288
doi:10.1016/j.ccep.2010.01.020
1877-9182/10/$ – see front matter

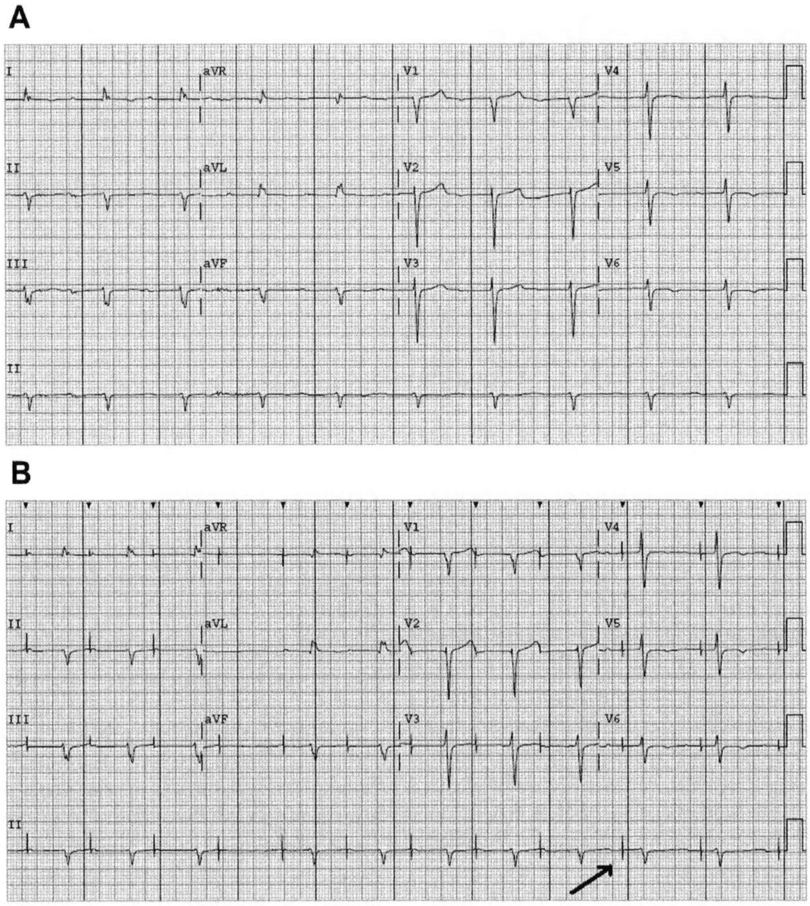

Fig. 1. (*A*) Tracing 1: 12-lead electrocardiogram shows normal sinus rhythm at a rate of 60 beats per minute with first-degree atrioventricular block (PR interval of 480 milliseconds). The programmed AV interval is 225 milliseconds. Despite the long PR interval, there is no evidence of ventricular pacing stimuli, and tracking function is not observed. (*B*) Tracing 2: 12-lead electrocardiogram shows atrial pacing stimuli and atrial capture. There is no evidence of ventricular pacing stimuli or capture throughout the tracing; the QRS complexes are native and are conducted from the atrial paced complexes. Near the end of the strip (*arrow*), the tracing shows P waves followed at regular intervals by pacing stimuli that do not depolarize tissue. The P-to-stimulus interval being constant, the diagnosis of the rhythm is appropriate atrial sensing with appropriate tracking, but no evidence of ventricular capture.

with atrial capture (ie, P wave) noted on external lead (**Fig. 4**).

To confirm right ventricular lead dislodgement into the right atrium, the patient was sent for a posterior-anterior (PA) and lateral chest radiograph (**Fig. 5**). Close inspection of the PA chest radiograph revealed that the right ventricular lead had indeed migrated into the right atrium. The patient was scheduled for lead repositioning. After successful repositioning of the lead into the right ventricular apex, malfunction of the lead was no longer observed. (A video of this can be accessed online at http://www.cardiacep.theclinics.com/.)

Correct interpretation of all the data in this case of right ventricular lead dislodgement begins with electrocardiogram tracings. In tracing 1, the sinus rate is just above the programmed base rate of 55 bpm, and as a result atrial pacing stimulus output is inhibited. The ventricular lead, being displaced into the atrium, over senses atrial activity (P wave over sensing) and therefore ventricular output is also inhibited. In tracing 2, atrial pacing from the atrial lead predominates, with resultant intrinsic conduction; there is no visible ventricular output, likely caused by over sensing of atrial pacing stimuli or paced P waves

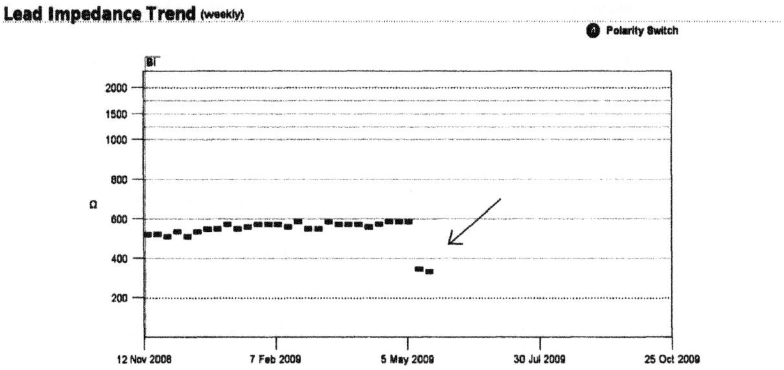

Fig. 2. Pacemaker interrogation report showing stable ventricular lead impedance (ohms) until an acute decrease on recent measurement (*arrow*).

by the ventricular lead displaced into the atrium. Later in tracing 2 (arrow), as the sinus rate increases, appropriate atrial sensing occurs and as a result an appropriately timed ventricular pacing stimulus at the sensed AV delay is triggered; the ventricular stimuli do not capture the ventricle because of the ventricular lead displacement into the atrium.

Interpretation of pacemaker interrogation begins with appreciating a sudden decline in ventricular lead impedance from previous values (see **Fig. 2**), as well as an abrupt decrease in the amplitude of sensed ventricular activity to the lower levels expected in the atrium (see **Fig. 3**). Although these findings can suggest lead insulation breach, ventricular lead migration should also be considered. Based on these findings, after programming the device to VOO mode of function (see **Fig. 4**) and using the information from the external electrocardiogram, marker channels, and intracardiac electrograms, it is apparent that ventricular lead output is nearly simultaneously sensed on the atrial intracardiac electrogram, suggesting that both leads are located in the same chamber. In addition, ventricular lead stimulus output is seen to result in atrial pacing on the surface electrocardiogram, confirming the diagnosis of ventricular dislodgement into the atrium.

Pacing lead dislodgement is defined as a change in lead position that may or may not affect the functionality of the pacing system. Only those dislodgements that result in a malfunction of the pacemaker system are clinically relevant. There are 2 time periods after pacing system implantation during which lead migration may occur: early (within 6 weeks of implantation) and late (after the first 6 weeks of implantation). Early lead dislodgement is more common than late lead dislodgement.[1] In dual-chamber systems, the atrial lead is most often the lead displaced, particularly in the early period.[2–4]

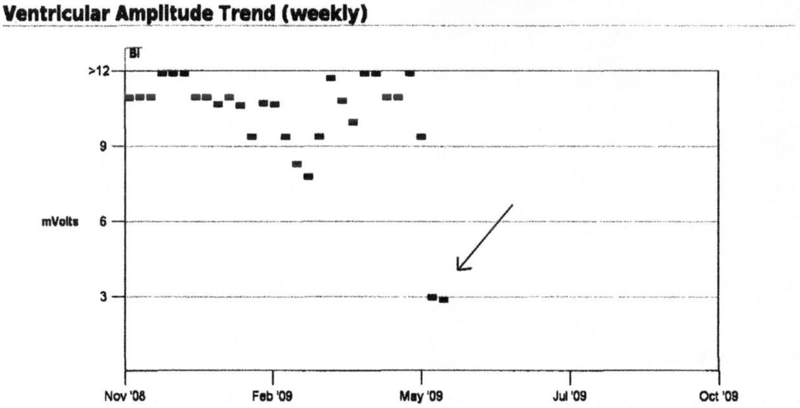

Fig. 3. Pacemaker interrogation report depicting stable ventricular sensed amplitude (millivolts) with an acute decrease on recent measurement (*arrow*).

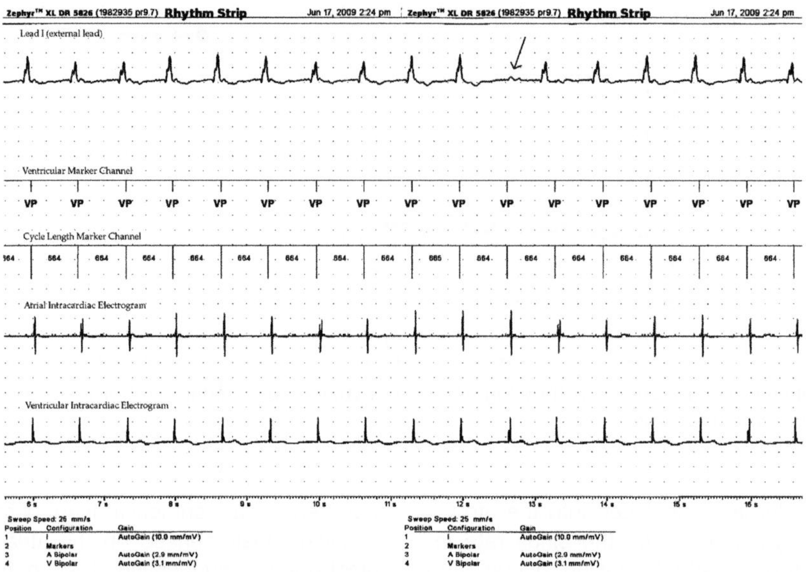

Fig. 4. Pacemaker interrogation rhythm strip during VOO mode operation with lower rate of 90 ppm. The first line represents lead I from external leads placed on the patient. The second line shows the ventricular markers and cycle length markers. The third line represents the atrial bipolar intracardiac electrogram, and the bottom line shows the ventricular bipolar intracardiac electrogram. With V pacing, there are atrial electrograms that occur immediately after each ventricular lead stimulus. Ventricular lead stimulus output is also seen to result in atrial pacing on the surface electrocardiogram (*arrow*).

The most useful and cost-effective means to diagnose pacemaker lead dislodgements are the 12-lead electrocardiogram and chest radiography. In addition, lead integrity can be investigated by device interrogation through the programmer, with focus on measuring lead impedance, sensed amplitude, and pacing threshold measurement.[1]

The approach to treatment of lead dislodgement will vary according to severity of malfunction of the pacing system, pacemaker dependency, the lead displaced, and time since implantation. If detected early, most lead dislodgements are amenable to revision by reopening the pacemaker pocket and repositioning the lead, as long as the distal end has not been fixed by the endocardial fibrous reaction.[5]

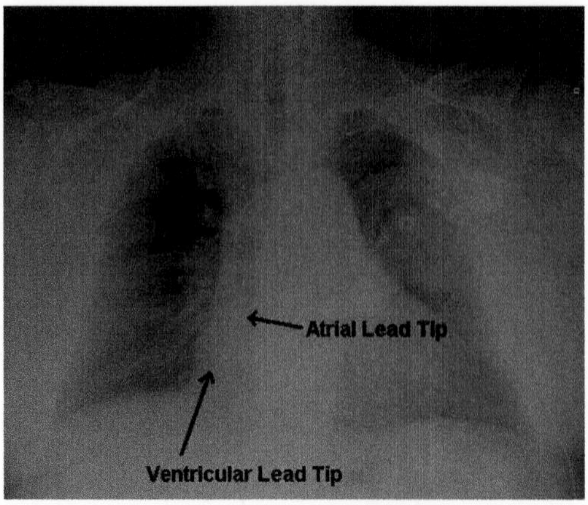

Fig. 5. PA chest radiograph showing the atrial lead in the right atrial appendage and the ventricular lead folded back proximally into the right atrium.

REFERENCES

1. Fuertes B, Toquero J, Arroyo-Espliguero R, et al. Pacemaker lead displacement: mechanisms and management. Indian Pacing Electrophysiol J 2003; 3(4):231–8.
2. Chauhan A, Grace AA, Newell SA, et al. Early complications after dual chamber versus single chamber pacemaker implantation. Pacing Clin Electrophysiol 1994;17(11 Pt 2):2012–5.
3. Greenspon AJ, Cox J, Greenberg RM. Atrial lead dislodgement with a DDD pacemaker. Pacing Clin Electrophysiol 1986;9(3):436–40.
4. Stark S, Farshidi A, Hager WD, et al. Unusual presentation of DDD pacemaker system malfunction. Pacing Clin Electrophysiol 1985;8(2):255–60.
5. Nawa S, Shimizu N, Kino K, et al. Spontaneous secure reimplantation of a dislodged pacemaker electrode onto the right ventricular outflow tract, reestablishing a sufficient pacing condition. Clin Cardiol 1993;16(3):267–9.

Ablation of Complex Atrial Flutters

Gregory M. Marcus, MD, MAS

KEYWORDS

• Catheter ablation • Atrial flutter • Atypical flutter

Atrial flutter is a common arrhythmia that can substantially reduce a patient's quality of life and increase the risk of stroke. There are estimated to be approximately 200,000 new atrial flutter (AFL) cases in the United States annually.[1] Fortunately, most of these cases can be cured with catheter ablation. The most common form is typical cavo-tricuspid isthmus (CTI)–dependent flutter, resulting in either a counterclockwise (most common) or clockwise circuit around the tricuspid annulus that can be interrupted and subsequently prevented by contiguous ablation from the tricuspid annulus to the inferior vena cava.

Typical CTI-dependent flutter makes up at least 90% of cases of atrial flutter, but several other circuits can be responsible.[2] Recognizing common patterns can help the electrophysiologist map and often cure these atypical flutters. For example, some less common atrial flutters that may not demonstrate the classic intracardiac activation sequence observed in typical CTI-dependent atrial flutter can still be addressed by ablation in the CTI. Lower loop reentry is CTI dependent, but breaks across the crista terminalis, resulting in a circuit confined to the lower right atrium that essentially travels around the inferior vena cava. Intra-isthmus reentry occurs as a result of micro-reentry within the CTI, most commonly in the medial portion.

Additional right atrial circuits have been well described, including upper loop reentry, which uses the upper right atrium, traveling across a conduction break in the mid to upper crista terminalis and around the superior vena cava. Scar-related atrial flutter can also be seen in the right atrium, either as a result of previous surgery or spontaneously, and forms a discrete area of slow conduction; if that conduction is slow enough that the surrounding myocardium repolarizes before exit from the scar, atrial flutter can occur.

Left atrial flutters are becoming more common as a result of the growing number of patients undergoing left atrial ablations for atrial fibrillation. In many cases, these flutters likely occur because of either incomplete ablation lines or recovery of conduction across previously ablated areas. Mitral annular flutter is one of the most common, representing a circuit that traverses around the mitral annulus; ablation across what has been deemed the "mitral isthmus," from the left lower pulmonary vein to the mitral isthmus, can address this arrhythmia.[3] Many other scar and pulmonary vein–related circuits have also been described.[3]

Successful and efficient ablation of these atypical flutters requires the use of multiple tools and techniques. Specifically, entrainment mapping can be used to quickly narrow down the general area of the circuit and ultimately can help to identify the specific and best place to deliver ablation lesions. There are several caveats related to entrainment mapping that must be kept in mind. First, one may inadvertently terminate the circuit; this is no small matter as it may be difficult to reinitiate the clinically relevant flutter, particularly in a patient with complex scar and multiple potential circuits. Second, although entrainment mapping can essentially confirm that one is "in" the circuit, it does not by itself reveal the critical isthmus or the best place to perform ablation. This decision requires in part an understanding of concealed versus manifest fusion, and interpretation of the

Disclosures: Dr Marcus has received research support from St Jude Medical and Atricure and speaker fees from St Jude Medical and Biotronik.
Division of Cardiology, Electrophysiology Section, University of California, 500 Parnassus, MUE 434, San Francisco, CA 94143-1354, USA
E-mail address: marcusg@medicine.ucsf.edu

Card Electrophysiol Clin 2 (2010) 289–290
doi:10.1016/j.ccep.2010.01.016
1877-9182/10/$ – see front matter

type of fusion can be difficult given often small surface electrocardiogram flutter waves that are frequently buried in the QRS or T wave. Third, effective entrainment mapping requires electrical capture of the myocardium, a necessity that may be difficult in the midst of a scar. Therefore, entrainment mapping, although an invaluable tool, must be performed in concert with other techniques.

Three-dimensional electroanatomic mapping is helpful in delineating the activation sequence of the circuit and the location of potentially important anatomic landmarks (such as the mitral valve annulus and pulmonary veins) as well as scar. However, like entrainment mapping, even a perfect map of an atrial flutter circuit does not show the protected isthmus or the best place to deliver ablations. A common misconception is that "early meets late" points to the responsible area, but in fact the location of that observation within the circuit is somewhat arbitrary. If early does meets late, that provides good evidence that the tacharrhythmia is not focal in origin, but a combination of knowledge regarding anatomic barriers, concealed versus manifest fusion during entrainment, and interpretation of the local electrograms are important in determining the optimal ablation site. In addition, apparent focal activation may in fact represent micro-reentry, where entrainment can still prove useful.

Careful attention to the local electrogram is required. Particularly when dealing with scar-based atrial flutter, complex, fractionated mid-diastolic signals are often found at the successful ablation site. However, there can be more than one scar and interpretation of the meaning of the intracardiac electrogram must be considered along with data gleaned from entrainment and the electroanatomic map.

REFERENCES

1. Granada J, Uribe W, Chyou PH, et al. Incidence and predictors of atrial flutter in the general population. J Am Coll Cardiol 2000;36(7):2242–6.
2. Lee KW, Yang Y, Scheinman MM. Atrial flutter: a review of its history, mechanisms, clinical features, and current therapy. Curr Probl Cardiol 2005;30(3): 121–67.
3. Jais P, Shah DC, Haissaguerre M, et al. Mapping and ablation of left atrial flutters. Circulation 2000;101(25): 2928–34.

Multiple Interrelated Right Atrial Flutters

Gregory M. Marcus, MD, MAS

KEYWORDS

• Catheter ablation • Atrial flutter • Lower loop • Upper loop

CASE PRESENTATION

An 82-year-old man developed presyncope associated with dyspnea while playing basketball. A 12-lead electrocardiogram demonstrated atrial flutter consistent with a typical cavotricuspid isthmus–dependent circuit. He was referred for electrophysiology study, with a plan for curative ablation.

A duodecapolar catheter was placed around the tricuspid annulus (TA), a quadripolar catheter was positioned in the His bundle region, and a decapolar catheter was positioned in the coronary sinus (CS). The initial atrial activation sequence was consistent with typical, counterclockwise, atrial flutter (**Fig. 1**); this was confirmed after entrainment from the cavotricuspid isthmus revealed a postpacing interval that was nearly identical to the tachycardia cycle length.

Subsequently, the activation sequence spontaneously changed (**Fig. 2**). An attempt to entrain this tachycardia from the apparent earliest location (TA 9–10) resulted in a change to a third atrial flutter (**Fig. 3**). This third tachycardia then spontaneously changed to a fourth atrial flutter (**Fig. 4**). An attempt to entrain the fourth tachycardia resulted in termination.

A successful cavotricuspid isthmus ablation was then performed, with confirmation of bidirectional conduction block. No subsequent atrial flutter could be induced despite aggressive pacing from multiple sites.

DISCUSSION

Based on the expected activation sequence and entrainment mapping, the first atrial flutter observed was typical counterclockwise atrial flutter. This initial atrial flutter then spontaneously changed to a different atrial flutter in which the midlateral right atrium seemed to be activated earliest. Note that the electrograms recorded along the TA spread out from the midlateral right atrium, such that the upper lateral wall was being activated in a superior and septal direction (in a clockwise direction) while the lower lateral wall was activated in an inferior and septal direction (in the counterclockwise direction). Activation of the proximal CS followed shortly after the lateral cavotricuspid annulus (TA 1–2). This pattern of activation is most consistent with a lower loop flutter (**Fig. 5**).[1]

The development of typical counterclockwise atrial flutter is believed to require an arc of conduction block across the crista terminalis, with the wave front spreading just superior to and then lateral to that line of block.[2] However, some patients can exhibit a break in this arc of conduction block, enabling the wave front to traverse the high, mid, or low crista terminalis during atrial flutter. When the wave front travels across the posterior right atrium and through the crista terminalis with subsequent anterior activation along the cavotricuspid isthmus, lower loop atrial flutter is occurring; the path is essentially identical to typical counterclockwise atrial flutter, but the posterior aspect travels lower and breaks across the crista terminalis. The diagnosis is confirmed when entrainment from the cavotricuspid isthmus reveals a postpacing interval equal to the tachycardia cycle length with concealed fusion. Lower loop atrial flutter can be cured with the classic cavotricuspid isthmus ablation.

Disclosures: Dr Marcus has received research support from St Jude Medical and Atricure and speaker fees from St Jude Medical and Biotronik.

Division of Cardiology, Electrophysiology Section, University of California, 500 Parnassus, MUE 434, San Francisco, CA 94143-1354, USA
E-mail address: marcusg@medicine.ucsf.edu

Card Electrophysiol Clin 2 (2010) 291–294
doi:10.1016/j.ccep.2010.01.023

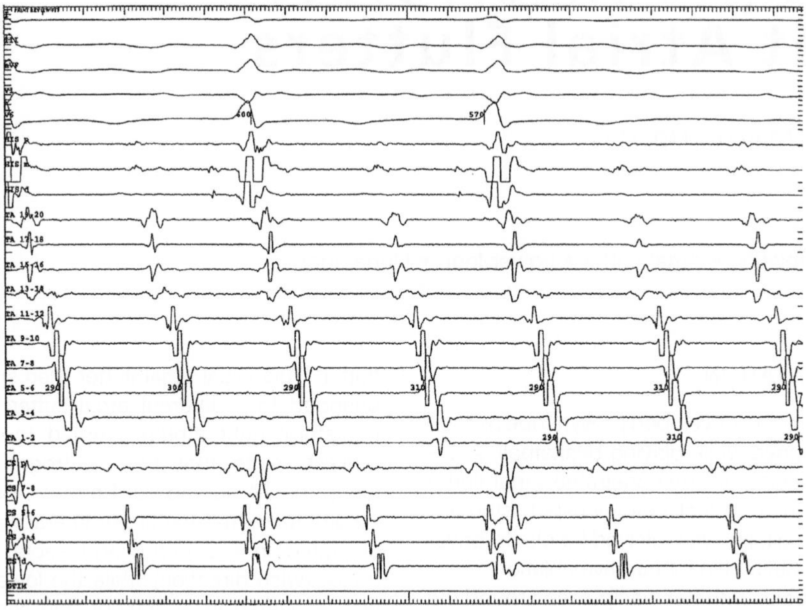

Fig. 1. Intracardiac electrograms showing an activation sequence consistent with typical counterclockwise atrial flutter. Surface leads I, III, aVF, V1, and V6 are shown. His, His bundle; p, proximal; m, mid; d, distal. TA, duodecapolar around the tricuspid annulus with 1, 2 as most distal (lateral to the cavotricuspid isthmus) and 19, 20 as most proximal. CS, coronary sinus with 1, 2 as most distal and 9, 10 as most proximal.

An attempt to entrain the apparent lower loop flutter resulted in a pattern most consistent with typical counterclockwise flutter. This then spontaneously changed to a fourth atrial flutter. The tricuspid annulus activation during the fourth atrial flutter is similar to the apparent lower loop atrial flutter, again with the midlateral tricuspid annulus activated first. However, a crucial difference is that the proximal CS was on time with the lateral cavotricuspid isthmus (TA 1–2); therefore, this cannot be traversing across the cavotricuspid isthmus (in which case one would expect

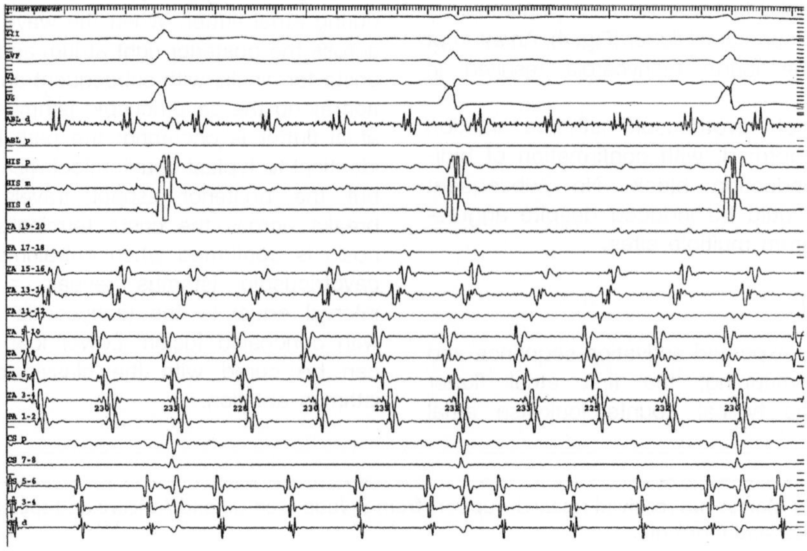

Fig. 2. Intracardiac electrograms showing an activation sequence consistent with lower loop atrial flutter (see text). Surface leads I, III, aVF, V1, and V6 are shown. His, His bundle; p, proximal; m, mid; d, distal. TA, duodecapolar around the tricuspid annulus with 1, 2 as most distal (lateral to the cavotricuspid isthmus) and 19, 20 as most proximal. CS, coronary sinus with 1, 2 as most distal and 9, 10 as most proximal.

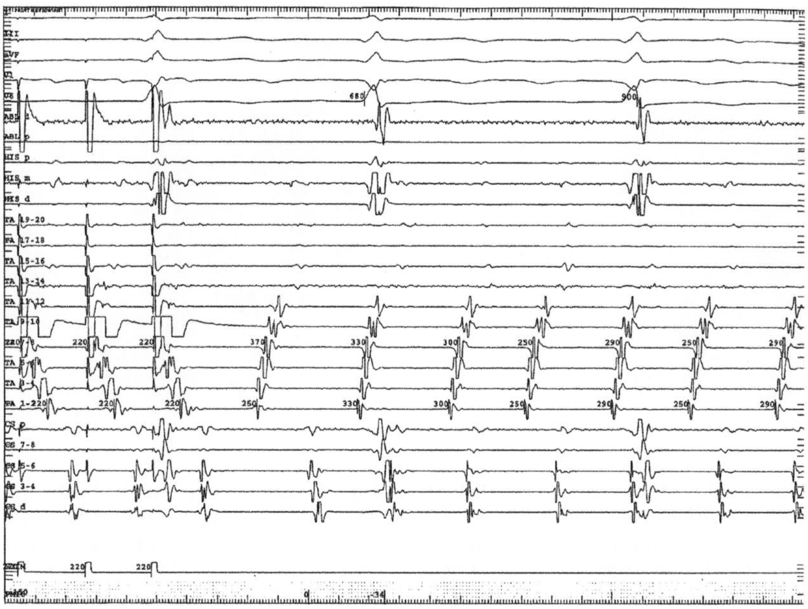

Fig. 3. Pacing from TA 9, 10 during the lower loop flutter changes the activation sequence to one most compatible with clockwise typical atrial flutter. Surface leads I, III, aVF, V1, and V6 are shown. His, His bundle; p, proximal; m, mid; d, distal. TA, duodecapolar around the tricuspid annulus with 1, 2 as most distal (lateral to the cavotricuspid isthmus) and 19, 20 as most proximal. CS, coronary sinus with 1, 2 as most distal and 9, 10 as most proximal.

sequential activation from the lateral side to the proximal coronary sinus), meaning it cannot be lower loop flutter.

Note that there is some variation in the tachycardia cycle length. Changes in the midlateral tricuspid annulus (TA 5–6 and TA 7–8) precede changes in the CS, suggesting that coronary sinus activation occurs relatively late in the circuit. The most likely explanation is that this is an upper loop flutter.[1] Some have used this term to describe

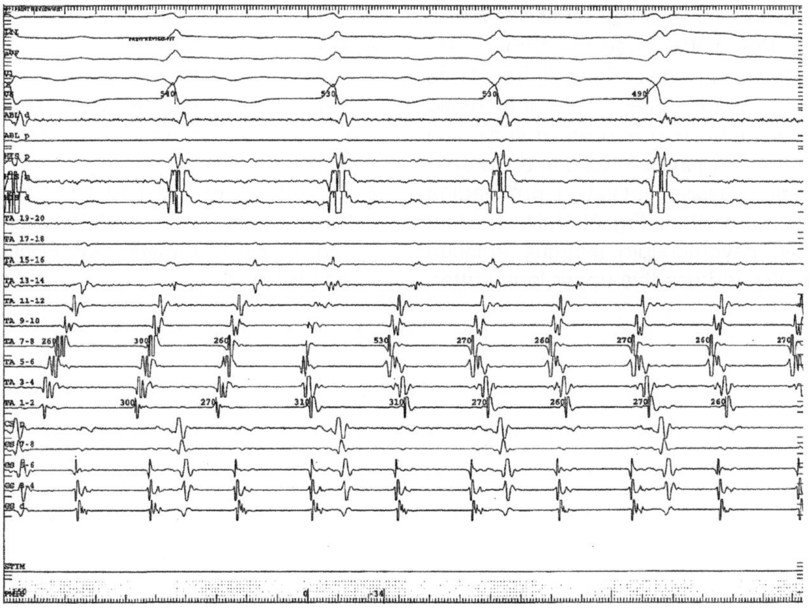

Fig. 4. The clockwise atrial flutter spontaneously changes to an apparent upper loop atrial flutter (see text). Surface leads I, III, aVF, V1, and V6 are shown. His, His bundle; p, proximal; m, mid; d, distal. TA, duodecapolar around the tricuspid annulus with 1, 2 as most distal (lateral to the cavotricuspid isthmus) and 19, 20 as most proximal. CS, coronary sinus with 1, 2 as most distal and 9, 10 as most proximal.

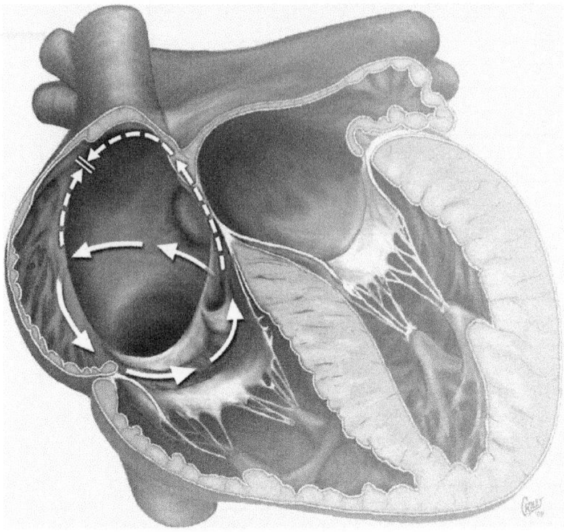

Fig. 5. Lower loop atrial flutter involves a circuit that uses the cavotricuspid isthmus in a lateral to septal direction and then crosses through a break in the line of conduction block that normally occurs along the crista terminalis as it travels septal to lateral along the posterior right atrium. The dashed lines demonstrate passive activation not integral to the circuit. (Illustration by David Criley.)

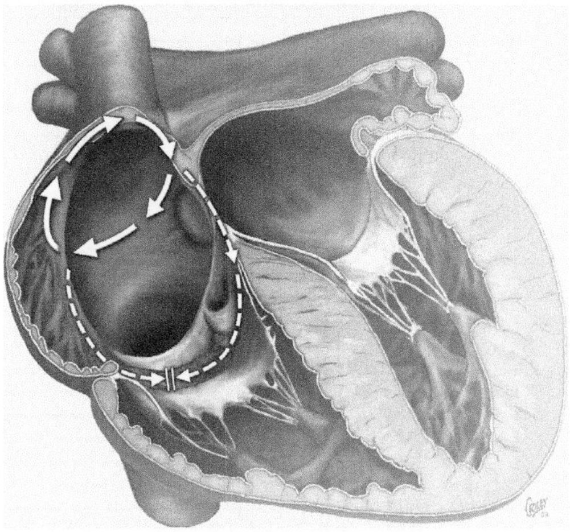

Fig. 6. Upper loop atrial flutter traverses across a break in the line of conduction block that normally occurs along the crista terminalis, travels in a lateral to septal direction (clockwise) just superior to the crista terminalis, down the septum, and then across the posterior right atrial wall until it continues through the same crista terminalis break again. The dashed lines demonstrate passive activation not integral to the circuit. (Illustration by David Criley.)

a circuit that travels around and just inferior to the superior vena cava. However, the term is also used to describe a circuit that traverses across a break in the crista terminalis, travels in a lateral to septal direction (clockwise) just superior to the crista terminalis, down the septum, and then across the posterior right atrial wall until it continues through the same crista terminalis break again. It seems that this upper loop flutter used the same crista terminalis break as the lower loop flutter. Note that conduction along the inferior-lateral tricuspid annulus (TA 3–4 to TA 1–2) is passive activation following the crista terminalis break, and CS activation represents passive activation proceeding down the right atrial septum (**Fig. 6**). Unlike the first 3 atrial flutters, cavotricuspid isthmus ablation would not directly address this upper loop flutter. However, failure to re-induce the upper loop flutter after successful cavotricuspid isthmus ablation suggests that it was likely a tachycardia-induced tachycardia (specifically, the clockwise flutter may have been necessary first to set up the upper loop flutter).

REFERENCES

1. Yang Y, Cheng J, Bochoeyer A, et al. Atypical right atrial flutter patterns. Circulation 2001;103(25):3092–8.
2. Olgin JE, Kalman JM, Lesh MD. Conduction barriers in human atrial flutter: correlation of electrophysiology and anatomy. J Cardiovasc Electrophysiol 1996;7(11):1112–26.

A Case of Atrial Arrhythmia After Lung Transplant

Duy Thai Nguyen, MD, Gregory M. Marcus, MD, MAS*

KEYWORDS

- Catheter ablation • Micro-reentry
- Atrial tachycardia • Lung transplant

CLINICAL PRESENTATION

A 71-year-old male with a history of double lung transplant for pulmonary fibrosis 2 months previously presented with shortness of breath and presyncope. He was found to be in a regular narrow-complex tachycardia (**Fig. 1**). The patient had no pretransplant history of arrhythmias. Attempts to rate control the arrhythmia were limited by labile blood pressures. The patient underwent cardioversion and loading of amiodarone. However, after the arrhythmia recurred with significant symptoms, the patient was referred for electrophysiologic study and ablation.

ELECTROPHYSIOLOGIC STUDY AND TREATMENT

Multipolar catheters were placed in the right atrium (RA), His-bundle region, right ventricle (RV), and coronary sinus (CS). At baseline, the patient was in a supraventricular tachycardia with a tachycardia cycle length (TCL) of 260 ms. There was 2:1 atrioventricular (AV) block, thus ruling out AV reentrant tachycardia. AV nodal reentrant tachycardia with lower common pathway block is rare and was essentially excluded by the eccentric atrial activation pattern (**Fig. 2**). Hence, atypical atrial flutter was the most likely diagnosis. Entrainment from the lateral RA and from the cavotricuspid isthmus showed that these areas were out of the tachycardia circuit; entrainment from the right atrial septum also resulted in a post-pacing interval (PPI) that was substantially longer than the TCL, but the PPI minus TCL in this area was the shortest found in the right atrium. Given these findings, as well as a distal to proximal CS atrial activation, a left atrial origin was suspected. A transseptal puncture for left atrial access was performed.

In the left atrium (LA), pacing from the mitral annulus, distal CS, lateral wall, and posterior wall showed that these areas were out of the circuit. Superior to the left atrial appendage, highly fractionated multicomponent potentials were found. This area corresponded to the presumed anastomosis site between the donor and recipient left atria. In this operation, the donor's 4 pulmonary veins and associated posterior left atrium are sutured to the anterior recipient left atrium. Pacing attempts were unsuccessful because of an inability to capture. Initial attempts to perform radiofrequency ablation superior to the left atrial appendage were unsuccessful because of an inability to generate adequate power and temperatures despite good tissue contact; it was assumed that this area may have had suture material that was not heating as expected. Subsequently, highly fractionated mid-diastolic potentials spanning more than half the TCL were

Disclosures: Dr Nguyen has received funding to attended educational events sponsored by Medtronic, Boston Scientific & St Jude Medical.
Dr Marcus has received research support from St Jude Medical and Atricure and speaker fees from St Jude Medical and Biotronik.
Cardiac Electrophysiology, Cardiology Division, University of California, San Francisco, 500 Parnassus Avenue, MU East 434, Box 1354, San Francisco, CA 94143, USA
* Corresponding author.
E-mail address: marcus@medicine.ucsf.edu

Card Electrophysiol Clin 2 (2010) 295–298
doi:10.1016/j.ccep.2010.01.017
1877-9182/10/$ – see front matter

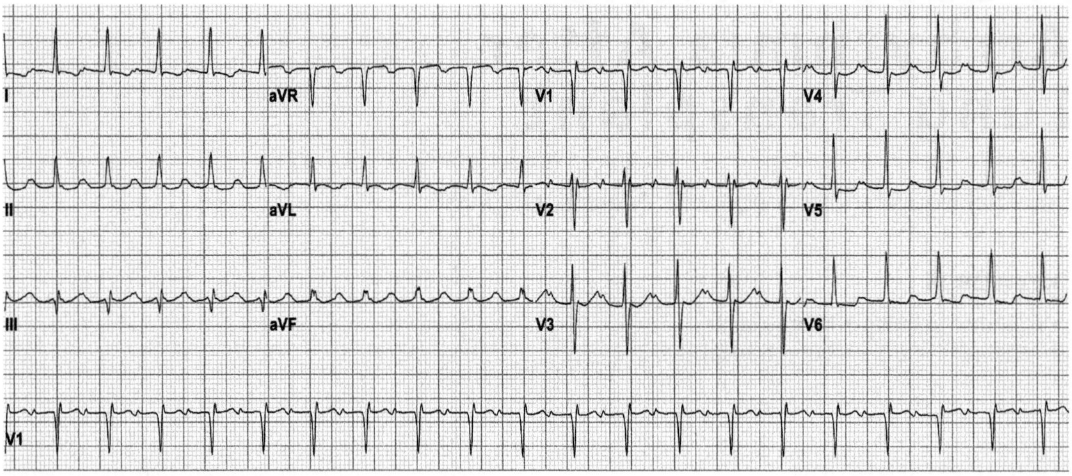

Fig. 1. Twelve-lead electrocardiogram of a regular narrow-complex tachycardia with a flutter wave midway between QRS complexes.

observed between the left upper pulmonary vein and the left atrial appendage (**Fig. 3**). Pacing from this site showed that the PPI minus TCL was zero and there was concealed fusion. The three-dimensional electroanatomic map (Ensite System, St Jude Medical) showed an apparent focal source, consistent with a micro-reentrant circuit (**Fig. 4**). Ablation at this site terminated the tachycardia (see **Fig. 4**), and the tachycardia could not be reinduced with atrial burst pacing or multiple extrastimuli. An ablation line was drawn from just posterior to the left atrial appendage to

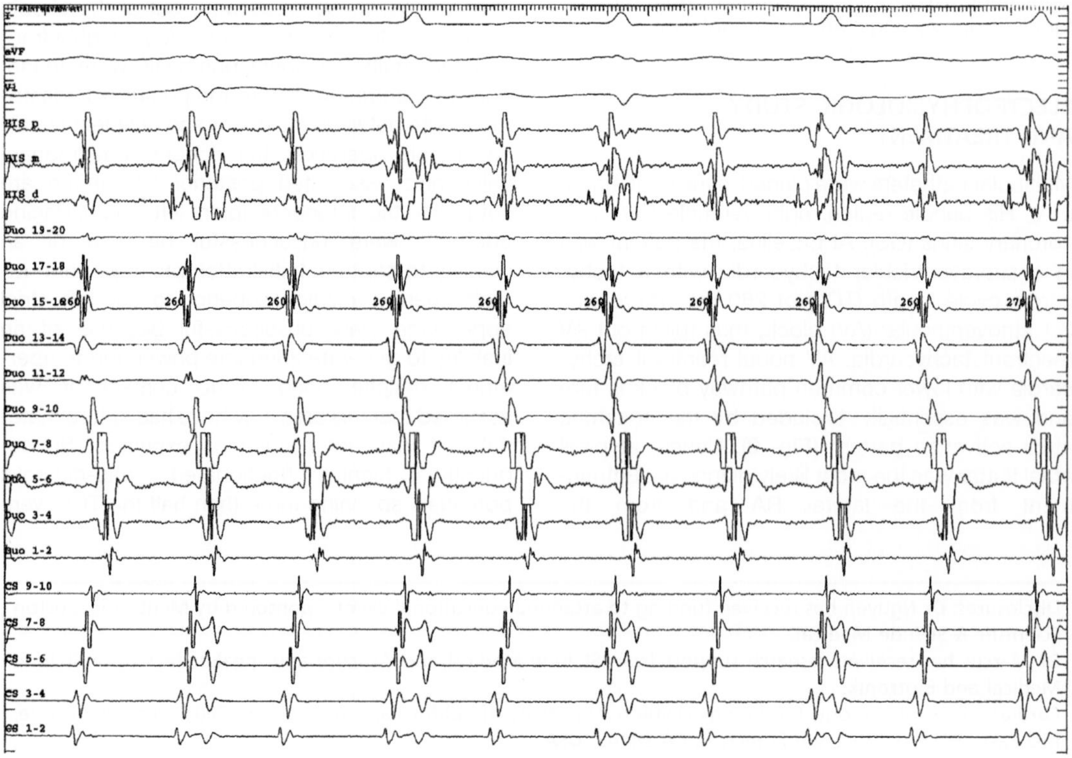

Fig. 2. Atrial tachycardia with 2:1 AV block with an atypical right atrial activation pattern. HIS, His bundle; p, proximal; m, mid; d, distal; Duo, duodecapolar around the tricuspid annulus, with 1-2 as most distal and 19-20 as most proximal; CS, coronary sinus, with 1-2 as most distal and 9-10 as most proximal.

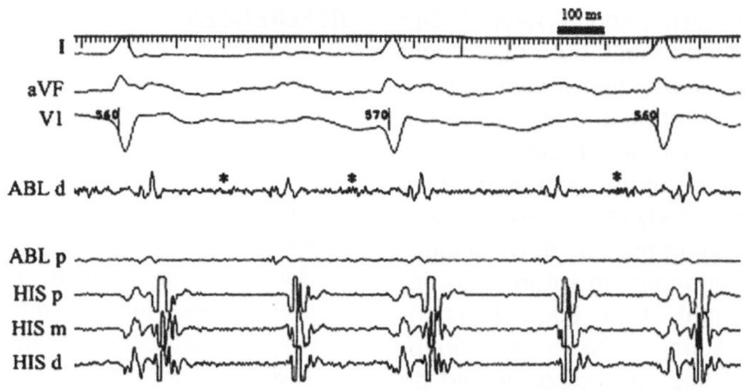

Fig. 3. Mid-diastolic complex fractionated signals (*) found between the left upper pulmonary vein and left atrial appendage. ABL, ablator; d, distal; p, proximal, HIS, His bundle; p, proximal; m, mid; d, distal.

the lateral mitral annulus. The patient has not had recurrence of this tachycardia for more than 6 months.

DISCUSSION

Atrial arrhythmias occur commonly after lung transplant, but surprisingly little is known about their pathophysiology, clinical features, or mechanisms of action.[1] Nielsen and colleagues[2] studied atrial arrhythmias after lung transplant, but grouped atrial fibrillation and atrial flutter together and reported a 14-day postoperative incidence of 39% (out of 200 patients). Data from the pediatric literature found an 11.3% incidence of atrial flutter in patients after lung transplant.[3] Less is known about the long-term incidence, management, and pathophysiology of atrial arrhythmias after lung transplant. Whether they are short-term or long-term sequelae, atrial arrhythmias following lung transplant seem to be associated with significant morbidity and mortality.[2,4]

The mechanism responsible for atrial flutter or atrial tachycardia after lung transplant has been reported to be macro-reentry around the anastomosis or suture lines between donor and recipient left atria.[5] Reentry involving the donor

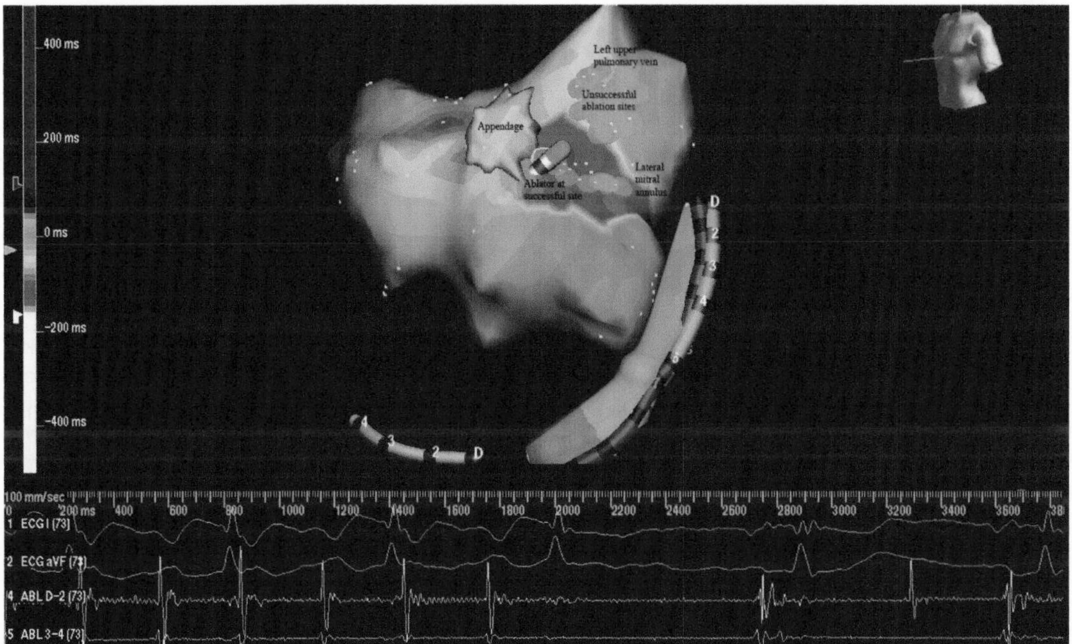

Fig. 4. Navix/ESI map (St Jude Medical) showing successful site of ablation just posterior to the left atrial appendage. Despite proof that the circuit was reentrant by entrainment mapping, the map suggests a focal source; this is most consistent with micro-reentry. The surface electrocardiograph leads and intracardiac electrograms below the map show termination of tachycardia. The unsuccessful ablation sites superiorly over presumed suture material are also shown.

pulmonary veins has also been reported.[6] Our patient's tachycardia was focal, but entrainment mapping proved that the mechanism was micro-reentrant tachycardia. It appeared to involve the anastomosis between donor and recipient left atria just anterior to the left upper pulmonary vein. As the surgery was relatively recent, the authors suspect that it involved an area of slow conduction caused by scar secondary to suturing and/or handling of the recipient tissue edge. Presumably, electrical connection between the donor and recipient atria at this early stage would be unlikely.

In summary, the key features of this case are relevant to most atypical flutters. A combination of entrainment and electroanatomic mapping can help to efficiently identify the culprit area. The target is typically a long mid-diastolic fractionated potential shown to be integral to the circuit by entrainment mapping. A micro-reentrant circuit may appear to be focal by the electroanatomic map, but entrainment techniques can still be used to localize the tachycardia.

REFERENCES

1. Lazaro MT, Ussetti P, Merino JL. Atrial fibrillation, atrial flutter, or both after pulmonary transplantation. Chest 2005;127(4):1461–2 [author reply: 1462].
2. Nielsen TD, Bahnson T, Davis RD, et al. Atrial fibrillation after pulmonary transplant. Chest 2004;126(2): 496–500.
3. Gandhi SK, Bromberg BI, Mallory GB, et al. Atrial flutter: a newly recognized complication of pediatric lung transplantation. J Thorac Cardiovasc Surg 1996;112(4):984–91.
4. Mason DP, Marsh DH, Alster JM, et al. Atrial fibrillation after lung transplantation: timing, risk factors, and treatment. Ann Thorac Surg 2007;84(6):1878–84.
5. Gandhi SK, Bromberg BI, Schuessler RB, et al. Left-sided atrial flutter: characterization of a novel complication of pediatric lung transplantation in an acute canine model. J Thorac Cardiovasc Surg 1996; 112(4):992–1001.
6. Sacher F, Vest J, Raymond JM, et al. Incessant donor-to-recipient atrial tachycardia after bilateral lung transplantation. Heart Rhythm 2008;5(1):149–51.

An Atrial Flutter Circuit Within the Cavotricuspid Isthmus

Yanfei Yang, MD*, Melvin Scheinman, MD

KEYWORDS

• Atrial flutter • Catheter ablation • Reentrant tachycardia

CLINICAL PRESENTATION

A 69-year-old man with hypertension and diabetes was admitted to our center for recurrent palpitations and documented atrial flutter (AFL). His surface electrocardiogram (ECG) suggested a typical counterclockwise (CCW) AFL, with negative flutter waves in the inferior leads (II, III, and aVF) and positive flutter waves in lead V_1. He had no prior history of cardiac surgery or ablation. Echocardiography showed mild left atrial (LA) enlargement and left ventricular (LV) hypertrophy, with a normal LV ejection fraction. After persistent symptoms on administration of β-blockers and recurrences despite amiodarone and electrical cardioversion, he was referred for electrophysiologic (EP) study and ablation.

ELECTROPHYSIOLOGIC STUDY AND ABLATION

The patient arrived in the EP laboratory in sinus rhythm. Electrogram recordings were obtained from a decapolar catheter positioned in the coronary sinus (CS), a quadripolar catheter at His bundle region, a duodecapolar catheter placed along the tricuspid annulus (TA) with its distal electrode at low lateral TA, and a rove catheter for mapping and ablation. Tachycardia was induced by atrial overdrive pacing, with the tachycardia cycle length (TCL) of 275 milliseconds and the 12-lead surface ECG identical to his clinical ECG of AFL (**Fig. 1**). Reentrant mechanism of the tachycardia was demonstrated by manifest entrainment at different overdrive pacing cycle lengths during the tachycardia. The intracardiac recordings as well as an electroanatomic mapping (EAM) by CARTO system (Biosense Webster, Inc, Diamond Bar, CA, USA) during the tachycardia showed a typical CCW activation pattern along the TA with "early-meets-late" within the cavotricuspid isthmus (CTI) (**Fig. 2**). Entrainment pacing from septal CTI (4-o'clock to 6-o'clock position in the left anterior oblique [LAO] view) and CS os showed "in circuit" response with the difference of post-pacing interval (PPI) and the TCL less than 30 milliseconds (**Fig. 3**). However, entrainment pacing from the anteroinferior CTI (6:00 to 7:00 in the LAO view) revealed it to be "out" of the circuit with the PPI-TCL greater than 30 milliseconds (see **Fig. 3**). Also, multiple sites along the TA and distal CS were demonstrated "out of the circuit" response with the PPI-TCL greater than 30 milliseconds (see **Fig. 2**). Of interest, during the tachycardia, spontaneous change of activation sequence along the TA from a CCW pattern to a simultaneous pattern was observed, but the TCL remained identical (**Fig. 4**). Fractionated potentials (FPs) and double potentials (DPs) were recorded within the region of septal CTI and CS os. Delivery of RF energy at the septal CTI area with maximal duration of FPs (138 milliseconds) terminated the tachycardia without reinducibility.

Division of Cardiology, Cardiac Electrophysiology Section, University of California San Francisco, 500 Parnassus Avenue, MU East 4S, Box 1354, San Francisco, CA 94143-1354, USA
* Corresponding author.
E-mail address: yang@medicine.ucsf.edu

Card Electrophysiol Clin 2 (2010) 299–303
doi:10.1016/j.ccep.2010.01.018
1877-9182/10/$ – see front matter

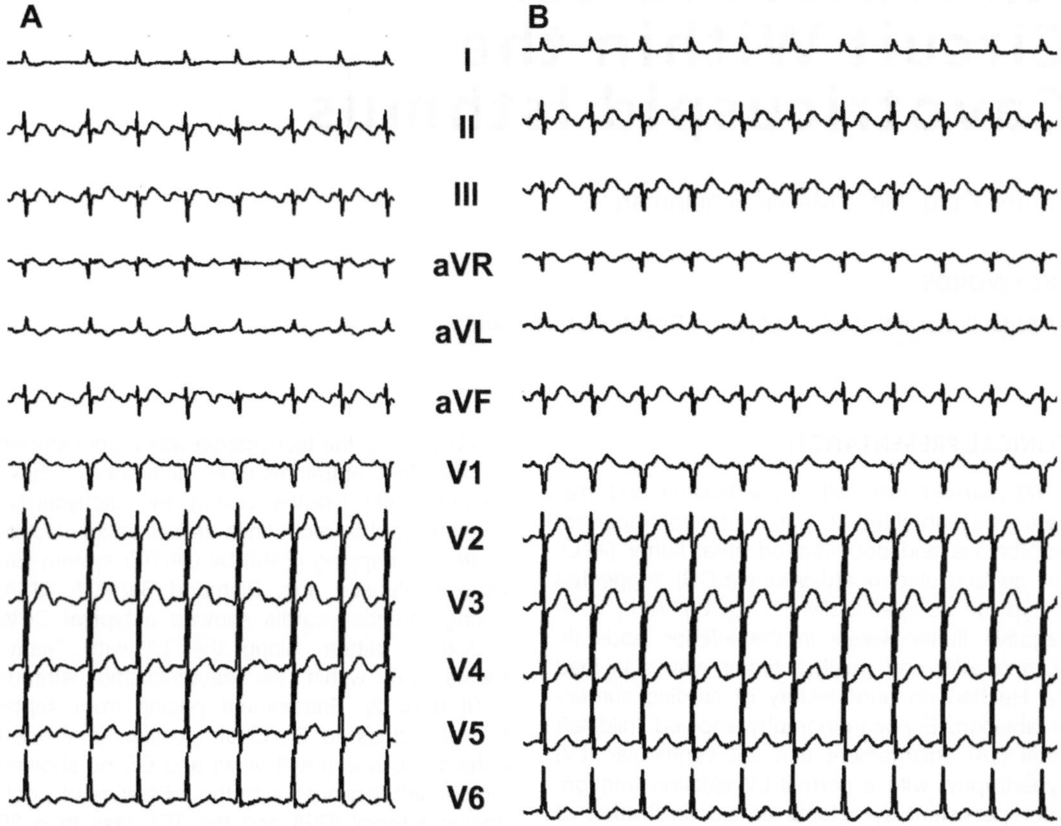

Fig. 1. Simultaneous recordings from 12-lead surface ECGs during tachycardia with 2 different activation patterns recorded from the intracardiac electrograms and an identical TCL (275 ms). Panel A shows the surface ECG during a CCW activation pattern; *Panel B* shows the 12 leads during simultaneous activation pattern. However, the F-wave morphology (negative in the inferior leads and positive in V1) in 12 leads in both panels is similar and indicates a typical CCW AFL.

DISCUSSION

CTI-dependent AFL has been well described, including the most common forms, typical CCW and clockwise reentrant circuits around the TA, which are readily appreciated and cured by the CTI ablation. However, the CTI-dependent AFL can also have other atypical forms, such as lower loop reentry with its reentrant circuit around the inferior vena cava and atypical activation pattern around the TA, for which a complete line of the CTI lesion can terminate the reentrant circuit.[1,2] Although the atypical forms of CTI-dependent AFL can easily be cured by the CTI ablation, it is of clinical importance to recognize these forms of AFL because they often show atypical activation patterns in the right atrium, which can mimic non–CTI-dependent AFL, LA flutter, or sometimes even atrial fibrillation (AF).

Although the entire reentrant circuit could not be illustrated by the available techniques (including the EAM), based on the entrainment mapping in this case, it was speculated that this was a localized reentrant circuit within the vicinity of the septal CTI. As previously described, the circuit was most likely intra-isthmus reentry.[3] This case has several remarkable diagnostic features and clinical implications. First, in this case, the typical ECG of AFL did not use a typical circuit. Previous studies have shown that the typical CTI-dependent AFL can have variable, sometimes even atypical ECG characteristics, especially in patients with diseased atria or post-AF ablation.[4,5] However, the surface ECG in this patient suggested a typical CCW AFL, but the EPS clearly showed that the tachycardia was not a typical CCW circuit around the TA, because entrainment mapping demonstrated that the low lateral TA was out of the circuit as well as other TA sites. Second, although the EAM demonstrated a CCW activation pattern along the TA, entrainment mapping revealed that most of the TA sites were not involved in the reentrant circuit; only the region of septal

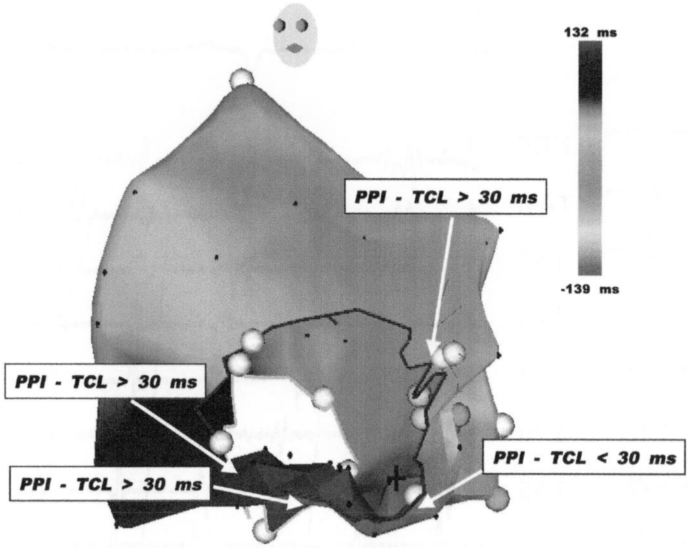

Fig. 2. EAM by CARTO system during the tachycardia, with a CCW activation pattern around the TA during tachycardia. In the left anterior oblique view, the map showed a typical CCW AFL pattern, with the earliest activation from the septal CTI, the latest activation at the anteroinferior CTI, and the "early-meets-late" at CTI. The mapped cycle length almost spanned the whole TCL (275 milliseconds)—99% of the TCL. Postpacing interval–TCL of entrainment pacing at different TA sites were marked at relevant sites in this map, which showed that only the septal CTI region was in the circuit, while the rest of right atrium was all out of the circuit.

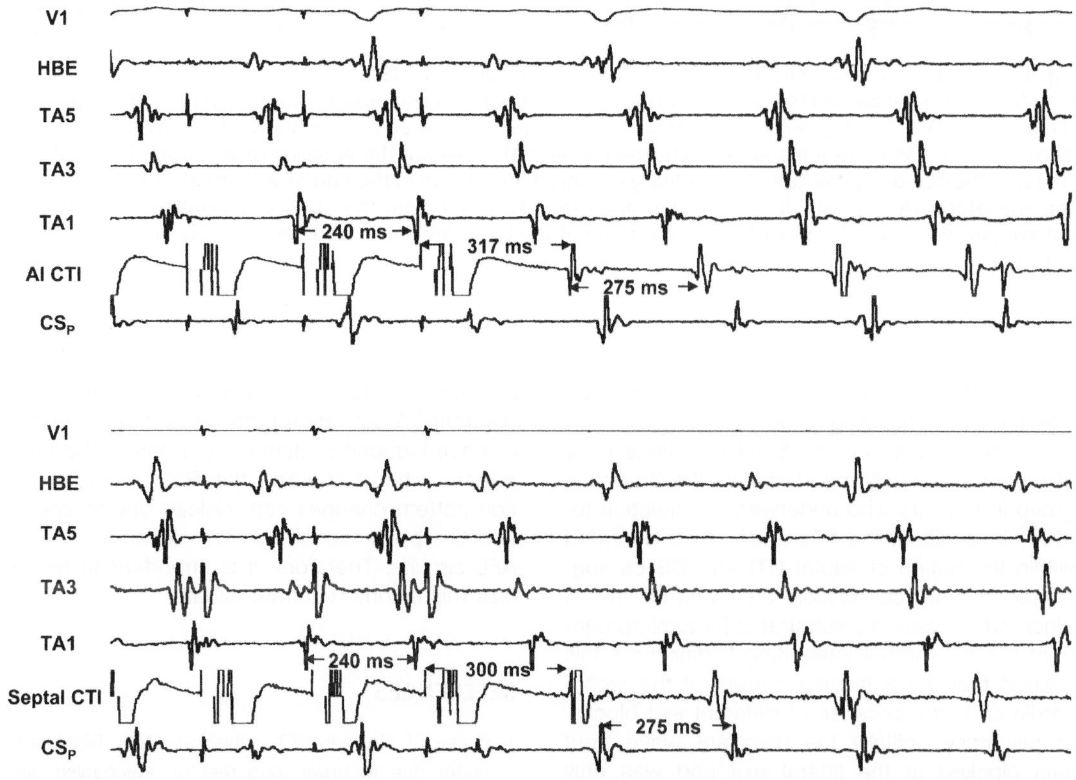

Fig. 3. Simultaneous recordings from surface ECG V_1, the His catheter (HBE) and a duodecapolar catheter along the TA with the distal bipole (TA1) at the low lateral TA and proximal bipole (TA10) close to the high septum of the right atrium. A CCW activation pattern along the TA is observed. (*Upper panel*) Entrainment from the anteroinferior CTI showed that this site of the isthmus was out of the circuit, with a TCL of 275 milliseconds and PPI of 317 milliseconds. (*Lower panel*) Entrainment from the septal CTI shows that this site of the isthmus was in the circuit, with PPI of 300 milliseconds.

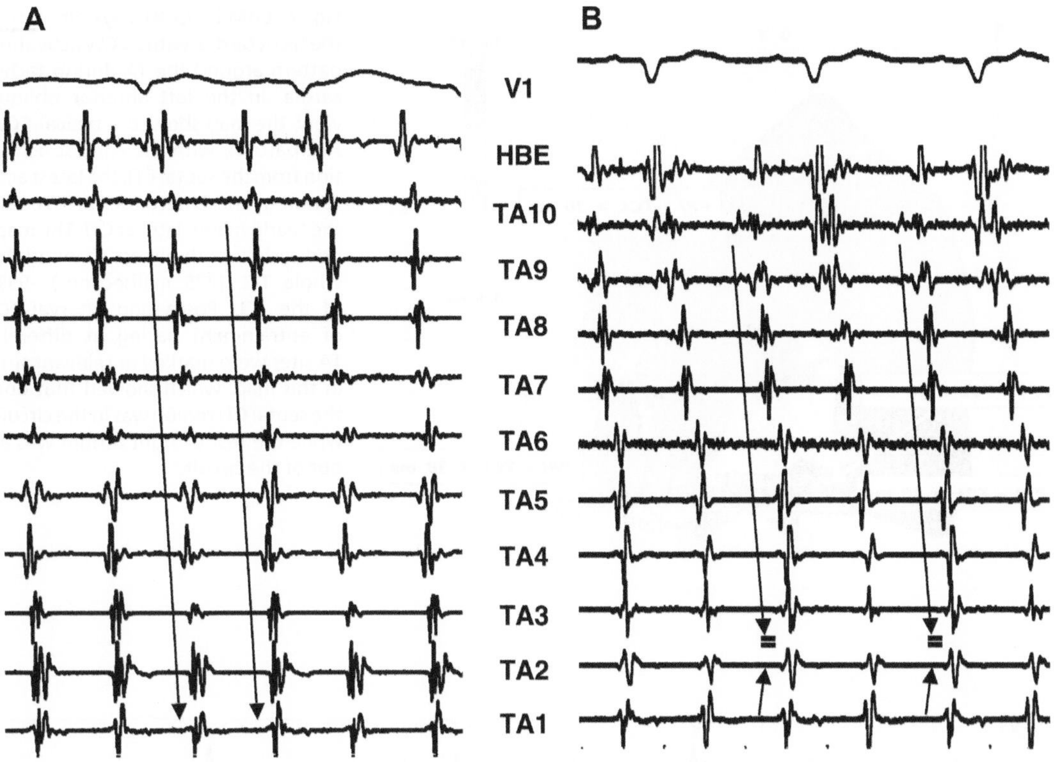

Fig. 4. Simultaneous recordings from surface lead V1, a His catheter (HBE), and a duo-decapolar catheter along the TA with its distal bipole (TA1) at the 7-o'clock position on the TA and proximal bipole (TA10) at the high septal region during AFL. This figure shows a spontaneous change of activation pattern during the tachycardia. The AFL started with a CCW pattern along the TA (*arrows*) (*panel A*). However, the signals recorded from the distal electrodes of the duo-decapolar catheter gradually advanced (not shown in the figure). As the early breakthrough at the low lateral TA gradually increased, the tachycardia switched from the CCW to a simultaneous activation pattern (*arrows*) along the TA without interruption of the tachycardia or change in the tachycardia cycle length (*panel B*).

CTI and CS os was in the circuit. Therefore, EAM may have a limited diagnostic capability for small or microreentrant circuits. Similar findings have also been previously reported from the Bordeaux group in patients who underwent LA ablation for AF.[6,7] In addition, the FPs and/or DPs recorded within the region of septal CTI and CS os suggested a slow conduction area and/or line of block, which were the substrates for a microreentrant circuit. Another interesting finding from this case is that the activation pattern of the tachycardia can vary because of different exit blocks. In this case, initially the reentrant wave front was blocked at the lateral exit and was only exited from the septal side of the circuit, hence a CCW activation pattern along the TA was presented; however, later the lateral exit block abated and the wave front slowly conducted through the anteroinferal CTI, resulting in a simultaneous activated pattern along the TA. In their previous study, the authors have described different TA activation patterns and spontaneous or pace-induced switching from one to the other pattern without affecting the TCL.[3] Such activation pattern changes can mislead one to speculate the presence of non–CTI-dependent or LA AFL circuits. Therefore, it is important to recognize this unique reentrant circuit.

REFERENCES

1. Cheng J, Cabeen WR, Scheinman MM. Right atrial flutter due to lower loop reentry: mechanism and anatomic substrates. Circulation 1999;99:1700–5.
2. Yang Y, Cheng J, Bochoeyer A, et al. Atypical right atrial flutter patterns. Circulation 2001;103:3092–8.
3. Yang Y, Varma N, Keung EC, et al. Reentry within the cavotricuspid isthmus: an isthmus dependent circuit. Pacing Clin Electrophysiol 2005;28:808–18.

4. Milliez P, Richardson AW, Obioha-Ngwu O, et al. Variable electrocardiographic characteristics of isthmus-dependent atrial flutter. J Am Coll Cardiol 2002;40:1125–32.
5. Chugh A, Latchamsetty R, Oral H, et al. Characteristics of cavotricuspid isthmus–dependent atrial flutter after left atrial ablation of atrial fibrillation. Circulation 2006;113:609–15.
6. Sanders P, Hocini M, Jais P, et al. Characterization of focal atrial tachycardia using high-density mapping. J Am Coll Cardiol 2005;46:2088–99.
7. Jais P, Sanders P, Hsu LF, et al. Flutter localized to the anterior left atrium after catheter ablation of atrial fibrillation. J Cardiovasc Electrophysiol 2006;17:279–85.

Ablation of Atrial Flutter in Congenital Heart Disease

Colleen Johnson, MD, MS*, Randall Lee, MD, PhD

KEYWORDS

• Transposition of the great arteries • Mustard correction
• Electrophysiology • Radiofrequency ablation

A 42-year-old woman with a history of D-transposition of the great arteries (TGA) and a Mustard correction at age 5 years presented to an outside hospital with palpitations and chest pain. She was found to be in a narrow complex regular tachycardia with a ventricular rate of approximately 230 beats per minute. She was electrically cardioverted and discharged. She then presented to another outside hospital while on vacation with the same symptoms. She was again in a narrow complex tachycardia with a ventricular rate of approximately 200 beats per minute. She was treated with intravenous diltiazem that slowed her ventricular rate to approximately 115 beats per minute. She has continued to have episodes of palpitations and chest pain. A transthoracic echocardiogram revealed severe right atrial and right ventricular enlargement as well as mild tricuspid regurgitation and a baffle lead. She was thus referred for electrophysiology study and possible ablation.

ELECTROPHYSIOLOGY STUDY

At baseline, the patient was in a narrow complex supraventricular tachycardia with an atrial cycle length of 270 milliseconds and 2-to-1 atrioventricular conduction, most consistent with atrial flutter given the cycle length and pattern of atrial depolarization (**Fig. 1**). Multipolar catheters were placed in the left atrium (LA) and the subpulmonic (left) ventricular apex (LVA) via the right femoral vein. An electroanatomic activation map of the right atrium was performed using the Biosense Webster CARTO system (Diamond Bar, CA, USA). Multiple attempts to cross the superiorly located baffle leak seen on transesophageal echocardiogram failed. As such, a 4-mm irrigated tip ablation catheter was advanced retrograde from the right femoral artery to the right atrium via the subaortic right ventricle and tricuspid valve. The electroanatomic activation map was then completed. Attempts to pace from the cavotricupsid isthmus were unsuccessful with only intermittent capture. Using the electroanatomic map and the surface electrocardiogram, we hypothesized atrial activation to be most consistent with counterclockwise atrial flutter using the cavotricuspid isthmus. Therefore, ablation of the cavotricuspid isthmus was pursued.

STRATEGY FOR RADIOFREQUENCY ABLATION

Selection of sites for ablation was based on an anatomic approach. Radiofrequency (RF) applications were given along the inferior aspect of the tricuspid annulus, the isthmus of atrial tissue between the tricuspid annulus and the inferior vena caval (IVC) orifice. The mid-to-anterior aspect of the cavotricuspid isthmus ablation was performed retrograde via the aorta to the systemic right ventricle and tricuspid annulus. A 4-mm irrigated tip ablation catheter was positioned at approximately 6 o'clock on the tricuspid annulus. Discrete RF applications targeting a power of 30 W and a 10% decrease in impedance were made from the tricuspid annulus posteriorly

Division of Cardiology, Cardiac Electrophysiology Department, University of California San Francisco, 500 Parnassus Avenue, MU 434, Box 1354, San Francisco, CA 94143, USA
* Corresponding author.
E-mail address: Colleen.J.Johnson@ucsfmedctr.org

Card Electrophysiol Clin 2 (2010) 305–308
doi:10.1016/j.ccep.2010.01.021
1877-9182/10/$ – see front matter

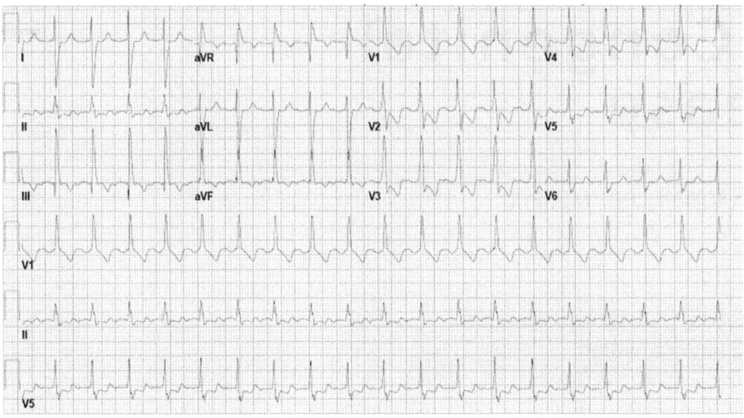

Fig. 1. Baseline electrocardiogram showing right ventricular hypertrophy with repolarization abnormality and a narrow complex supraventricular tachycardia most consistent with atrial flutter given the cycle length and pattern of atrial depolarization.

toward the IVC until the atrial baffle obstructed movement. The posterior aspect of the cavotricuspid isthmus ablation was performed by advancing the 4-mm ablation catheter to the juncture of the inferior vena cava and the atrial baffle. Discrete RF applications targeting a power of 30 W and a 10% decrease in impedance were made from the atrial baffle to the orifice of the IVC. A total of 22 discrete RF applications were made (**Fig. 2**). Although bidirectional conduction block could not be proved because of inability to pace, atrial flutter was terminated during RF ablation.

DISCUSSION

Sudden death is the leading cause of mortality in adult patients with TGA status after atrial switch correction. In a retrospective study of patients with TGA status after surgical baffling, only New York Heart Failure Association functional class and the development of supraventricular tachycardias were found to be independent risk factors for late mortality.[1] Supraventricular tachycardias have been shown to either degenerate into ventricular fibrillation resulting in sudden death or produce cardiogenic shock with subsequent death

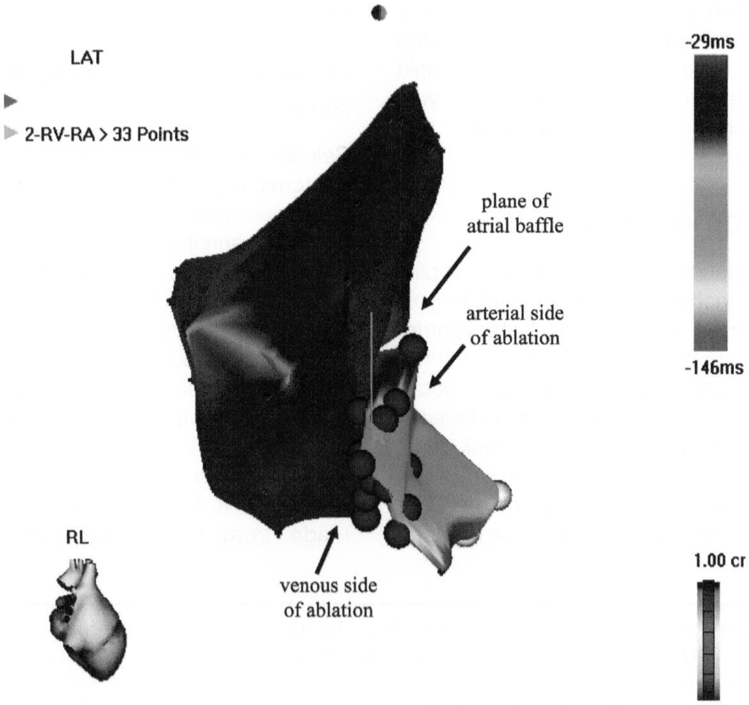

Fig. 2. Right lateral projection of electroanatomic map of atrial flutter and ablation sites (*red points*) on both sides of the atrial baffle.

secondary to rapid ventricular rates in the setting of right ventricular dysfunction.[1,2] Uncontrolled atrial flutter conferred a fourfold increase in 6-year mortality in patients with TGA status after Mustard correction.[3]

Atrial flutter is the most common tachyarrhythmia in the adult TGA population, the onset of which typically occurs long after surgical correction.[1,4] The mechanisms that predispose these patients to atrial flutter (altered hemodynamics, residual lesions, and surgical scars) are all inherent to the disease or the atrial switch correction.[4,5] Our patient had severe right atrial and ventricular dilation as well as mild tricuspid regurgitation and a baffle leak, all of which increase the likelihood of developing right-sided atrial flutter.

Given the prevalence of atrial flutter in patients with TGA status after surgical baffling and its risk for increase mortality, the eradication of this arrhythmia by means of intracardiac ablation is highly desirable. Although not all atrial flutters are typical in patients with TGA after surgical baffling, electroanatomic mapping confirms that most use the cavotricuspid isthmus as a region of critical conduction.[6,7] Therefore, ablation of the cavotricuspid isthmus is highly efficacious in curing reentrant atrial flutter in most of these patients. Unfortunately, ablation of the cavotricuspid isthmus is complicated by the bisection of the isthmus by the caval baffle.

Access to the caval and ventricular sides of the tricuspid annulus for radiofrequency ablation of atrial flutter can be achieved via different routes. The initial approach is to cross the atrial baffle at the site of a baffle leak. Unfortunately, as was the case in our patient, this is not always possible given the superior location and the size of the baffle leak. A similar approach involves puncture of the atrial baffle. The transseptal approaches across surgical baffles has been found to be very safe with an extremely low risk of residual shunts or other complications.[8,9] However, 2 cases in which there was residual shunt after baffle puncture were in patients with fenestrated atrial baffles.[9] Although our patient did not have a fenestrated baffle, she did have an existing baffle leak. As there are no data on whether baffle puncture would result in further residual shunt in a patient with a preexisting baffle leak, we decided the safest approach to the ventricular side of the tricuspid annulus would be a retrograde aortic approach.

A retrograde aortic approach is often used in catheter ablation of atrial arrhythmias, including atrial flutter and atrioventricular nodal reentrant tachycardia, in patients with TGA status after baffle procedures.[10] Kanter and colleagues[11] describe successful radiofrequency catheter ablation of atrial flutter in 8 patients with TGA status after atrial switch correction using a retrograde aortic approach with no complications. In 5 of the 8 patients in whom it was attempted, concealed entrainment of the atrial flutter could be shown on systemic and pulmonary venous sides of the atrial baffle. This finding underlines the importance of radiofrequency ablation of the cavotricuspid isthmus on both sides of the atrial baffle. This was the approach chosen for our patient, the success of which was demonstrated by termination of the tachycardia during ablation.

Given the preponderance of intraatrial reentry tachycardias and their risk of morbidity in the TGA status after atrial switch correction, definitive ablation of the arrhythmia is required. As the anatomic substrate has been altered because of the congenital disease and the surgical correction, electroanatomic mapping to ensure the area or critical conduction as well as novel approaches to these areas are necessary for success.

REFERENCES

1. Dos L, Teruel L, Ferreira IJ, et al. Late outcome of Senning and Mustard procedures for correction of transposition of the great arteries. Heart 2005; 91(5):652–6.
2. Silka M, Kron J, McAnulty J. Supraventricular tachyarrhythmias, congenital heart disease, and sudden cardiac death. Pediatr Cardiol 1992;13(2):116–8.
3. Garson A Jr, Bink-Boelkens M, Hesslein PS, et al. Atrial flutter in the young: a collaborative study of 380 cases. J Am Coll Cardiol 1985;6(4):871–8.
4. Li W, Somerville J. Atrial flutter in grown-up congenital heart (GUCH) patients. Clinical characteristics of affected population. Int J Cardiol 2000;75(2–3): 129–37 [discussion: 138–9].
5. Kanter RJ, Garson A Jr. Atrial arrhythmias during chronic follow-up of surgery for complex congenital heart disease. Pacing Clin Electrophysiol 1997; 20(2 Pt 2):502–11.
6. Zrenner B, Dong J, Schreieck J, et al. Delineation of intra-atrial reentrant tachycardia circuits after Mustard operation for transposition of the great arteries using biatrial electroanatomic mapping and entrainment mapping. J Cardiovasc Electrophysiol 2003;14(12):1302–10.
7. Sokoloski MC, Pennington JC 3rd, Winton GJ, et al. Use of multisite electroanatomic mapping to facilitate ablation of intra-atrial reentry following the Mustard procedure. J Cardiovasc Electrophysiol 2000;11(8):927–30.
8. Perry JC, Boramanand NK, Ing FF. "Transseptal" technique through atrial baffles for 3-dimensional

mapping and ablation of atrial tachycardia in patients with d-transposition of the great arteries. J Interv Card Electrophysiol 2003;9(3):365–9.
9. El-Said HG, Ing FF, Grifka RG, et al. 18-year experience with transseptal procedures through baffles, conduits, and other intra-atrial patches. Catheter Cardiovasc Interv 2000;50(4):434–9 [discussion: 440].
10. Khairy P, Van Hare GF. Catheter ablation in transposition of the great arteries with Mustard or Senning baffles. Heart Rhythm 2009;6(2):283–9.
11. Kanter RJ, Papagiannis J, Carboni MP, et al. Radiofrequency catheter ablation of supraventricular tachycardia substrates after Mustard and Senning operations for d-transposition of the great arteries. J Am Coll Cardiol 2000;35(2):428–41.

Atrial Flutter Late After Remote Tetralogy of Fallot Repair

David S. Kwon, MD, PhD, Gregory M. Marcus, MD, MAS*

KEYWORDS

• Atrial flutter • Tetralogy of Fallot • Catheter ablation
• Atrial arrhythmia

CLINICAL PRESENTATION

A 41-year-old male with a history of tetrology of Fallot (TOF) repair with an infundibular resection at 8 years of age developed sharp left-sided chest pain associated with dyspnea while changing his bicycle tire. The 12-lead electrocardiogram revealed typical clockwise appearing atrial flutter with variable conduction and a right bundle branch block. An echocardiogram was notable for a flail anterior tricuspid valve leaflet with accompanying severe tricuspid regurgitation and severe right atrial dilation. The patient was referred for electrophysiology study and ablation before surgical repair of his tricuspid valve.

ELECTROPHYSIOLOGY STUDY

The patient presented to the electrophysiology laboratory in atrial flutter. Multipolar catheters were placed in standard positions marking the right ventricular apex (RVA), His bundle (His), and the coronary sinus (CS). The 9, 10 bipole of the decapolar catheter was positioned at the CS ostium. A duodecapolar catheter was placed in the right atrium around the tricuspid annulus.

Based on the 20-pole catheter activation sequence, the arrhythmia appeared to be a typical clockwise atrial flutter. However, the activation sequence of the CS electrograms revealed a distal to proximal activation sequence (**Fig. 1**). Entrainment from the distal CS revealed a postpacing interval that was substantially longer than the tachycardia cycle length, demonstrating that the distal CS was out of the circuit. Despite this eccentric activation pattern in the CS, pacing within the cavotricuspid isthmus (CTI) resulted in entrainment with concealed fusion, and the difference between the postpacing interval and the tachycardia cycle length was 20 milliseconds, confirming clockwise CTI-dependent atrial flutter.

Pacing from the CTI revealed that CS activation was passive; the first return coronary sinus electrograms were at the pacing cycle length, and the following coronary sinus electrograms (after the first turnaround along the tricuspid annulus as seen in the duodecapolar signals) was then at tachycardia cycle length (**Fig. 2**).

As shown by the diminutive CS signals, fine voltage mapping in the region medial to the CTI revealed an area of scar. It was assumed that low septal scarring had occurred as part of the patient's previous TOF repair, resulting in conduction block from the right atrium into the proximal CS.

Ablation of this clockwise atrial flutter was accomplished successfully in the CTI with demonstration of bidirectional block. No atrial flutter could subsequently be induced.

Disclosures: Dr Marcus has received research support from St Jude Medical and Atricure and speaker fees from St Jude Medical and Biotronik; Dr Kwon is a member of the Electrophysiology Fellows Advisory Board for Medtronic.
Section of Cardiac Electrophysiology, Division of Cardiology, University of California, 500 Parnassus Avenue, MU 434, San Francisco, CA 94143, USA
* Corresponding author.
E-mail address: marcus@medicine.ucsf.edu

Card Electrophysiol Clin 2 (2010) 309–311
doi:10.1016/j.ccep.2010.01.022

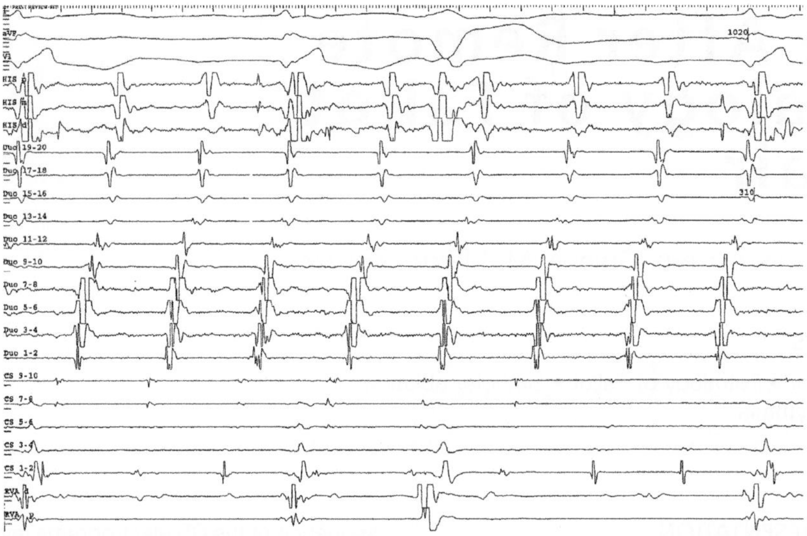

Fig. 1. Intracardiac electrograms of clockwise atrial flutter. The surface leads (I, avF, V1), His bundle intracardiac electrograms (proximal, mid, distal), duodecapolar catheter around the tricuspid annulus (1, 2, distal poles; 19, 20, proximal poles), CS (1, 2, distal poles; 9, 10, proximal poles), and RVA catheter (distal, proximal) are shown. The CS electrograms reveal a distal to proximal activation sequence in atrial flutter.

DISCUSSION

This case illustrates an atrial arrhythmia in a patient with repaired TOF, demonstrating that an atypical intracardiac electrogram activation sequence by itself does not exclude typical CTI-dependent flutter.

Much attention has been given to ventricular arrhythmias and the risk of sudden cardiac death in these patients, but the morbidity associated with atrial arrhythmias after TOF repair is becoming increasingly appreciated. Atrial tachyarrhythmias have been observed in as many as 34% of these patients, with atrial fibrillation or atrial

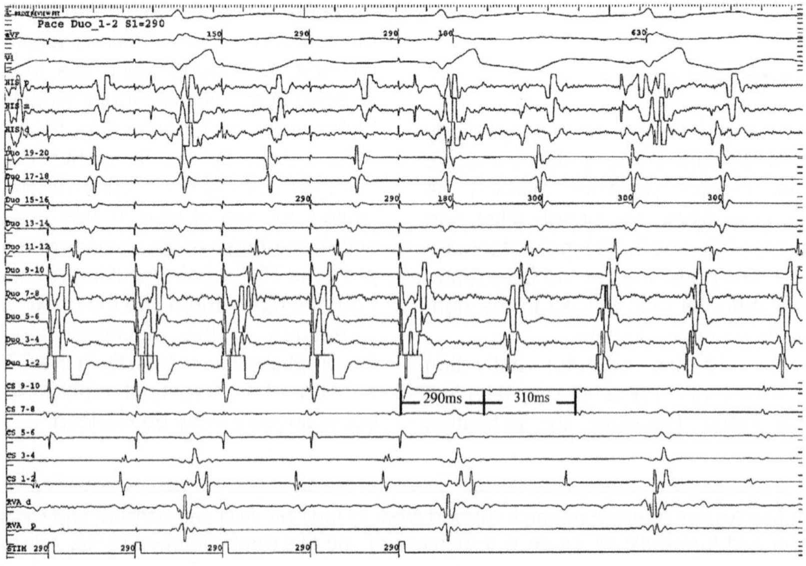

Fig. 2. The surface leads (I, avF, V1), His bundle intracardiac electrograms (proximal, mid, distal), duodecapolar catheter around the tricuspid annulus (1, 2, distal poles; 19, 20, proximal poles), CS (1, 2, distal poles; 9, 10, proximal poles), and RVA catheter (distal, proximal) are shown. Pacing from the duodecapole catheter (bipole 1, 2) at 290 milliseconds entrains the atrial flutter tachycardia with concealed fusion. Proximal CS activation (9, 10) occurs after activation of bipole 19, 20 on the duodecapole catheter (final paced beat at 290 milliseconds) with return to the tachycardia cycle length on the ensuing beat (310 milliseconds).

flutter comprising 23%.[1,2] In some studies, further categorization of these repaired patients has revealed the tendency for older patients to present with atrial tachyarrhythmias, presumably because of the type of surgical repair.[3–5] For example, Gatzoulis and colleagues[6] reported that patients who had been repaired with a transannular patch repair were not as likely to develop atrial fibrillation or atrial flutter but were more likely to develop sustained ventricular arrhythmias.

One critical feature of these repaired patients is the amount and pattern of atrial scarring. Scarring itself may be a nidus of atrial arrhythmias, especially for atypical flutter circuits, such as lower loops and intraisthmus variants.[7] The nature of this scarring may also explain how differences in surgical approaches manifest as atrial arrhythmias. Marine and colleagues[8] proposed, from a small series of 9 patients, how CS activation patterns may occur depending on whether the atrial flutter proceeds in a counterclockwise or clockwise fashion. Their goal was to fully interrogate CS activation by capturing the earliest atrial signal, yet in all patients with clockwise atrial flutter, they did not observe a completely distal to proximal CS activation pattern, as was observed in this case presentation. In 7 of 9 patients, they observed a fused CS pattern and in 2 of 9 patients a proximal to distal pattern remained, demonstrating that conduction from the CS ostium was involved in left atrial activation. In this case of atrial flutter after TOF repair, we observed that likely surgical scarring on the medial aspect of the CTI near the coronary sinus ostium created conduction block, resulting in the unusual distal to proximal pattern of CS activation.

An increasing number of patients with congenital heart disease are surviving well into adulthood, and with the variety of potential instigators for atrial arrhythmias, the modern day electrophysiologist must be prepared to carefully map and ablate these arrhythmias. As demonstrated by this case, even atypical intracardiac electrograms can be observed in typical atrial flutter.

REFERENCES

1. Roos-Hesselink J, Perlroth MG, McGhie J, et al. Atrial arrhythmias in adults after repair of tetralogy of Fallot. Circulation 1995;91:2114–8.
2. Perloff JK, Natterson PD. Atrial arrhythmia in adults after repair of tetralogy of Fallot. Circulation 1995; 91:2118–9.
3. Harrison DA, Siu SC, Hussain F, et al. Sustained atrial arrhythmias in adults late after repair of tetralogy of Fallot. Am J Cardiol 2001;87:584–8.
4. Lip GYH, Singh SP. Arrhythmias in adults following repair of tetralogy of Fallot. Am J Cardiol 2001; 88:936.
5. McRae ME. Repaired tetralogy of Fallot in the adult. Prog Cardiovasc Nurs 2005;20(3):104–10.
6. Gatzoulis MA, Balaji S, Webber SA, et al. Risk factors for arrhythmia and sudden cardiac death late after repair of tetralogy of Fallot: a multicentre study. Lancet 2000;356:975–81.
7. Yang Y, Varma N, Keung EC, et al. Reentry within the cavotricuspid isthmus: an isthmus dependent circuit. Pacing Clin Electrophysiol 2005;28:808–18.
8. Marine JE, Korley VJ, Obioha-Ngwu O, et al. Different patterns of interatrial conduction in clockwise and counterclockwise atrial flutter. Circulation 2001;104: 1153–7.

Supraventricular Tachycardia After Atrial Fibrillation Ablation

Duy Thai Nguyen, MD, Randall Lee, MD, PhD,
Zian H. Tseng, MD, MAS*

KEYWORDS

- Catheter ablation • Atypical atrial flutter
- Mitral annulus • Coronary sinus

CLINICAL PRESENTATION

A 68-year-old woman, with a history of paroxysmal atrial fibrillation (AF), was status post wide area circumferential ablation and electrical isolation of her pulmonary veins at a different institution 6 months before current presentation. Three months after ablation, she developed an atrial arrhythmia requiring cardioversion and oral amiodarone. She presented again with palpitations, exertional dyspnea, and was found to be in an atrial arrhythmia with rapid ventricular rate (**Fig. 1**). Continuous activation of the P waves suggested a macroreentrant tachycardia (as opposed to a clear isoelectric baseline between P waves, which would be more suggestive of a focal source). Upright P waves in V1 coinciding with an initial upright deflection of the P waves in the inferior leads indicated that typical atrial flutter was less likely, although cavotricuspid isthmus (CTI)–dependent atrial flutter may appear atypical in patients with atrial disease or who are status post left atrial ablation.[1] Because of difficulty with rate control and arrhythmia recurrence despite treatment with amiodarone, she was referred to our center for electrophysiologic (EP) study and ablation.

EP STUDY AND TREATMENT

At EP study, multipolar catheters were placed in the right atrium (RA), His bundle region (His), right ventricle (RV), and coronary sinus (CS). At baseline, the patient was tachycardic, with an atrial tachycardia cycle length (TCL) of 220 milliseconds and 2:1 atrioventricular (AV) block, thus ruling out AV reentrant tachycardia (**Fig. 1**). Although atrial activation during 2:1 block was mid-RP (**Fig. 2**), typical AV nodal reentrant tachycardia with lower common pathway block is rare and was excluded by an eccentric CS atrial activation pattern and by entrainment maneuvers (see later) indicating that mid and distal CS were part of the tachycardia circuit.

Activation of the tricuspid annulus as recorded by the duodecapolar catheter suggested CTI block (discontinuous activation between bipole 3, 4 lateral to the CTI and bipole 1, 2 positioned in the CS os). Entrainment of the lateral RA, CTI, proximal CS, and right atrial septum resulted in postpacing intervals (PPIs) that were substantially longer than the TCL. However, entrainment of the CS at CS bipoles 7, 8 and more distally (to CS 1–2) resulted in PPIs 30 milliseconds or less than TCL, consistent with a macroreentrant left atrial tachycardia (AT).

Disclosures None.

Cardiac Electrophysiology, Cardiology Division, University of California, San Francisco, 500 Parnassus Ave, MU East 4, Box 1354, San Francisco, CA 94143, USA
* Corresponding author.
E-mail address: zhtseng@medicine.ucsf.edu

Card Electrophysiol Clin 2 (2010) 313–316
doi:10.1016/j.ccep.2010.01.024

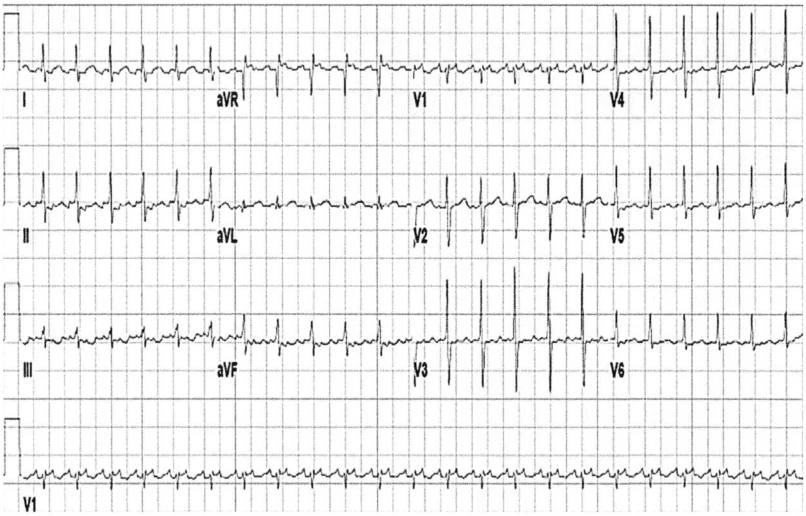

Fig. 1. Twelve-lead electrocardiogram of patient's presenting arrhythmia.

Hence, a transseptal puncture was performed for left atrial mapping.

In the left atrium, entrainment at the roof, septum, and right-sided pulmonary veins resulted in PPIs longer than TCL by greater than 30 milliseconds; these areas were thus out of the tachycardia circuit. Entrainment of various locations around the mitral annulus (**Fig. 3**) demonstrated that all these areas were in the circuit. Electroanatomic mapping confirmed a macroreentrant tachycardia, with the activation time around the mitral annulus equal to the TCL. Furthermore, the site of latest activation met the site of earliest activation in the region of the mitral annulus near CS 5, 6 (early meets late). Thus, it was concluded that the patient had a mitral annular AT.

Ablation was targeted at the mitral isthmus between the mitral annulus and the left lower pulmonary vein. Despite 2 complete lines of ablations along the mitral isthmus, with good electrical signal attenuation during ablation, the tachycardia persisted. Hence, the open irrigated-tip catheter (Thermocool, Biosense Webster) was inserted into the CS and an epicardial ablation line was drawn from CS 1, 2 (most distal) to CS 7, 8, adjacent to the endocardial mitral isthmus line. At this point, the tachycardia terminated and could not be re-induced. Four months after ablation, the patient has done well without recurrence.

DISCUSSION

The incidence, mechanism of tachycardia, and approach to diagnosis and treatment of atrial arrhythmias occurring after AF ablation depend in large part on the strategy used in the initial AF ablation.[2] If the initial AF ablation used an anatomic and substrate-based approach to create circumferential ablation lesions around pulmonary veins, the incidence of postablation ATs can be as high as 24% and the tachycardia mechanism is most likely to be macroreentrant around anatomic barriers or within scar channels.[3,4] If using a circular mapping catheter to guide electrical isolation of pulmonary veins (PVs), the risk of developing postablation AT is estimated at less than 5% and the tachycardia mechanism is more likely to be focal and arise from near the ostia of reconnected pulmonary veins.[5] At the referring institution, this patient underwent a hybrid AF ablation approach, with wide area circumferential ablation lines created around her pulmonary veins but also using a circular mapping catheter to confirm PV electrical isolation. Hence, she was at risk of developing either focal or macroreentrant tachycardia; her 12-lead electrocardiogram suggested a macroreentrant circuit, later confirmed by the EP study.

The approach to suspected atrial arrhythmias after AF ablation should use a combination of entrainment and electroanatomic activation mapping.[6] Pacing and attempted entrainment of the tachycardia from several sites in the RA, including the CTI, should first be performed to assess for typical or atypical right atrial flutters. If the response to pacing and entrainment suggests macroreentrant tachycardia and no site in the RA is found to be in the circuit, entrainment from the atrial septum and from the CS should be done to assess for left atrial (LA) tachycardias.

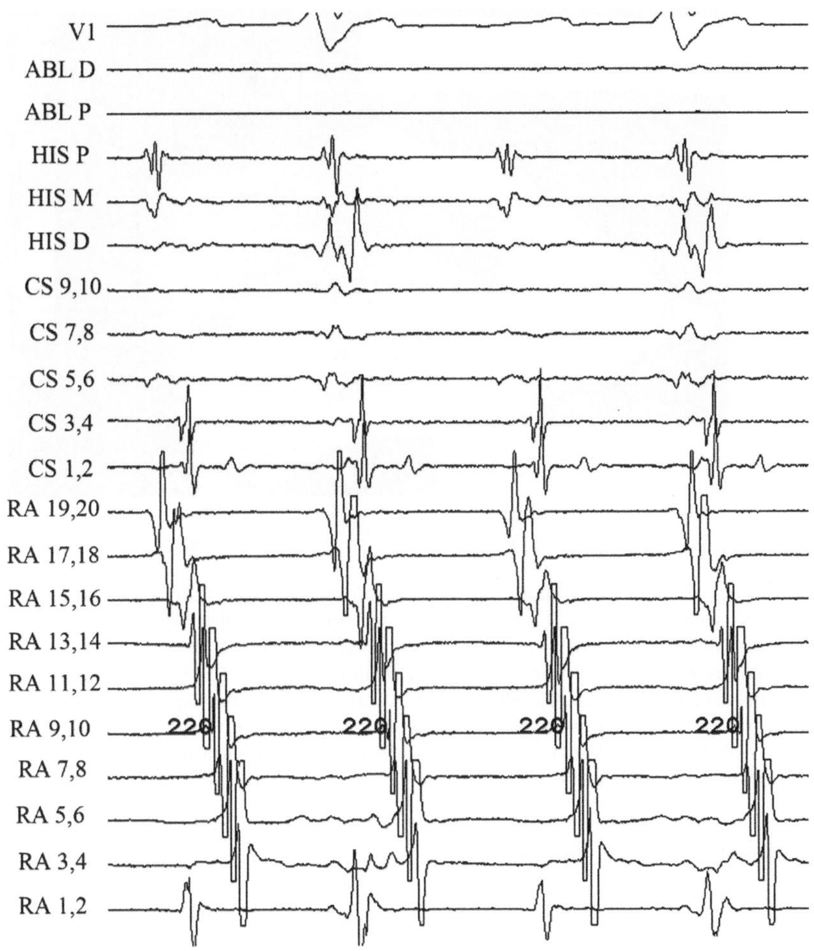

Fig. 2. Baseline intracardiac electrograms during tachycardia. ABL, ablator; P, proximal; D, distal; His, His bundle; M, mid. RA, duodecapolar positions around the tricuspid annulus with 1, 2 as most distal and 19, 20 as most proximal. RA (duodecapolar) bipole 1, 2 is positioned into the CS os. CS, coronary sinus with 1, 2 most distal and 9, 10 most proximal.

In the left atrium, pacing at several cycle lengths from several sites around the mitral annulus, from the LA septum, and from the LA roof can be quickly performed to assess for macroreentrant circuits versus focal tachycardias. Focal tachycardias should be suspected if there is significant variability in the TCL, if the activation map does not account for most of the TCL, if there is lack of early meets late activation, or if there is an inability to show that 2 sites more than 2 cm apart are part of the tachycardia circuit.[7] Assessment for pulmonary vein reconnection should also be performed. Electroanatomic mapping can be used to delineate complex circuits and to confirm that the activation time of the circuit encompassing large areas in the LA is similar to the TCL, that is, that the tachycardia is macroreentrant, as opposed to focal in nature (typically resulting in a map with the earliest area much less than 50% of TCL).

Mitral annular ATs are the most common macroreentrant circuits after AF ablation.[2,4] In this patient, entrainment from several sites around the mitral annulus resulted in PPIs similar to the TCL. In addition, activation time around the mitral annulus was similar to the TCL, and the site of early meets late activation was at the mitral annulus. The narrowest anatomic region for ablation of a mitral annular flutter is between the left lower pulmonary vein and the mitral annulus, otherwise known as the mitral isthmus. Linear ablation at the mitral isthmus is thus performed for mitral annular tachycardias. Not uncommonly, epicardial ablation via the CS adjacent to the mitral isthmus is necessary to terminate the tachycardia,[8] as in this case. This is because muscle

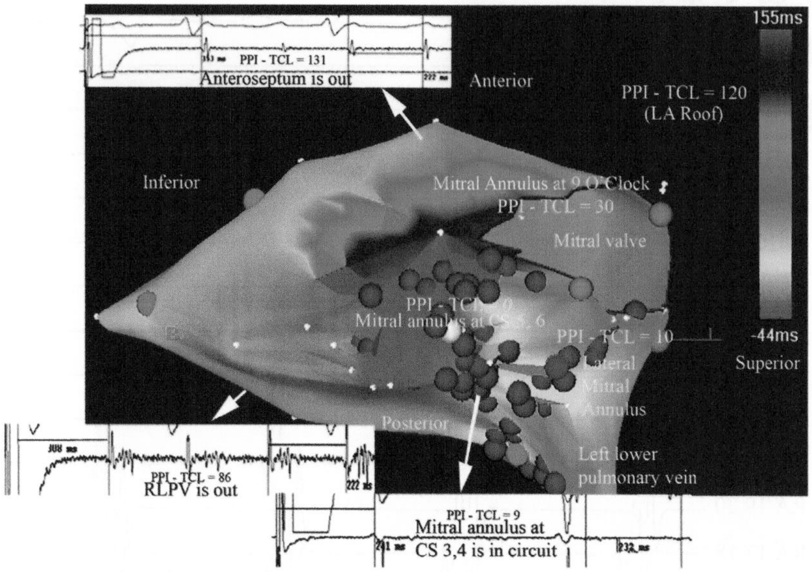

Fig. 3. Inferolateral view of Carto electroanatomic map (Biosense Webster) of the left atrium. Postpacing interval minus tachycardia cycle length (PPI−TCL) was calculated for the left atrial (LA) roof, anteroseptum, and right lower pulmonary vein (RLPV), which were all out of the tachycardia circuit. PPI minus TCL was also derived for the lateral mitral annulus, mitral annulus near CS 3, 4, mitral annulus near CS 5, 6, and mitral annulus at 9 o'clock. These were all in the circuit (PPI−TCL<30 milliseconds). Atrial activation timing was also obtained, with red as earliest activation and purple as latest activation. The tachycardia circuit revolved counterclockwise around the mitral annulus, with the site of latest activation meeting the site of earliest activation in the mitral annulus near CS 5, 6. Sites of ablation are shown as red circles.

connections from the CS muscle to the LA are part of the circuit.

SUMMARY

Atrial arrhythmias occur commonly after AF ablation. Initial conservative management with medical therapy and cardioversion is reasonable, particularly in the early period (first 3 months) after ablation, because many of these arrhythmias remit over time.[3] However, definitive therapy with ablation may be required, depending on the clinical circumstances, and should focus on the putative mechanism of tachycardia and its likely location, both of which can be suggested by the initial AF ablation strategy. Response to pacing, entrainment, and electroanatomic activation mapping are useful to confirm the mechanism, define complex circuits, and guide ablation targets.

REFERENCES

1. Chugh A, Latchamsetty R, Oral H, et al. Characteristics of cavotricuspid isthmus-dependent atrial flutter after left atrial ablation of atrial fibrillation. Circulation 2006;113(5):609–15.
2. Gerstenfeld EP, Marchlinski FE. Mapping and ablation of left atrial tachycardias occurring after atrial fibrillation ablation. Heart Rhythm 2007;4(Suppl 3):S65–72.
3. Chugh A, Oral H, Lemola K, et al. Prevalence, mechanisms, and clinical significance of macroreentrant atrial tachycardia during and following left atrial ablation for atrial fibrillation. Heart Rhythm 2005;2(5):464–71.
4. Mesas CE, Pappone C, Lang CC, et al. Left atrial tachycardia after circumferential pulmonary vein ablation for atrial fibrillation: electroanatomic characterization and treatment. J Am Coll Cardiol 2004; 44(5):1071–9.
5. Gerstenfeld EP, Callans DJ, Dixit S, et al. Mechanisms of organized left atrial tachycardias occurring after pulmonary vein isolation. Circulation 2004;110(11): 1351–7.
6. Jais P, Hocini M, Weerasoryia R, et al. Atypical left atrial flutters. Card Electrophysiol Rev 2002;6(4): 371–7.
7. Roberts-Thomson KC, Kistler PM, Kalman JM. Atrial tachycardia: mechanisms, diagnosis, and management. Curr Probl Cardiol 2005;30(10):529–73.
8. Jais P, Hocini M, Hsu LF, et al. Technique and results of linear ablation at the mitral isthmus. Circulation 2004;110(19):2996–3002.

Supraventricular Tachycardia in Pulmonary Hypertension

Duy Thai Nguyen, MD*, Melvin Scheinman, MD

KEYWORDS
- Catheter ablation • Pulmonary hypertension
- Atrial tachycardia • Supraventricular arrhythmia

CLINICAL PRESENTATION

A 48-year-old woman, with a history of primary pulmonary hypertension and right heart failure, was admitted with a supraventricular tachycardia (**Fig. 1**), hypotension, and congestive heart failure. She was on multiple central vasopressors and pulmonary vasodilators and was transferred to the authors' hospital for evaluation of emergent heart and lung transplant. The patient was previously diagnosed at another institution with typical atrial flutter; she required as many as 18 direct-current cardioversions, despite initiation of intravenous (IV) amiodarone, and had undergone an unsuccessful ablation of the cavotricuspid isthmus (CTI). Her echocardiogram showed massively enlarged right atrium (RA) and right ventricle (RV). The authors were asked to consider a repeat electrophysiology (EP) study and ablation to provide her with some cardiopulmonary reserve while she awaited her heart-lung transplant.

EP STUDY AND TREATMENT

At EP study, multipolar catheters were placed in the RA, His bundle region, RV, and coronary sinus (CS). At baseline, the patient had an atrial tachycardia cycle length (TCL) of 300 ms with 2:1 atrioventricular (AV) block, thus ruling out AV reentrant tachycardia. AV nodal reentrant tachycardia with lower common pathway block is rare and was essentially excluded by a high to low atrial activation pattern (**Fig. 2**). Furthermore, with the duodecapolar catheter located anteriorly around the tricuspid annulus, the atrial activation pattern was not reflective of clockwise or counterclockwise typical atrial flutter. Hence, atypical atrial flutter was the most likely diagnosis. Entrainment from the CS (proximal and distal), atrial septum, superior RA, and CTI showed that these areas were out of the tachycardia circuit (**Fig. 3**).

Entrainment from the midlateral wall of the RA showed that the postpacing interval minus TCL was 3 ms, and there was concealed fusion (see **Fig. 3**). Furthermore, highly fractionated mid-diastolic potentials spanning more than half the TCL were observed in this midlateral RA region (**Fig. 4**A). In addition, the 3-D electroanatomic map (EnSite Sytem, St Jude Medical) demonstrated an apparent focal source because there was no evidence that the site of latest activation met the site of earliest activation and the activation map spanned less than 60% of the TCL. Radiofrequency (RF) was applied with a standard 4-mm catheter in the midlateral RA, with immediate termination of the tachycardia (see **Fig. 4**B). The tachycardia could not be reinduced post ablation. After the successful ablation and in concert with

Dr Nguyen has received grants to attend educational events sponsored by Boston Scientific, St Jude Medical, and Medtronic.
Cardiac Electrophysiology, Division of Cardiology, University of California, San Francisco, 500 Parnassus Avenue, MU East 4, Box 1354, San Francisco, CA 94143, USA
* Corresponding author.
E-mail address: nguyend@medicine.ucsf.edu

Card Electrophysiol Clin 2 (2010) 317–319
doi:10.1016/j.ccep.2010.01.025

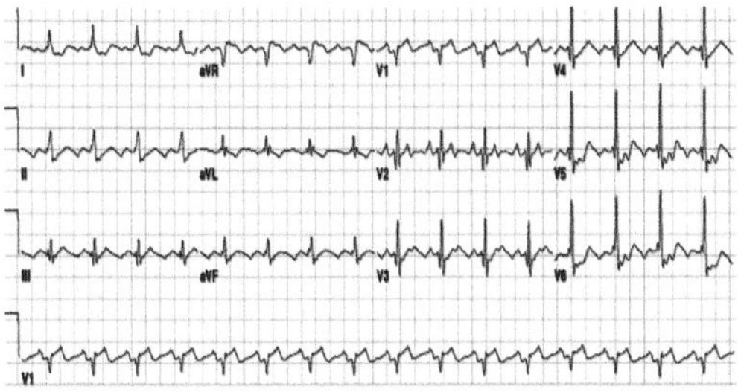

Fig. 1. 12-Lead EKG of patient's presenting arrhythmia.

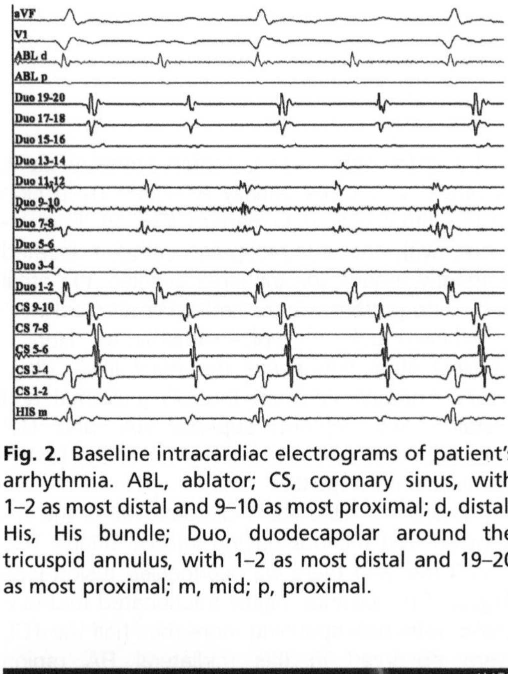

Fig. 2. Baseline intracardiac electrograms of patient's arrhythmia. ABL, ablator; CS, coronary sinus, with 1–2 as most distal and 9–10 as most proximal; d, distal; His, His bundle; Duo, duodecapolar around the tricuspid annulus, with 1–2 as most distal and 19–20 as most proximal; m, mid; p, proximal.

continued heart failure therapy, the patient did remarkably well. She was weaned off all vasopressors and antiarrhythmics. She was discharged from the hospital on pulmonary vasodilators and has continued to improve such that heart-lung transplant was no longer being considered. She has remained free of arrhythmias for more than 4 months.

DISCUSSION

Pulmonary hypertension, primary or secondary, is a disease with significant morbidity and mortality. It is characterized by right-sided volume and pressure overload, which leads to structural changes and fibrosis in the RA, thus predisposing to supraventricular arrhythmias.

In the authors' patient, the surface P waves showed a pattern consistent with typical flutter; however, this did not turn out to be the arrhythmia, as the CTI was out of the circuit. Hence, the patient did not have P waves typical for the site of successful ablation. Thus, using the P-wave morphology to actually localize the origin of arrhythmia can be challenging in patients with pulmonary hypertension, because studies assessing P-wave configuration during atrial arrhythmias were done in structurally normal atria and cannot be extrapolated to the authors' patient's abnormal atria.[1]

Mapping of the authors' patient's tachycardia suggested that it was focal, because the activation map spanned less than 60% of the TCL and there was no evidence that the site of latest activation

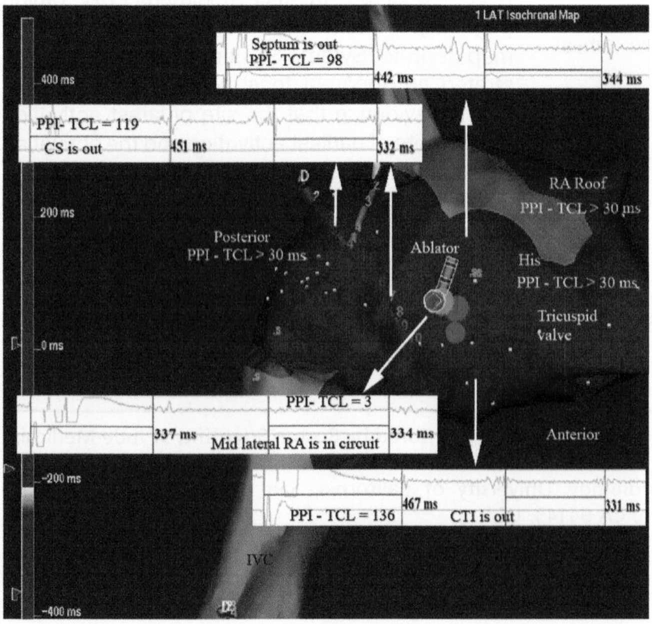

Fig. 3. Lateral view of ESI Navix map (St Jude Medical) of RA. Postpacing interval minus TCL (PPI-TCL) is given for coronary sinus (CS), right atrial (RA) septum, CTI, and midlateral RA wall (where PPI-TCL = 3). PPI-TCL was also noted to be greater than 30 ms at the RA roof, posterior wall, and near the His region. Note that the His catheter (yellow catheter) was displaced in this image, and the proper location of the His is noted. Also shown is the ablator at the successful ablation site where one RF application immediately terminated tachycardia.

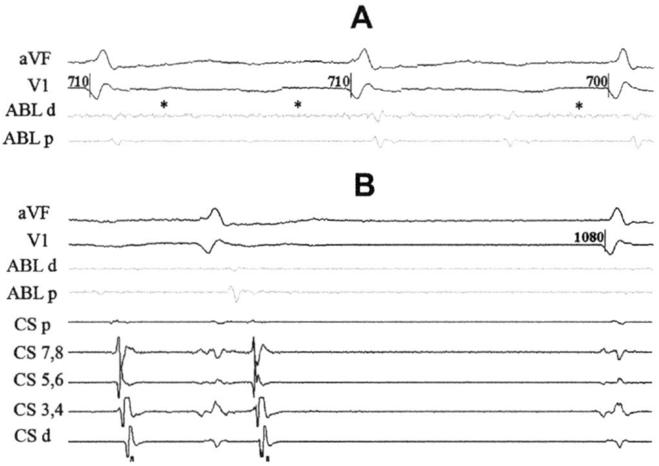

Fig. 4. (*A*) Fractionated, low-amplitude potentials (*asterisks*) on ABL d noted in midlateral right atrial wall, spanning more than half the TCL. (*B*) Termination of tachycardia. ABL, ablator; CS, coronary sinus, with 1–2 as most distal and 9–10 as most proximal; d, distal; p, proximal.

met the site of earliest activation. Focal tachycardias can be triggered, automatic, or microreentrant. Because the tachycardia was entrainable in only 1 discrete location, the mechanism was microreentry.[2] Furthermore, the fact that the tachycardia terminated with one RF application in one location further supported this diagnosis.

The origin of this patient's arrhythmia in the midlateral RA was anterior to the crista terminalis, where about one-third to one-half of all right atrial tachycardias arise in structurally normal hearts.[3] The crista terminalis is a region of the RA with marked anisotropy, sluggish transverse conduction, and swift linear conduction, all substrates for microreentry.[4,5] In structurally abnormal and remodeled atria, areas other than the crista terminalis can also develop nonuniform anisotropy and conduction blocks and can, therefore, predispose to microreentry.[6]

In summary, patients with pulmonary hypertension and right-sided volume overload are susceptible to right atrial tachycardias. Typical P-wave morphology rules to localize an arrhythmia may not be reliable in structurally abnormal atria. A focal atrial tachycardia should be suspected if activation mapping does not encompass the TCL and if there is no evidence of a late meets early activation. Entrainment mapping can still be used to localize certain focal tachycardias if microreentry is involved. The target is typically a multifractionated, mid-diastolic potential that is integral to the microreentrant circuit by entrainment mapping. In the authors' patient, the electrogram recordings over the successful site were nondescript and could have been easily overlooked; however, the consistent fractionated potentials and the concealed entrainment at the site directed the successful ablation attempt.

REFERENCES

1. Kistler PM, Kalman JM. Locating focal atrial tachycardias from P-wave morphology. Heart Rhythm 2005; 2(5):561–4.
2. Roberts-Thomson KC, Kistler PM, Kalman JM. Focal atrial tachycardia I: clinical features, diagnosis, mechanisms, and anatomic location. Pacing Clin Electrophysiol 2006;29(6):643–52.
3. Kalman JM, Olgin JE, Karch MR, et al. "Cristal tachycardias": origin of right atrial tachycardias from the crista terminalis identified by intracardiac echocardiography. J Am Coll Cardiol 1998;31(2):451–9.
4. Roberts-Thomson KC, Kistler PM, Kalman JM. Atrial tachycardia: mechanisms, diagnosis, and management. Curr Probl Cardiol 2005;30(10): 529–73.
5. Saffitz JE, Kanter HL, Green KG, et al. Tissue-specific determinants of anisotropic conduction velocity in canine atrial and ventricular myocardium. Circ Res 1994;74(6):1065–70.
6. de Bakker JM, van Rijen HM. Continuous and discontinuous propagation in heart muscle. J Cardiovasc Electrophysiol 2006;17(5):567–73.

Index

Note: Page numbers of article titles are in **boldface** type.

Card Electrophysiol Clin 2 (2010) 321–323
doi:10.1016/S1877-9182(10)00053-5

Printed and bound by CPI Group (UK) Ltd, Croydon, CR0 4YY
03/10/2024
01040355-0017

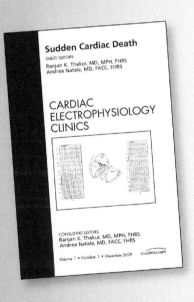